Food Lipids and Health

ift Basic Symposium Series

Edited by
INSTITUTE OF FOOD TECHNOLOGISTS
221 N. LaSalle St.
Chicago, Illinois

Food Lipids and Health

edited by

Richard E. McDonald

National Center for Food Safety and Technology
Food and Drug Administration
Summit-Argo, Illinois

David B. Min

Department of Food Science and Technology
The Ohio State University
Columbus, Ohio

Marcel Dekker, Inc.   New York • Basel • Hong Kong

Library of Congress Cataloging-in-Publication Data

Food lipids and health/edited by Richard E. McDonald, David B. Min.
    p.   cm.—(IFT basic symposium; 11)
    Based on the 19th annual symposium.
    Includes index.
    ISBN: 0-8247-9712-4 (alk. paper)
    1. Lipids in human nutrition—Congresses.   2. Food—Lipid content—
Congresses.   I. McDonald, Richard E.   II. Min, David B.   III. Series.
QP751.F654   1996
612.3'97—dc20   96-18488
                                                                    CIP

The publisher offers discounts on this book when ordered in bulk quantities. For more information, write to Special Sales/Professional Marketing at the address below.

This book is printed on acid-free paper.

Marcel Dekker, Inc.
270 Madison Avenue, New York, New York 10016

Current printing (last digit):
10 9 8 7 6 5 4 3 2 1

PRINTED IN THE UNITED STATES OF AMERICA

Preface

The Institute of Food Technologists (IFT) and the International Union of Food Science and Technology (IUFoST) began sponsoring an annual basic symposium in 1976. Each year the IFT Basic Symposium Committee chooses a topic of major importance to the food industry, then facilitates a two-day symposium designed to present an in-depth fundamental treatise of a single subject. The primary emphasis of each symposium is to apply basic aspects and applications of fundamental ideas to the solution of a major problem. Internationally recognized speakers at the forefront of their specialties are invited to participate. The monographs that result from these annual symposia represent the only books sponsored by IFT.

This book presents the Nineteenth Basic Symposium, Food Lipids and Health, held June 1 and 2, 1995, prior to the IFT Annual Meeting in Anaheim, California. This symposium brought together experts from the food industry, academia, and government agencies to discuss the latest developments in lipid chemistry and nutrition.

There is a general consensus that fat intake should be controlled to help maintain an active and healthy lifestyle. However, the relationship of dietary lipids to human health is a complicated issue that has sparked some controversy. Consumer health consciousness, concerns about cholesterol, and the types and content of dietary fat have resulted in a great deal of research. Several food products have been reformulated to increase unsaturated fat while reducing total fat content. However, these products are more susceptible to oxidation. In response to consumer surveys, low-fat and even no-fat products are being marketed to replace high-fat products. Some of these fat-reduced products have little resemblance to their high-fat counterparts since fat makes an important contribution to the desirable texture and flavor of many food products.

This book provides an in-depth discussion of recent developments in lipid chemistry and nutrition and how these developments affect the food industry. The major lipid health issues are presented including dietary recommendations, atherosclerosis, cancer, immune response, and bone health. The more controversial issues discussed include health effects of saturated fat, *trans* fatty acids, fat substitutes, cholesterol oxidation products, and frying oils. Other discussions include lipid contributions to flavor and functionality, enzyme modification of lipids, natural antioxidants, and evaluation of lipid quality and stability. Recent developments concerning the use of lipids in food products are described, including the application of plant biotechnology to edible oils, current developments of fat substitutes, and the use of lipids in medical and designer foods. New findings are described regarding biochemical and physiological factors that affect dietary lipid intake in humans.

In summary, this book provides a state-of-the-art review of each subject and reflects the latest scientific thinking on food lipids and health. These reviews will give the reader an appreciation of the complexities of lipid chemistry and nutrition. Many unresolved issues are identified that will demand additional research. The goal of this book is to help serve as a catalyst for additional research to improve the functionality, flavor, and nutritional properties of processed lipid-containing food products and ingredients.

The editors would like to acknowledge the help of the IFT Basic Symposium Committee, who initiated the idea for the symposium and made several suggestions that were incorporated into the symposium. John Klis, IFT Director of Publications; Anna May Schenck, an IFT Scientific Editor; and others on the IFT staff made significant contributions including organization, publicity, facility planning, and editorial assistance. The symposium and this book would not have been possible without their help.

The editors gratefully acknowledge the contributing authors who successfully met the numerous deadlines that were imposed on their already busy schedules. In particular, we deeply appreciate the contribution of Dr.

Thomas Smouse, author of Chapter 11, who died of cancer less than three months after the symposium. Tom's presentation, "Significance of Lipid Oxidation to Food Processors," was extremely well received and he was an active participant during the numerous discussions that took place. We had the privilege of collaborating and serving with Tom in various capacities and knew him as a highly respected scientist, colleague, and friend.

Richard E. McDonald
David B. Min

Contributors

Paul B. Addis   Department of Food Science and Nutrition, University of Minnesota, St. Paul, Minnesota

Robert Aeschbach   Nestec Ltd., Nestlé Research Centre, Lausanne, Switzerland

Casimir C. Akoh   Department of Food Science and Technology, The University of Georgia, Athens, Georgia

William E. Artz   Department of Food Science and Human Nutrition, University of Illinois, Urbana, Illinois

Rafael Codony   Nutrition and Food Science Unit, Faculty of Pharmacy, University of Barcelona, Barcelona, Spain

Kobra Eghtedary   Department of Nutrition and Food Science, Wayne State University, Detroit, Michigan

Francesco Guardiola   Nutrition and Food Science Unit, Faculty of Pharmacy, University of Barcelona, Barcelona, Spain

Steven L. Hansen   Bunge Foods, Bradley, Illinois

David M. Klurfeld   Department of Nutrition and Food Science, Wayne State University, Detroit, Michigan

David Kritchevsky   The Wistar Institute, Philadelphia, Pennsylvania

Pierre Lambelet   Nestec Ltd., Nestlé Research Centre, Lausanne, Switzerland

Hyung-Ok Lee   Department of Food Science and Technology, The Ohio State University, Columbus, Ohio

Jürg Löliger   Nestec Ltd., Nestlé Research Centre, Lausanne, Switzerland

Jane Love   Department of Food Science and Human Nutrition, Iowa State University, Ames, Iowa

Richard D. Mattes   Department of Foods and Nutrition, Purdue University, West Lafayette, Indiana

Richard E. McDonald   National Center for Food Safety and Technology, Food and Drug Administration, Summit-Argo, Illinois

David B. Min   Department of Food Science and Technology, The Ohio State University, Columbus, Ohio

Magdi M. Mossoba   Center for Food Safety and Applied Nutrition, Food and Drug Administration, Washington, D.C.

Michael W. Pariza   Food Research Institute, Department of Food Microbiology and Toxicology, University of Wisconsin—Madison, Madison, Wisconsin

Peter W. Park   Technical Affairs Division, Crown Laboratories, Inc., Las Vegas, Nevada

Edward G. Perkins   Department of Food Science and Human Nutrition, University of Illinois, Urbana, Illinois

Elizabeth M. Prior   Nestec Ltd., Nestlé Research Centre, Lausanne, Switzerland

Mary K. Schmidl   Humanetics Corporation, St. Louis Park, Minnesota

Mark F. Seifert   Department of Anatomy, Indiana University School of Medicine, Indianapolis, Indiana

Thomas H. Smouse[†]   Archer Daniels Midland Company, Decatur, Illinois

---

[†]Deceased.

John E. Vanderveen   Center for Food Safety and Applied Nutrition, Food and Drug Administration, Washington, D.C.

Toni Voelker   Calgene Inc., Davis, California

Kathleen Warner   Food Quality and Safety Research, National Center for Agricultural Utilization Research, Agricultural Research Service, U.S. Department of Agriculture, Peoria, Illinois

Bruce A. Watkins   Department of Food Science, Lipid Chemistry and Metabolism Laboratory, Purdue University, West Lafayette, Indiana

Contents

Food Lipids and Health

1

Dietary Recommendations for Lipids and Measures Designed to Facilitate Implementation

John E. Vanderveen

Food and Drug Administration
Washington, D.C.

Foods containing high levels of lipids have long been considered to have special importance in the diet. For example, the Navy Ration Law of 1794 required that each sailor be provided 2 ounces of butter or a gill of oil as part of his ration (USC, 1794). Although this law was amended several times, the requirement for butter and oil remained in effect for nearly 180 years. It was not until early 1990, when the Department of Defense was trying to lower the amount of saturated fat in the diets of enlisted personnel by substituting margarine for butter, that the law was changed (USC, 1990). Clearly the requirement in the Navy Ration Law reflected the perceived importance in that period of time of providing some fat in the diet, but the amounts were established more for economic reasons than for health purposes.

During the first half of this century, nutritionists made some recommendations about the amount of fat that should be consumed in the diet. In an 1894 publication, W. O. Atwater, working for the U.S. Department of Agriculture (USDA), recommended that the level of fat be approximately 33% of calories (Atwater, 1894). In a revised version of the publication (Atwater,

1901), he simply recommended a specific amount of protein and indicated that energy requirements should be supplied by fat and carbohydrates in amounts necessary to meet work needs. Atwater clearly viewed fat as a dense source of calories and a substance that provided palatability to food.

In 1917, the Division of the Army Surgeon General's Office implemented a series of nutrition surveys in several army camps to collect data necessary to establish ration allowances. The data obtained from these surveys were reviewed by a group of eminent nutrition experts, who acted as an Advisory Council to the Army (Murlin and Miller, 1919). A major finding of these surveys was that the ration contained too much fat. The Advisory Council recommended that a diet that supplied 12.5% of calorie needs from protein, 25% in the form of fats, and 62.5% in the form of carbohydrates was more healthful. The rationale given for these recommendations was that "muscular work is done with less effort if there is a plentiful supply of carbohydrates" and that "carbohydrate is a cheaper source of muscular energy than is fat."

Judging from the claims made in advertisements for fat products in the first half of the century, however, food scientists and most nutritionists viewed the role of lipids in foods primarily as a source of calories and a factor in food acceptance. Meat animals were bred for high levels of carcass fat. Dairy cattle were selected for the fat content of their milk; a premium price was paid for milk with the highest fat content. Even low-fat foods such as potatoes and other vegetables prepared by frying or cooking with animal fats were considered to have added value because of the flavor and taste.

Acceptance by scientists of a diet with higher levels of fat seemed to be evident by the early 1940s. One of the publications most quoted by nutrition experts and also most reflective of the general consensus of the nutrition community through the years is the *Recommended Dietary Allowances* publication of the National Academy of Sciences. In May 1941, the Committee on Food and Nutrition of the National Research Council issued the first *Recommended Dietary Allowances* (NRC, 1941). This report made recommendations for calories, protein, calcium, iron, and six vitamins for various age/sex groups. Although the report did not contain recommendations about fat, a dietary "pattern" was presented that would provide the recommended levels of nutrients, and a model menu was included. The fat level in this model menu was calculated to be 35% of calories.

The revised *Recommended Dietary Allowances* published by the Food and Nutrition Board of the National Research Council in January 1943 again did not address requirements for fat (NAS-NRC, 1943). However, the 1945 revision contained a footnote about fat under the title Further Recommendations (NAS-NRC, 1945). Citing a "paucity of information" on human fat requirements and noting that fat allowances at the time were "based more on food habits than on physiological requirements," the report did point out that linoleic and arachidonic acids requirements had been shown to be requirements for experimental animals. On that basis, the report then stated that it was desirable to include fat in the diet to the extent of at least 20–25% of total calories with at least 1% of total calories in the form of "essential" unsaturated fatty acids. The report further stated that for those who require diets with high levels of calories (4500 calories) for physical work and in diets for children and adolescents it was desirable that 30–35% of the calories be derived from fat.

There was no change in the third revision (NAS-NRC, 1948), but the fourth revision of the *Recommended Dietary Allowances* acknowledged that fat consumption had increased from 32 to 40% between 1909 and 1952 (NAS-NRC, 1953). In the fifth revision, the Food and Nutrition Board dropped any reference to a recommendation about the level of fat in the diet, drawing attention to the potential harmful effects of excessive intakes of fat or some kinds of fat. This revision took special note of the high rate of mortality due to coronary artery disease and cited broad proposals for correcting the diet. Concluding that it was not yet possible to definitively state a reasonable allowance for fat, the Board simply recommended that a diet selected from a wide variety of foodstuffs of both animal and vegetable origin would be most likely to maintain good health (NAS-NRC, 1958).

Although early in this century physicians observed that cardiovascular disease and other conditions were related to diet, these reports went largely unnoticed because they were published in obscure journals. For example, de Lange (1916) reported that natives from Indonesia had very low levels of serum cholesterol compared to Northern Europeans. He noted, however, that when these Indonesians became employed on ships and consumed western diets, their cholesterol levels increased and they developed cardiovascular disease like their Dutch counterparts (de Lange, 1922).

As the fourth decade of the century approached, some scientists who were engaged in research into the causes of chronic diseases began to study the relationships of the so-called western diets and these diseases. These studies tended to indicate that diets high in animal fats containing cholesterol were highly correlated with the incidence of coronary heart disease. However, it was the epidemiological studies by Keys (1957) linking the incidence of cardiovascular disease to the levels of fat in the diet that stirred great controversy among scientists in the early 1950s. Later studies by Hegsted et al. (1965), Keys et al. (1965), and others showed that serum cholesterol levels were raised when certain saturated fatty acids made up a significant portion of the diet. These studies also showed that addition of unsaturated fatty acids to the diet tended to lower serum cholesterol levels. *Trans* fatty acids and monounsaturated fatty acids showed no effect and therefore were considered neutral.

Both Hegsted and Keys used their data to develop predictive equations

for effects on serum cholesterol of adding various fatty acids and cholesterol
to human diets (Keys et al., 1957; Hegsted et al., 1986). However, it was only
when data from large population studies were published that such predictive equations could be put to use in assessing the impact of specific diets on
the risk of developing heart attacks. Even the results of these studies were
not uniformly accepted by all scientists in the field. Some researchers
pointed out that there were many variables in this study that could have
explained the results. Furthermore, not all clinical studies designed to show
the relationship between dietary saturated fats and serum cholesterol levels
yielded the same results. This lack of consistency led to significant debate
among investigators in the lipid field.

At the time of the White House Conference on Health and Nutrition in
late 1969, the debate was still very evident (White House Conference, 1970).
It was agreed, however, that some consumers wanted information about the
lipid content of foods so that they could comply with their physicians'
recommendations to consume diets containing lower levels of saturated fats
and cholesterol. Manufacturers of products derived from plant oils began
listing the levels of polyunsaturated fatty acids on the labels of their products. Some members of the public health community applauded this action,
but there was no uniformity in the way the products were labeled, and often
the labeling did not contain information on total fat and saturated fat.

Attempting to provide uniformity to such information, the Food and
Drug Administration (FDA) promulgated voluntary labeling regulations,
which allowed the listing of amounts of total fat and optional listing of both
unsaturated and saturated lipids and/or cholesterol. When information on
fatty acid and cholesterol content was listed as part of nutrition labeling, the
regulations required that a statement accompany the nutrition labeling
panel, explaining that the information on fatty acid content was provided to
help consumers comply with the advice of their physicians. At that time,
many investigations believed that the effect of dietary saturated fatty acids
and cholesterol on blood cholesterol levels was influenced significantly by
the individuals' genetics and therefore that most individuals were not affected. Hearings held by the Senate Select Committee on Nutrition and
Human Needs had a significant impact on demonstrating a need to provide
guidance to the public on this important issue (USC, 1977).

In the late 1970s, the U.S. Department of Health and Humans Services
and the USDA joined forces in providing advice about diet to normal,
healthy consumers. The result of this effort was the development of a
pamphlet entitled *Nutrition and Your Health: Dietary Guidelines for Americans*
(USDA-DHEW, 1980). Most commonly referred to simply as *Dietary Guidelines for Americans* or *Dietary Guidelines*, this pamphlet has since been revised
and published in 1985 (USDA) and again in 1990 (USDA). A new revision is

to be released in early 1996. One of the specific guidelines in this pamphlet addresses the consumption of fat, saturated fat, and cholesterol. The condensed advice given in each of these editions is reproduced in Table 1.1. The only difference between the recommendations of the first and second editions was that the second edition recommended using skim milk and skim milk products. The text of both editions indicates that there was still controversy about what recommendations are appropriate for healthy Americans. It is also interesting to note that both the first and second editions focus recommendations about fat only on maintaining cardiovascular health.

Also in the late 1970s, hearings were held jointly by the FDA, USDA, and Federal Trade Commission (FTC) to determine the need for changes in food labeling and advertising. In December 1979, the three agencies published the tentative conclusions from these hearings in the *Federal Register* (FDA-FTC-USDA, 1979). Among the positions was the intent to proceed with rule-making on defining nutrient content claims for fats and to eliminate the required statement associated with fatty acid labeling, but the rule-making was delayed because of a change in administration.

In retrospect the delay may have been fortunate because a great deal of consensus building in the area of diet and health occurred during the 1980s. At the start of the decade, consensus was limited to certain relationships between diet and specific diseases (i.e., blood cholesterol levels were shown to be a risk factor for coronary heart disease and certain saturated fatty acids raised blood cholesterol levels, whereas certain polyunsaturated fatty acids lowered blood cholesterol). However, the advice during the 1970s to raise consumption of polyunsaturated fatty acids was contrary to some observations of the relationship between dietary fat intake and the risk of certain forms of cancer. Similarly, the observed relationships between diet and other chronic diseases were not always consistent with those observed for coronary heart disease.

Two major efforts sought to bring about consensus on dietary advice to the population. The U.S. Department of Health and Human Services initiated work on *The Surgeon General's Report on Nutrition and Health* (DHHS, 1988). This report brought together the latest information on reducing the risk of chronic disease through dietary measures. It concluded that high fat intake is associated with risk of obesity, some types of cancer, and possibly gallbladder disease. It also concluded that there is strong consistent evidence for the relationship between saturated fat intake, high blood cholesterol levels, and increased risk of coronary heart disease. Finally, the report concluded that dietary cholesterol raises blood cholesterol levels, but the effect is less pronounced than that for saturated fat. The overall advice on lipids in the Surgeon General's report was as follows:

Fats and cholesterol: Reduce consumption of fat (especially saturated fat) and cholesterol. Choose foods relatively low in these substances, such as vegetables, fruits, whole grain foods, fish, poultry, lean meats, and low-fat dairy products. Use food preparation methods that add little or no fat.

At the same time, the National Academy of Sciences (NAS) Food and Nutrition Board assembled a committee to prepare a report entitled "Diet and Health: Implications for Reducing Chronic Disease" (NAS, 1989). The NAS report, like the Surgeon General's report, concluded that total amounts and types of fats and other lipids in the diet influence the risk of atherosclerotic cardiovascular disease, certain forms of cancer, and possibly obesity. The authors failed to establish a direct link with gallbladder disease but indicated that it is associated with obesity. The NAS report narrowed concerns about intakes of saturated fatty acids and the rise in levels of serum

TABLE 1.1   Lipid Consumption Advice from USDA *Dietary Guidelines*

1980—AVOID TOO MUCH FAT, SATURATED FAT, AND CHOLESTEROL
  Choose lean meat, fish, poultry, dry beans, and peas as your protein sources.
  Moderate your use of eggs and organ meats (such as liver).
  Limit your intake of butter, cream, hydrogenated margarines, shortenings, and coconut oil and foods made from such products.
  Trim excess fat off meats.
  Broil, bake, or boil rather than fry.
  Read labels carefully to determine both amount and types of fat contained in foods.
1985—AVOID TOO MUCH FAT, SATURATED FAT, AND CHOLESTEROL
  Choose lean meat, fish, poultry, and dry beans and peas as protein sources.
  Use skim or low-fat milk and milk products.
  Moderate your use of egg yolks and organ meats.
  Limit your intake of fats and oils, especially those high in saturated fat, such as butter, cream, lard, heavily hydrogenated fats (some margarines), shortenings, and foods containing palm and coconut oils.
  Trim fat off meats.
  Broil, bake, or boil rather than fry.
  Moderate your use of foods that contain fat, such as breaded and deep-fried foods.
  Read labels carefully to determine both amount and type of fat present in foods.

Table 1.1   Continued

1990—CHOOSE A DIET LOW IN FAT, SATURATED FAT, AND CHOLES-
TEROL
Fats and oils
  Use fats and oils sparingly in cooking.
  Use small amounts of salad dressings and spreads, such as butter,
    margarine, and mayonnaise. One tablespoon of most of these spreads
    provides 10–11 grams of fat.
  Choose liquid vegetable oils most often because they are lower in
    saturated fat.
  Check labels on foods to see how much fat and saturated fat are in a
    serving.
Meat, poultry, fish, dry beans, and eggs
  Have two or three servings, with a daily total of about 6 ounces. Three
    ounces of cooked lean beef or chicken without skin—the size of a
    deck of cards—provides about 6 grams of fat.
  Trim fat from meat, take skin off poultry.
  Have cooked dry beans and peas instead of meat occasionally.
  Moderate the use of egg yolks and organ meats.
Milk and milk products
  Have two to three servings daily. (Count as a serving: 1 cup of milk or
    yogurt or about 1½ ounces of cheese.)
  Choose skim or low-fat milk and fat-free of low-fat yogurt and cheese
    most of the time. One cup of skim milk has only a trace of fat, 1 cup
    of 2% fat milk has 5 grams of fat, and 1 cup of whole milk has 8 grams
    of fat.

Source: USDA, 1980, 1985, 1990.

total and low-density lipoprotein (LDL) cholesterol to intake of saturated
fatty acids 12 to 16 carbon atoms in length. The report stated that reductions in these saturated fatty acids will likely reduce coronary heart disease.
    The authors of the NAS report also stated that there were indications that
the levels of saturated fat together with total fat were associated with higher
incidence of and mortality from cancers of the colon, prostate, and breast.
The report concluded that when polyunsaturated fatty acids are substituted
for saturated fat in the diet, omega-6 polyunsaturated fatty acid lowers total
serum cholesterol and LDL cholesterol and lowers some high-density lipoprotein (HDL) cholesterol to a lesser extent. The report also indicated that
omega-6 polyunsaturated fatty acids promote certain cancers in animals,
but no human data show such an association. It was concluded that omega-3

polyunsaturated fatty acids lower plasma triglycerides and increase blood clotting time. The report stated that monounsaturated fatty acids lower LDL cholesterol when substituted for saturated fatty acids.

Concerning dietary cholesterol, the report concluded that inter- and intraindividual response varies substantially, but that dietary cholesterol raises serum total and LDL cholesterol and increases the risk of coronary heart disease. Finally, the report concluded that *trans* fatty acids and their *cis* isomers have similar effects on plasma lipids. The finding was consistent with that of a select panel of investigators convened by the Life Sciences Research Office of the Federation of American Societies for Experimental Biology (Senti, 1985); their report indicated that, based on available data, *trans* fatty acids in the diet had no effect on health. The NAS report recommended that Americans limit dietary fat to 30% and saturated fat to 10% of calories per day and limit their intake of cholesterol to not more than 300 mg per day.

The third edition of the *Dietary Guidelines* was also being prepared late in 1989. As shown in Table 1.1, the key difference in the third edition (USDA, 1990) from the two previous editions was the incorporation of more quantitative guidance. For example, three servings of protein foods per day totaling 6 ounces and two to three 1-cup servings of milk and milk products were recommended. Specific limits of total fat and saturated fat were recommended: the limits were not more than 30% of calories from fat and not more than 10% of calories from saturated fat in the diet. During 1989, hearings on food labels were again held jointly by FDA, FTC, and USDA in various locations across the country. Based on these hearings, it was decided that a comprehensive rule-making should be undertaken to revise nutrition labeling, revise and expand food content claims, and make provisions for health claims.

While the FDA undertook the drafting of proposed rules (FDA, 1990), an independent study commissioned jointly by the U.S. Department of Health and Human Services and the USDA was conducted by the Food and Nutrition Board of the NAS. The purpose of this study was to assess which information was essential to consumers in planning healthful diets and to advise the government on how best to present the information. During this same period, the Congress held hearings designed to determine whether the Federal Food, Drug, and Cosmetic (FD&C) Act provided the agency with authority to require mandatory nutrition labeling and to permit the use of health claims on food labeling. Although the FDA contended that it had the authority under the FD&C Act, a bill was introduced entitled the Nutrition Labeling and Education Act (NLEA) of 1990, which was designed to require mandatory nutrition labeling, make provisions for regulations on both nutrient content claims and health claims, and require national uniformity for all food-labeling provisions, except that states could require special warning statements in situations in which the warning statements would inform consumers about harmful substances in foods.

In the summer of 1990, the FDA published proposed rules and indicated that the report of the NAS study would be considered as comments. The NAS report was completed in October (NAS, 1990). Before the comment period for the proposal was closed, however, the Congress passed and the president signed the NLEA into law (USC, 1990). The complete provisions of this act are too extensive to cover in this chapter, however, the act has had enormous impact on how lipids must be addressed in nutrition labeling, nutrient content claims, and health claims.

Regulations that implement the NLEA (FDA, 1993) require that total calories from fat, the total content of fat and cholesterol, and the amounts of saturated fat must be included in all foods covered by mandatory nutrition labeling. The amounts must be listed on a per-serving basis. In addition, manufacturers can voluntarily label both polyunsaturated and monounsaturated fats, but if either is labeled, the other must also be labeled. The information is mandatory for most processed foods sold at retail in the United States. The amounts of these nutrients must be listed in grams for total fat and saturated fat (poly- and monounsaturated fat when listed) and in milligrams for cholesterol. These values must also be expressed as a percentage of the daily values: 65 g for total fat, 20 g for saturated fat, and 300 mg for cholesterol per 2000-calorie diet. No daily values were established for poly- or monounsaturated fats (see Fig. 1.1).

It is important to note the definitions for each of these terms. Total fat is defined as the sum of all fatty acids expressed as triglycerides. Previous nutrition-labeling regulations relied on the method of the Association of Official Analytical Chemists (AOAC) for determining fat content of foods, which did not always include all fatty acids. Calories from fat are calculated by multiplying grams of total fat by 9 calories. The definition of saturated fat includes all fatty acids containing no double bonds. The previous definition included only four saturated fatty acids: lauric (C-12), myristic (C-14), palmitic (C-16), and stearic (C-18). Polyunsaturated fatty acids include only those unsaturated fatty acids that have *cis-cis* methylene–interrupted bonds. Monounsaturated fatty acids include only the *cis* forms. Although not defined, all fatty acids with a *trans* configuration are considered *trans* fatty acids, even if a *cis* linkage is also present.

The NLEA did not address the question of *trans* fatty acids but provided authority for the Secretary of Health and Human Services to require that additional nutrients be included in nutrition labeling if such information would help consumers select a healthful diet. The NLEA provisions for nutrient content and health claims established certain requirements before

Nutrition Facts

Serving Size ½ cup (114g)
Servings Per Container 4

Amount Per Serving

Calories 260   Calories from Fat 120

	% Daily Value*
Total Fat 13g	**20%**
Saturated Fat 5g	**25%**
Cholesterol 30mg	**10%**
Sodium 660mg	**28%**
Total Carbohydrate 31g	**11%**
Dietary Fiber 0g	**0%**
Sugars 5g	
Protein 5g	

Vitamin A 4%	•	Vitamin C 2%
Calcium 15%	•	Iron 4%

* Percent Daily Values are based on a 2,000 calorie diet. Your daily values may be higher or lower depending on your calorie needs:

		Calories:	2,000	2,500
Total Fat	Less than		65g	80g
Sat Fat	Less than		20g	25g
Cholesterol	Less than		300mg	300mg
Sodium	Less than		2,400mg	2,400mg
Total Carbohydrate			300g	375g
Dietary Fiber			25g	30g

Calories per gram:
Fat 9 • Carbohydrate 4 • Protein 4

FIG. 1.1   An example of the new food label.

these claims could be included on food labeling. The most fundamental of these is that all claims must be established through the rule-making process before they can be included on the label. Both types of claims are also subject to provisions, which are influenced by the composition of the food as well.

In the case of nutrient content claims, the labeling must contain, prominently and in immediate proximity, a referral statement directing consumers to the nutrition information panel. However, nutrient content claims made for foods that contain amounts of a nutrient exceeding a level determined to increase the risk of a disease or condition must make a disclosure statement, instead of the referral statement, that directs the consumer to specific information in the nutrition information panel about the nutrient (e.g., "See side panel for information on fat and other nutrients"). In the following three circumstances, the disclosure statement must be modified to include the amount of a particular nutrient present: (1) fiber claims for products that are not low in fat must state the amount of fat present; (2) cholesterol claims for products that contain fat at levels exceeding the disclosure levels must state the amount of fat present; and (3) saturated fat claims for products that are not cholesterol-free must state the amount of cholesterol present and, if the product is not free of or low in fat, must state the amount of total fat present.

Health claims cannot be made for a food that contains levels of a nutrient that would make it difficult for a consumer to construct a daily diet that conforms with widely accepted guidelines for reducing the risk of a disease or condition. The levels of such nutrients (i.e., "disclosure levels" for nutrient content claims and "disqualifying levels" for health claims) are shown in Table 1.2.

FDA regulations have provided for 13 nutrient content claims for lipids. They are listed in Table 1.3 together with the necessary requirements for individual foods, main dishes, and meals. In some cases synonyms can be used for the adjective descriptor, e.g., "zero," "no," or "without" can be used for "free." These nutrient content claims were carefully established through the notice and comment rule-making process so that consumers could have confidence that the claims always have the same definition when used on food labels. For example, a serving of low-fat cookies would have the same maximum fat content as a serving of low-fat cake, etc. Any party can petition the FDA to create an additional nutrient content claim which, if properly supported with necessary scientific data, can be established through notice and comment rule-making.

FDA regulations have provided for five health claims involving the lipid content of foods (Table 1.4). Table 1.4 also includes information on food requirements, claim requirements, and the model claim statement. As noted above, these claims cannot be used if the food contains an amount equal to or more than the nutrient amount shown in Table 1.2. The model claim statement does not have to be used verbatim but can be reworded, provided that all elements of the statement are conveyed and the revised

TABLE 1.2 Specified Levels of Nutrients for Disclosure (Nutrient Content Claims) and Disqualification (Health Claims)

Nutrient	Individual foods	Main dishes	Meats
Fat (g)	13	19.5	26
Saturated fat (g)	4	6	8
Cholesterol (mg)	60	90	120
Sodium (mg)	480	720	960

TABLE 1.3   Requirements for Nutrient Content Claims

Claim	Individual food (per reference amount)[a,b]	Meal and main dishes (per labeled serving)[b]
Fat free	<0.5 g fat	<0.5 g fat
Low fat	≤3 g fat	≤3 g fat/100 g ≤30% of calories from fat
Reduced fat	25% less fat	25% less fat
Saturated fat free	<0.5 g saturated fat <0.5 g *trans* fatty acids	<0.5 g saturated fat <0.5 g *trans* fatty acids
Low saturated fat	≤1 g saturated fat ≤15% of calories from saturated fat	≤1 g saturated fat/100 g <10% of calories from saturated fat
Reduced saturated fat	25% less saturated fat	25% less saturated fat
Cholesterol free	<2 mg cholesterol ≤2 g saturated fat	<2 mg cholesterol ≤2 g saturated fat
Low cholesterol	<20 mg cholesterol ≤2 g saturated fat	≤20 mg cholesterol/100 g ≤2 g saturated fat/100 g
Reduced cholesterol	25% less cholesterol ≤2 g saturated fat	25% less cholesterol ≤2 g saturated fat
Lean	<10 g total fat ≤4.5 g saturated fat <95 mg cholesterol	<10 g total fat ≤4.5 g saturated fat <95 mg cholesterol
Extra lean	<5 g total fat <2 g saturated fat <95 mg cholesterol	<5 g total fat <2 g saturated fat <95 mg cholesterol
Light/lite (in fat)	50% less fat	Low fat
Healthy	Low fat Low saturated fat ≤60 mg cholesterol	Low fat Low saturated fat ≤90 mg cholesterol
Healthy game or seafood	Extra lean	

[a]All free claims except cholesterol must also be per labeled serving.
[b]All lean and extra lean must also be per 100 grams.

statement has the same meaning. As with the nutrient content claims, new health claims can be the subject of a citizen's petition but must be substantiated by scientific data. If the petition has merit, the FDA will then have to submit the proposed claim to notice and comment rule-making.

Several issues concerning the labeling of fats have remained under active discussion since the completion of final NLEA-implementing rules. Among these are how to address the labeling and claims of fats with low bioavailability, how to label saturated fats that do not raise blood cholesterol levels, and what labeling, if any, is needed to inform consumers about *trans* fatty acids.

During the late 1980s, three studies were performed in the Netherlands as reported by Katan and coworkers (Mensink and Katan, 1990; Mensink et al., 1992; Zock and Katan, 1992). These studies indicated that the addition of *trans* fatty acids to the diets of adult humans raised blood cholesterol levels. Because these studies involved the use of *trans* fatty acids that were not common to U.S. diets and because the levels of *trans* fatty acids in the studies were higher than those common in U.S. diets, some investigators questioned the relevance of these studies to the U.S. situation. Other investigators maintained that the studies were relevant (Willett and Ascherio, 1994). Consequently, the USDA conducted a clinical study designed to determine whether *trans* fatty acids found in the U.S. diet raised blood cholesterol levels. Unfortunately, the results of the USDA study were not published until 1994 (Judd et al., 1994), well after the NLEA-implementing regulations were completed.

In the preamble to these regulations, the FDA indicated that there were insufficient data to determine if consumers need information on *trans* fatty acid levels in foods to plan healthful diets. FDA has since received a petition from the Center for Science in the Public Interest (CSPI) requesting that the agency include *trans* fatty acids in the definition of saturated fats. The petition also requested that the level of *trans* fatty acids be a factor in criteria for claims. In a letter, the Malaysian Palm Oil Promotion Council supported the CSPI petition but offered an alternative in which *trans* fatty acids would be listed in a separate line of the nutrition labeling panel as *trans* fat. Both organizations contend that the recent metabolic studies of Katan and co-workers and of Judd et al. demonstrate that *trans* fatty acids raise serum LDL cholesterol levels, and that information about the levels of *trans* fatty acids needs to be factored into the nutrition information used by consumers to plan their diets.

These issues will be addressed as quickly as permitted by available resources and competing priorities for those resources. However, the federal agencies that have roles in disease prevention and health promotion are involved with private sector organizations in making use of the new label

TABLE 1.4 Health Claims Relating to Lipid Content

Approved claims	Food requirements	Claim rquirements	Model claim statements
Dietary saturated fat and cholesterol and risk of coronary heart disease (21 CFR 101.75)	Low saturated fat, low cholesterol, and low-fat fish and game meats: "Extra Lean"	Required terms: "Saturated fat and cholesterol"; "Coronary heart disease" or "Heart disease"; includes physician statement (individuals with elevated blood total or LDL cholesterol should consult their physicians) if claim defines high or normal blood total and LDL cholesterol	While many factors affect heart disease, diets low in saturated fat and cholesterol may reduce the risk of this disease.
Fruits, vegetables, and grain products that contain fiber, particularly soluble fiber, and risk of coronary heart disease (21 CFR 101.77)	A fruit, vegetable, or grain product that contains fiber, low saturated fat, low cholesterol, low fat, at least 0.6 g of soluble fiber per RA (without fortification), and soluble fiber content provided on label	Required terms: "Fiber," "Dietary fiber," "Some types of dietary fiber," "Some dietary fibers," or "Some fibers"; "Saturated fat" and "Cholesterol"; "Heart disease" or "Coronary heart disease"; includes physician statement (individuals with elevated blood total or LDL cholesterol should consult their physicians) if claim defines high or normal blood total and LDL cholesterol	Diets low in saturated fat and cholesterol and rich in fruits, vegetables, and grain products that contain some types of dietary fiber, particularly soluble fiber, may reduce the risk of heart disease, a disease associated with many factors.

Dietary fat and cancer (21 CFR 101.73)	Low fat fish and game meats: "Extra Lean"	Required terms: "Total fat" or "Fat"; "Some types of cancers" or "Some cancers"; does not specify types of fats or fatty acids that may be related to risk of cancer	Development of cancer depends on many factors. A diet low in total fat may reduce the risk of some cancers.
Fiber-containing grain products, fruits, and vegetables and cancer (21 CFR 101.76)	A grain product, fruit, or vegetable that contains dietary fiber, low fat, and good source of dietary fiber (without fortification)	Required terms: "Fiber," "Dietary fiber," or "Total dietary fiber"; "Some types of cancer" or "Some cancers"; does not specify types of dietary fiber that may be related to risk of cancer	Low-fat diets rich in fiber-containing grain products, fruits, and vegetables may reduce the risk of some types of cancer, a disease associated with many factors.
Fruits and vegetables and cancer (21 CFR 101.78)	A fruit or vegetable, low fat, and good source (without fortification) of at least one of the following: vitamin A, vitamin C, or dietary fiber	Required terms: "Fiber," "Dietary fiber," or "Total dietary fiber"; "Total fat" or "Fat"; "Some types of cancer" or "Some cancers"; characterizes fruits and vegetables as "Foods that are low in fat and may contain vitamin A, vitamin C, and dietary fiber"; characterizes specific food as a "good source" of one or more of the following: dietary fiber, vitamin A, or vitamin C; does not specify types of fats or fatty acids or types of dietary fiber that may be related to risk of cancer	Low-fat diets rich in fruits and vegetables (foods that are low in fat and may contain dietary fiber, vitamin A, or vitamin C) may reduce the risk of some types of cancer, a disease associated with many factors. Broccoli is high in vitamins A and C and is a good source of dietary fiber.

information in informing the public. These efforts are being directed at all segments of the U.S. population in a variety of forms and ways, including electronic media, print media, teaching curricula, and one-on-one counseling.

It is recognized that additional scientific information is needed to fully understand the role of lipids in health and disease and that the message may need to be fine-tuned in the future. There has also been significant recognition on the part of producers, manufacturers, retailers, and others who have a role in shaping the food supply. New foods with altered lipid contents which help consumers plan healthier diets have been developed and marketed. The success of these efforts will likely take years to determine, and a continued desire by consumers to maintain and improve their health is essential to this success.

REFERENCES

Atwater, W. O. 1948. *Foods: Nutritive Value and Cost.* USDA Farmers' Bulletin No. 23. Washington, DC.

Atwater, W. O. 1901. *Principles of Nutrition and Nutritive Value of Food.* USDA Farmers' Bulletin No. 142. Washington, DC.

de Langen, C. D. 1916. Cholesterine-stofwisseling en Rassen-patholgie. *Geneeskd. Tijdschr. Ned. Indie.* 56: 1–34.

de Langen, C. D. 1922. Het Cholesterinegehalte van het Bloed in Indic. *Geneeskd. Tijdschr. Ned. Indie.* 62: 1–4.

DHHS. 1988. *The Surgeon General's Report on Nutrition and Health.* U.S. Department of Health and Human Services, Public Health Service, DHHS (PHS) Publ. No. 88-50210. Superintendent of Documents, Stock No. 017-001-00465-1. U.S. Government Printing Office, Washington, DC.

FDA-FTC-USDA. 1979. Food labeling: Tentative position of agencies. *Fed. Reg.* 44: 75990–76020.

FDA. 1990. Food labeling; mandatory status of nutrition labeling and nutrient content revision; proposed rule. *Fed. Reg.* 55: 29487.

FDA. 1993. Food labeling; general provisions; nutrition labeling; label format; nutrient content claims; health claims; ingredient labeling; state and local requirements; and exemptions; 1993 final rules. *Fed. Reg.* 58: 2079–2964.

Hegsted, D. M., McGrandy, R., Myers, M. L., et al. 1965. Quantitative effects of dietary fat on serum cholesterol in man. *Am. J. Clin. Nutr.* 17: 281–295.

Hegsted, D. M. 1986. Serum-cholesterol responses to dietary cholesterol: A re-evaluation. *Am. J. Clin. Nutr.* 44: 299–305.

Judd, J. T., Clevidence, B. A., Muesing, R. A., Wittes, J., Sunkin, M. E., and

Podczasy, J. J. 1994. Dietary *trans* fatty acids: Effects on plasma lipids and lipoproteins of healthy men and women. *Am. J. Clin. Nutr.* 59: 861–868.

Keys, A. 1957. Diet and the epidemiology of coronary heart disease. *J. Am. Med. Assoc.* 164: 1912–1919.

Keys, A., Anderson, J. T., and Grande, F. 1957. Prediction of serum-cholesterol responses of man to changes in fats in the diet. *Lancet* 2: 959–966.

Keys, A., Anderson, J. T., and Grande, F. 1965. Serum cholesterol response to changes in the diet. IV. Particular saturated fatty acids in the diet. *Metabolism* 14: 776–787.

Mensink, R. P., and Katan, M. B. 1990. Effect of dietary *trans* fatty acids on high-density and low-density lipoprotein cholesterol levels in healthy subjects. *N. Engl. J. Med.* 323: 439–445.

Mensink, R. P., Zock, P. L., Katan, M. B., and Hornstra, G. 1992. Effect of dietary *cis* and *trans* fatty acids on serum lipoprotein[a] levels in humans. *J. Lipid Res.* 33: 1493–1501.

Murlin, J. R. and Miller, C. W. 1919. Preliminary results of nutritional surveys in United States army camps. *Am. J. Public Health* 9(6): 401–413.

NAS. 1989. *Diet and Health: Implications for Reducing Chronic Disease Risk.* National Academy Press, Washington, DC.

NAS. 1990. *Nutrition Labeling—Issues and Directors for the 1990s.* National Academy Press, Washington, DC.

NAS-NRC. 1943. *Recommended Dietary Allowances.* Publ. No. 115. Food and Nutrition Board, National Academy of Sciences-National Research Council, Washington, DC.

NAS-NRC. 1945. *Recommended Dietary Allowances.* Publ. No. 122. Food and Nutrition Board, National Academy of Sciences-National Research Council, Washington, DC.

NAS-NRC. 1948. *Recommended Dietary Allowances.* Publ. No. 129. Food and Nutrition Board, National Academy of Sciences-National Research Council, Washington, DC.

NAS-NRC. 1953. *Recommended Dietary Allowances.* Publ. No. 302. Food and Nutrition Board, National Academy of Sciences-National Research Council, Washington, DC.

NAS-NRC. 1958. *Recommended Dietary Allowances.* Publ. No. 589. Food and Nutrition Board, National Academy of Sciences-National Research Council, Washington, DC.

NRC. 1941. *Recommended Dietary Allowances.* Committee on Food and Nutrition, National Research Council, Washington, DC.

Senti, F. R. (Ed.). 1985. *Health Aspects of Dietary trans Fatty Acids.* Life Sciences Research Office, Federation of American Societies for Experimental Biology, Bethesda, MD. (Tentitive Position)

USC. 1794. Navy Ration Law. United State Congress, Washington, DC.

USC. 1977. Final Report, U.S. Congress Senate Select Committee on Nutrition and Human Needs, 95th Congress, First Session.

USC. 1990. Navy Rations, United States Congress, Washington, DC. Title 10: Section 6082.

USC. November 8, 1990. Nutrition Labeling and Education Act of 1990. Public Law 101-535, 104 Stat. 2353, 21 USC, 301 note, 321, 337, 343, 343 notes, 343-1, 343-1 note, 345, 371.

USDA. 1985. *Nutrition and Your Health: Dietary Guidelines—Guidelines for Americans.* 2nd ed. USDA Home and Garden Bulletin No. 232. U.S. Government Printing Office, Washington, DC.

USDA. 1990. *Nutrition and Your Health: Dietary Guidelines for Americans.* 3rd ed. USDA Home and Garden Bulletin No. 232. U.S. Government Printing Office, Washington, DC.

USDA-DHEW. 1980. *Nutrition and Your Health: Dietary Guidelines for Americans.* USDA and U.S. Dept of Health, Education, and Welfare, Washington, DC.

White House Conference on Food, Nutrition and Health. 1970. Final Report. Superintendent of Documents (1970; 0-378-473). Government Printing Office, Washington, DC.

Willett, W. C., and Ascherio, A. 1994, *Trans* fatty acids: Are the effects only marginal? *Am. J. Public Health* 84: 722–724.

Zock, P. L., and Katan, M. B. 1992. Hydrogenation alternatives: Effects of *trans* fatty acids and stearic acid versus linoleic acid on serum lipids and lipoproteins in humans. *J. Lipid Res.* 33:399–410

2
Food Lipids and Atherosclerosis

David Kritchevsky

The Wistar Institute
Philadelphia, Pennsylvania

ATHEROSCLEROSIS

The term atherosclerosis was coined in 1904 and was intended to describe the gruel-like consistency of early lipid deposits in the artery. Atherosclerosis is derived from the Greek word for porridge and was meant to describe in one word the early aortic fatty deposits (athero) and later hardening (sclerosis). Early lipid deposits eventually accumulate fibrous tissue, complex carbohydrates, blood products, and calcium. Atherosclerosis, strictly speaking, is one of several changes that occur in the artery. In current usage, however, it is an inclusive, popular term for all arterial changes. Davignon (1978) has devised a representation of the many factors—extrinsic, hormonal, and lipid content of the blood and arterial wall metabolism—all of which contribute to this condition. It has been characterized as a lifestyle disease, meaning a disease of multiple etiology. In the absence of an unequivocal test for impending heart attack, we allude to a variety of indicators of increased risk. These indicators, designated as risk factors, offer a statistical diagnosis, which is a statement of odds. At this moment the major risk factors are male gender, obesity, cigarette smoking, hypertension, and hyper-cholesterolemia. Family history and gender are beyond medical control, but the other major risk factors are amenable to medical or behavioral alteration. Hopkins and Williams (1981) identified 246 risk factors for cardiovascular disease. Risk factors for coronary disease begin to manifest their potential for lesion development even in young subjects (Strong, 1995).

Early studies in which dietary cholesterol was shown to produce atherosclerotic lesions in the arteries of rabbits (Anitschkow, 1913) implicated sterol as a prime suspect. Serum or plasma levels reflect the availability of cholesterol to the arterial tissue, and measurement of plasma cholesterol has become a standard medical protocol. Gofman et al. (1950) revolutionized our concepts of circulating lipids by providing a means of separating the different lipoproteins, lipid-protein aggregates, which are the vehicle for transporting fats in the blood. The lipoproteins are characterized by their hydrated densities, and the lighter materials are richer in triglycerides. Low-density lipoprotein (LDL) is characterized as the "bad" cholesterol because it is generally associated with increased risk. The protein-rich high-density lipoprotein (HDL) is popularly recognized as "the good cholesterol." As research continues, the lipoprotein area is subjected to increasing fine-tuning. Molecular size influences the ease with which LDL molecules enter the arterial wall (Stender and Zilversmit, 1981). Krauss and Burke (1982) identified a number of subclasses of human LDL. Austin et al. (1988) analyzed the subclass of LDL in 109 cases of myocardial infarction and 121 controls and observed that the LDL pattern characterized by increased levels of small, dense particles was associated with a threefold increased risk of myocardial infarction. The correlation was independent of age, sex, or relative weight. Total plasma cholesterol levels in cases and controls were not significantly different (226 ± 47 vs. 215 ± 40 mg/dL), but triglyceride levels were significantly ($p < 0.001$) higher in the cases (214 ± 104 vs. 157 ± 68 mg/dL). Polymorphism of apolipoprotein E offers an opportunity to segregate subjects according to their susceptibility to successful treatment of lipidemia (Utermann et al., 1977). Another relatively new factor in the lipoprotein family is lipoprotein (a) [Lp(a)], which was first described by Berg in 1963. Lp(a) is an LDL whose apoprotein (apoB) is linked to apoprotein (a) via a disulfide bridge. Lp(a) interferes with normal fibrinolytic processes and is thought to offer an especially high risk for myocardial infarction.

The most common screening method is simple assessment of serum cholesterol. It must then be recognized that a single reading may not be a true indicator of risk. Plasma/Serum cholesterol values may fluctuate diurnally and seasonally. Recent articles have pointed up the seasonal variability of cholesterol (Kritchevsky, 1985; Gordon et al., 1988; Robinson et al., 1992). Hegsted and Nicolosi (1987) emphasized the need for basing diagnosis on more than one measurement. Harlap et al. (1982) demonstrated seasonal fluctuations of lipids and lipoproteins in 5246 men and women in the Jerusalem Lipid Research Clinic. They concluded that "clinicians should take season into account when diagnosing hyperlipidemia and evaluating success or failure of its treatment." Gordon et al. (1988) analyzed seasonal lipid variations in 1446 hypercholesterolemic men who comprised the placebo group in the Lipid Research Clinics Coronary Primary Prevention Trial. They found highly significant seasonal cycles for total, LDL, and HDL cholesterol. Total and LDL cholesterol varied inversely with hours of daylight, and HDL cholesterol varied positively with ambient temperature.

FOOD LIPIDS

Cholesterol

Studies in rabbits, chickens, and other susceptible species show that dietary cholesterol can lead to atherosclerosis. The level of cholesterol fed in these studies is usually high, and there have been no attempts to establish a dose-response relationship.

Because of the presence of serum cholesterol in the risk factor spectrum and the evidence from animal studies, the general advice has been to reduce levels of dietary cholesterol. The advice is based partially on the fact that cholesterol in the diet is usually associated with saturated fat. However, studies of actual cholesterol intake as it affects cholesterol levels have yielded equivocal results.

Gertler et al. (1950) studied two groups of 40 men each taken from a larger study of heart disease. One group had coronary disease and the other was a control. The subgroups were those with the highest or lowest serum cholesterol levels or those who ingested the most or least cholesterol. While in every subgroup the men with heart disease had significantly higher cholesterol levels than the controls, there was no relationship between cholesterol intake and cholesterol level (Table 2.1). Several studies show that addition of eggs to the daily diet does affect cholesterolemia of free-living subjects (Slater et al., 1976; Kummerow et al., 1977; Porter et al., 1977; Dawber et al., 1982). Analysis of diets of the participants of three large population studies (Framingham, Puerto Rico and Hawaii) who did or did not have coronary incidents showed no relation to either fat or cholesterol content (Gordon et al., 1981). McNamara (1990) reviewed data from 68 clinical studies involving 1490 subjects and concluded that every 100 mg of

Table 2.1 Dietary and Serum Cholesterol in Control Subjects
or Subjects with Coronary Heart Disease (CHD) (10 men in
each subgroup)

| Subgroup | Group | | $p <$ |
	CHD	Control	
Lowest serum cholesterol			
Cholesterol (mg/dl)	196 ± 5	162 ± 2	0.001
Dietary cholesterol (g/week)	3.3 ± 0.5	3.8 ± 0.3	NS
Highest serum cholesterol			
Cholesterol (mg/dl)	416 ± 17	313 ± 3	0.001
Dietary cholesterol (g/week)	4.1 ± 0.6	4.3 ± 0.4	NS
Lowest cholesterol intake			
Cholesterol (mg/dl)	271 ± 14	222 ± 16	0.05
Dietary cholesterol (g/week)	1.3 ± 0.1	1.4 ± 0.1	NS
Highest cholesterol intake			
Cholesterol (mg/dl)	288 ± 22	213 ± 11	0.01
Dietary cholesterol (g/week)	5.7 ± 0.2	7.0 ± 0.3	0.01

NS, not significant.
Source: Modified from Gertler et al., 1950.

cholesterol ingested led to a plasma cholesterol increase of 2.3 ± 0.2 mg/ dL. Hopkins (1992) reviewed data from 27 studies in which diets were supplied by a metabolic facility kitchen and constructed a curvilinear (hyperbolic) relationship for the cholesterolemic effect dietary cholesterol. The magnitude of change is a function of the baseline dietary cholesterol with the greatest response being seen when dietary intake is near zero. The individual response is a function of the many complex mechanisms underlying cholesterol metabolism from absorption to bile acid synthesis. La Rosa (1993) has suggested that the dietary cholesterol effect on serum cholesterol is about one-fifth that of saturated fat.

There is now increasing interest in a possible correlation between low plasma cholesterol levels and noncoronary death. The causes of noncoronary deaths in the course of primary and secondary prevention trials have been reviewed (Muldoon et al., 1990; Holme, 1990; Criqui, 1991; Kritchevsky and Kritchevsky, 1992). A review of a large number of trials (yielding 68406 deaths) found that cholesterol levels below 160 mg/dL were not advantageous (Jacobs et al., 1992). Data from the Lipid Research Clinics program found that the risk of colon cancer was increased in men whose cholesterol levels were below 187 mg/dL (Cowan et al., 1990).

Fatty Acid Saturation

In 1954 we (Kritchevsky et al., 1954) reported that saturated fat was more atherogenic than unsaturated fat in cholesterol-fed rabbits. Subsequently we found that as fats became more saturated they became more atherogenic for rabbits. One fat that did not fit the observation was cocoa butter, and its anomalous effect was attributed to its high content of stearic acid.

In human studies, Ahrens et al. (1957) fed a number of subjects a formula diet containing 45% of energy as carbohydrate, 40% of energy as fat, and 15% of energy as protein. The standard fat was corn oil. In general, cholesterol levels rose as fat saturation increased. McNamara et al. (1987) fed subjects diets containing high or low levels of cholesterol (about 240 or 840 mg) and high or low in saturated fat (P/S about 0.29 or 1.63). When the P/S ratio was low, the difference in plasma cholesterol between subjects on high or low cholesterol intake was 5 mg/dL; when the P/S ratio was high, the difference was 6 mg/dL. However, going from high to low saturation increased cholesterol by 25 or 24 mg/dL in subjects fed low or high cholesterol, respectively (Table 2.2). Frantz et al. (1989) fed a cohort of more than 9000 institutionalized subjects diets predominating in saturated or unsaturated fat and showed that cholesterol levels were unchanged (+2%) on the former diet but fell by 14% on the latter. Cardiovascular deaths were the same in the two groups, but total deaths were 8.5% lower in the controls.

Keys et al. (1965) and Hegsted et al. (1965) developed formulas for predicting cholesterol levels based upon dietary changes. The Keys formula is:

$$\Delta C = 1.35(2\Delta S - \Delta P) + 1.5\Delta Z$$

where ΔC represents the change in cholesterol levels, ΔS and ΔP represent changes in levels of saturated and unsaturated fatty acids, and z is the square root of mg of dietary cholesterol per 1000 kcal. The Hegsted formula is:

$$\Delta C = 2.16\Delta S - 1.65\Delta P + 0.168\Delta C \ (mg/1000 \ kcal) + 85$$

In both cases they found that stearic acid did not fit the formula. Hegsted further opined that about two thirds of the hypercholesterolemic effect of saturated fat was due to myristic acid.

More recently it has become possible to provide coefficients for specific fatty acids. Thus Hayes et al. (1995) have derived the formula:

$$Cholesterol = 229 + 8E_{14:0} - 36 \log E_{18:2}$$

E represents the energy contribution of myristic and linoleic acids. It is Hayes' view that myristic acid is hypercholesterolemic at any level and linoleic acid is hypocholesterolemic until its concentration reaches 4–6% of

TABLE 2.2 Plasma Cholesterol Levels in Subjects Fed High or Low
Levels of Cholesterol with Saturated or Unsaturated Fat

Dietary fat	Fat (P/S)	Cholesterol Dietary (mg)	Plasma (mg/dl)	Plasma (mmol/L)
Low cholesterol				
Saturated	0.31 ± 0.18	288 ± 64	243 ± 50	6.28 ± 1.29
Unsaturated	1.90 ± 0.90	192 ± 60	218 ± 46	5.63 ± 1.19
High cholesterol				
Saturated	0.27 ± 0.15	863 ± 161	248 ± 51	6.41 ± 1.32
Unsaturated	1.45 ± 0.50	820 ± 102	224 ± 46	5.79 ± 1.19

Source: Modified from McNamara et al., 1987.

energy. Palmitic acid may raise cholesterol when fed as part of a high-cholesterol diet. Derr et al. (1993) have adduced the following formula:

$$\Delta C = 2.3 \, \Delta \, 14{:}0 + 3.0\Delta \, 16{:}0 - 0.8\Delta \, 18{:}0 - 1.0 \, PUFA$$

On the basis of their own analysis of the literature, Mensink and Katan (1992) proposed the formula:

$$\Delta C = 1.2 \, (1.8\Delta S - 0.1\Delta M - 0.5 \, \Delta P)$$

where C represents cholesterol, S is the sum of lauric, myristic, and palmitic acids, and M and P are monounsaturates and polyunsaturates, respectively.

Based on a review of 420 dietary observations in 141 groups of subjects, Hegsted et al. (1993) concluded that (1) saturated fatty acids are the primary determinants of serum cholesterol levels, (2) polyunsaturates lower serum cholesterol, and (3) monounsaturates have no independent effect. They also found that dietary cholesterol contributes to cholesterolemia.

In a review of fatty acid effects, Katan et al. (1994) conclude that under metabolic ward conditions, replacement of carbohydrate by lauric, myristic or palmitic acid raises both LDL and HDL cholesterol and that oleic and linoleic acids raise HDL and lower LDL slightly. Mattson and Grundy (1985) have shown that monounsaturated fat is as effective as unsaturated fat in lowering cholesterol levels in males.

As has already been noted, stearic acid does not affect lipidemia in the expected way. Experimental studies in rats, dogs, and hamsters show that triglycerides rich in stearic acid are not absorbed as efficiently as those containing the shorter-chain fatty acids. These observations may explain, in part, why stearic acid is not as atherogenic or cholesterolemic as might be expected (Kritchevsky, 1994).

Peanut oil is anomalous in being an unsaturated fat that is unexpectedly atherogenic for rats (Gresham and Howard, 1960), rabbits (Kritchevsky et al., 1971), and monkeys (Vesselinovitch et al., 1974; Kritchevsky et al., 1982). Peanut oil differs from most naturally occurring plant oils in that is contains about 4–6% very long-chain fatty acids (arachidic, behenic, and lignoceric). To test whether these fatty acids influence atherogenicity, we mixed three common fats to provide an oil whose composition resembled that of peanut oil minus arachidic and behenic acids. This new fat, designated as PGF, was no more atherogenic than corn oil. We then co-randomized PGF with arachidic and behenic acids to give a new fat whose fatty acid spectrum was virtually identical to that of peanut oil. This new fat (PGFR) was also no more atherogenic than corn oil. The fatty acid spectra of peanut oil and PGFR were very similar, but, due to randomization, the distribution of their fatty acids was different. The next step was to randomize peanut oil. Rearrangement of the naturally occurring triglyceride rendered the peanut oil significantly less atherogenic (Kritchevsky et al., 1973). The sequence of experiments and the results are described more fully by Kritchevsky (1988).

The double bonds in most naturally occurring unsaturated fats are in the *cis* configuration, although butter and meat may contain a small amount of fat whose double bonds are in the *trans* configuration (*trans* fat). Plant fats vary in their levels of *trans* fat, which can range from 1 to 72% (Sommerfeld, 1983). However, the principal source of *trans* fat in the diet of developed countries is hydrogenated fat present in margarines, shortenings, and cooking fats. *Trans* fats are, in general, metabolized like their *cis* unsaturated counterparts (Ono and Fredrickson, 1964; Anderson and Coots, 1967). When *trans* fats are fed to rats (Moore et al., 1980) or monkeys (Kritchevsky et al., 1984), they accumulate in blood and tissues but disappear after the dietary stimulus has been removed. Cholesteryl esters of *trans* fats are synthesized (Kritchevsky and Baldino, 1978) and hydrolyzed (Sgoutas, 1968) more slowly than those of *cis* fats. *Trans* fats inhibit fatty acid desaturation and elongation (Privett et al., 1967) but do not seem to affect hepatic enzymes not involved in lipid metabolism (Ruttenberg et al., 1983). *Trans* fatty acids are hypercholesterolemic when fed to rabbits in cholesterol containing or cholesterol-free diets but they are not more atherogenic (McMillan et al., 1963; Ruttenberg et al., 1983). When swine were fed diets containing 17% fat in which the level of *trans* fat ranged from 0 to 48% for 10 months, there were no effects on either cholesterolemia or atherosclerosis (Elson et al., 1981). The levels of *trans* fat in tissues of human subjects who die of coronary heart disease are no different than those of controls. Houtsmuller (1978) suggested that *trans* fat should be regarded as quasi saturated fats.

Two recent reports from The Netherlands (Mensink and Katan, 1990) and Australia (Nestel et al., 1992) have raised concerns that *trans* fat may elevate Lp(a) levels in humans. Several American studies have found no effect of *trans* fat on Lp(a) (Lichtenstein et al., 1983; Wood et al., 1993; Clevidence et al., 1995). The American studies were carried out with margarines that contained a wide spectrum of *trans* fatty acids, whereas the other studies used elaidic acid–rich fats. The metabolic role of specific *trans* fatty acids remains to be elucidated.

Triglyceride Structure

A summary of the structure of the major triglycerides of most natural oils and fats shows that virtually all of them carry either oleic or linoleic acid at the 2 position. This position is described stereochemically as SN2 (Small, 1991). There must be a teleological reason for this since the fatty acid in the SN2 position is 78% conserved during digestion (Mattson and Volpenhein, 1964; Kayden et al., 1967). Vander Wal (1955) suggested that triglyceride structure was dictated by the need to keep fats fluid in vivo.

The influence of randomization on the atherogenicity of peanut oil has been alluded to. As a consequence of our early studies of the effects of saturation on the atherogenicity of various fats, we thought that preparation of fats containing an excess of a specific saturated fatty acid might offer a clue to individual atherogenic effects. Accordingly we co-randomized corn oil with trilaurin, trimyristin, tripalmitin, or tristearin to provide fats containing a large excess of lauric, myristic, palmitic, or stearic acid. The atherogenic effects of the four synthetic fats were the same (Kritchevsky and Tepper, 1967). The feeding of similarly derived fats to hamsters showed that the stearic acid–rich fat led to lower plasma cholesterol levels. The results obtained with the other three fats were similar (Imaizumi et al., 1993).

After Hegsted et al. (1965) carried out their seminal studies of fat saturation on human cholesterolemia, they concluded that 67% of the variance could be explained by the presence of myristic acid and that 91% of the variance was due to myristic, palmitic, and unsaturated fatty acids and cholesterol. They then fed fats prepared by co-randomization of trilaurin, trimyristin, tripalmitin, and tristearin with safflower or olive oils, butter fat, or medium-chain triglycerides. Feeding of these new fats, which contained one predominant fatty acid, gave no differences in cholesterol level, and they also concluded that the position of a fatty acid in the triglyceride molecule may influence metabolism (McGandy et al., 1970).

Lard and tallow are used in experimental diets requiring animal fat. They carry about the same level of palmitic acid (22 ± 3%) but more than 95% of the palmitic acid in lard is in the SN2 position, whereas only about 15% of the palmitic acid of tallow is in the SN2 position. Lard is significantly more atherogenic than tallow in rabbits fed semi-purified diet containing 0.4% cholesterol. In three experiments lard was shown to be significantly more atherogenic (by 126%) than tallow (Table 2.3). After randomization, the percentage of palmitic acid at the SN2 position of lard and tallow was 7.6% and 8.5%, respectively. These values represent 34 and 35% of the total palmitic acid present in those fats. After two fats were randomized, their average atherogenicities were virtually the same. The atherogenicity of lard had been reduced by 103% and that of tallow increased by 10% (Kritchevsky et al., 1995) (Table 2.4). Since the serum cholesterol levels in the rabbits fed the various fats were similar, the effect may be due to LDL size and density. These observations should be considered when reviewing serum cholesterol data derived from human subjects fed randomized fats.

Other Aspects of the Diet

It has been shown that animal and vegetable proteins have different effects on plasma cholesterol levels. The same is true for different fibers, so that pectin and guar gum are hypocholesterolemic but bran is not. Studies in rabbits show that soy protein is much less cholesterolemic and less atherogenic than casein in diets containing cellulose but that the two proteins are equivalent when the fiber is alfalfa (Kritchevsky et al., 1977). Eventually we will have to assess the contributions of all dietary components and their interactions when considering the atherogenicity of any specific diet.

Summary and Conclusion

In the absence of an unequivocal test for the impending coronary, we must assess levels of risk. One of the major risk factors is the level of serum or

TABLE 2.3 Summary of Three Experiments Comparing Atherogenicity of Tallow and Lard

	Atherosclerosis	
	Aortic arch	Thoracic aorta
Lard (24/26)	1.85 ± 0.20	1.29 ± 0.16
Tallow (23/26)	0.87 ± 0.14	0.52 ± 0.12
$p <$	0.001	0.001

TABLE 2.4   Atherosclerosis in Rabbits Fed Native or
Randomized Lard or Tallow

	Aorta		
	Arch	Thoracic	Area (%)
Lard	2.69 ± 0.28	1.75 ± 0.28	25.0 ± 6.9
Randomized lard	1.50 ± 0.28	0.69 ± 0.19	10.8 ± 2.5
Tallow	1.29 ± 0.24	0.79 ± 0.26	9.0 ± 2.2
Randomized tallow	1.50 ± 0.53	0.79 ± 0.28	11.4 ± 4.0
(ANOV) p =	0.029	0.018	0.064

plasma cholesterol. The level of saturation of a dietary fat has greater influence on serum or plasma cholesterol than the amount of cholesterol in the diet. Further analysis of the dietary fat–cholesterol level data show that lauric acid, myristic acid, and palmitic acid may each exert a specific effect on cholesterol levels. Stearic acid, on the other hand, has very little influence on cholesterol level. *Trans* unsaturated fatty acids are of current interest. Generally their effect resembles that of saturated fatty acids. However, some investigators find that *trans* fats raise levels of Lp(a). Whether this effect can be generalized to all *trans* fats or if it is due to a specific *trans* unsaturated fatty acid remains to be resolved. The structure of dietary triglycerides, i.e., the specific position on the triglyceride molecule of specific fatty acids, may influence lipidemia and atherosclerosis. For instance, lard is significantly more atherogenic for rabbits than tallow, but when the fats are randomized (all fatty acids equally distributed among the three carbon atoms of glycerol) they become equally atherogenic with severity at the level of that of tallow. Thus there is need for more fine-tuning with regard to the cholesterolemic and atherogenic effects of dietary fat. The influences of other components of the diet (protein, carbohydrate, fiber) must also be elucidated in future studies.

Most dietary guidelines begin by suggesting that we eat a variety of foods and maintain desirable weight. The best dietary advice for most healthy people is moderation, balance, and variety.

ACKNOWLEDGMENT

This work was supported, in part, by a Research Career Award (HL00734) from the National Institutes of Health.

REFERENCES

Ahrens, E. H. Jr., Insull, W. Jr., Blomstrand, R., Hirsch, J., Tsaltas, T. T., and Peterson, M. L. 1957. The influence of dietary fats on serum lipid levels in man. *Lancet* 1: 943–953.

Anderson, R. L., and Coots, R. H. 1969. The metabolism of geometric isomers of uniformly ^{14}C labeled Δ^9 octadecenoic acid and uniformly ^{14}C labeled $\Delta^{9,12-}$ octadecadienoic acid by the fasting rat. *Biochim. Biophys. Acta* 144: 526–531.

Anitschkow, N. N. 1913. Über die Veränderungen der Kaninchenaorta bei experimenteller Cholesterinsteatose. *Beitr. Pathol. Anat. Allg. Pathol.* 56: 379–404.

Austin, M. A., Breslow, J. L., Hennekens, C. H., Buring, J. E., Willett, W. C., and Krauss, R. M. 1988. Low-density lipoprotein subclass patterns and risk of myocardial infarction. *J. Am. Med. Assoc.* 260: 1917–1921.

Berg, K. 1963. A new serum type system in man: the Lp(a) system. *Acta Pathol. Microbiol. Scand.* 59: 369–382.

Clevidence, B. A., Judd, J. T., Schaefer, E. J., McNamara, J. R., Muesing, R. A., Wittes, J., and Sunkin, M. E. 1995. Plasma lipoprotein (a) levels in subjects consuming trans fatty acids. *FASEB J.* 9: A579.

Cowan, L. C., O'Connell, D. I., Criqui, M. T., Barrett-Conner, E., Busch, T. L., and Wallace, R. B. 1990. Cancer mortality and lipid and lipoprotein levels: the Lipid Research Clinics Program Mortality Follow-up Study. *Am. J. Epidemiol.* 131: 468–482.

Criqui, M. H. 1991. Cholesterol, primary and secondary prevention and all-cause mortality. *Ann. Int. Med.* 115: 973–976.

Davignon, J. 1978. The lipid hypothesis: pathophysiological basis. *Arch. Surg.* 113: 28–34.

Dawber, T. R., Nickerson, R. J., Brand, F. N., and Pool, J. 1982. Egg vs. serum cholesterol and coronary heart disease. *Am. J. Clin. Nutr.* 36: 617–625.

Derr, J., Kris-Etherton, P. M., Pearson, T. A., and Seligson, F. H. 1993. The role of fatty acid saturation on plasma lipids, lipoproteins and apolipoproteins II. The plasma total and low density lipoprotein cholesterol response to individual fatty acids. *Metabolism* 42: 130–134.

Elson, C. E., Benevenga, N. J., Canty, D. J., Grummer, R. H., Lalich, J. J., Porter, J. W., and Johnson, A. E. 1981. The influence of dietary unsaturated cis and trans and saturated fatty acids on tissue lipids of swine. *Atherosclerosis* 40: 115–137.

Frantz, I. D. Jr., Dawson, E. A., Ashman, P. L., Gatewood, L. C., Barth, G. E.,

Kuba, K., and Brewer, E. L. 1989. Test of effect of lipid lowering by diet on cardiovascular risk. *Arteriosclerosis* 9: 129–135.

Gertler, M. M., Garn, S. M., and White, P. D. 1950. Serum cholesterol and coronary artery disease, *Circulation* 2: 696–702.

Gofman, J. W., Lindgren, F., Elliott, H., Mantz, W., Hewitt, J., Strisower, B., Herring, V., and Lyon, T. P. 1950. The role of lipids and lipoproteins in atherosclerosis. *Science* 111: 166–171.

Gordon, D. J., Hyde, J., Trost, D. C., Whaley, F. S., Hannan, P. J., Jacobs, D. R., and Ekelund, L. G. 1988. Cyclic seasonal variation in plasma lipid and lipoprotein levels: The Lipid Research Clinics Coronary Primary Prevention Trial Placebo Group. *J. Clin. Epidemiol.* 41: 679–689.

Gordon, T., Kagan, A., Garcia-Palmieri, M., Kannel, W. B., Zukel, W. J., Tillotson, J., Sorlie, P., and Hjortland, M. 1981. Diet and its relation to coronary heart disease and death in three populations. *Circulation* 63: 500–515.

Gresham, G. A., and Howard, A. N. 1960. The independent production of atherosclerosis and thrombosis in the rat. *Br. J. Exp. Pathol.* 41: 395–402.

Harlap, S., Kark, J. D., Baras, M., Eisenberg, S., and Stein, Y. 1982. Seasonal changes in plasma lipid and lipoprotein levels in Jerusalem. *Isr. J. Med. Sci.* 18: 1158–1165.

Hayes, K. C., Pronczuk, A., and Khosla, P. 1995. A rationale for plasma cholesterol modulation by dietary fatty acids: Modeling the human response in animals. *J. Nutr. Biochem.* 6: 188–194.

Hegsted, D. M., Ausman, L. M., Johnson, J. A., and Dallal, G. E. 1993. Dietary fat and serum lipids: An evaluation of experimental data. *Am. J. Clin. Nutr.* 57: 875–883.

Hegsted, D. M., McGandy, R. B., Myers, M. L., and Stare, F. J. 1965. Quantitative effects of dietary fat on serum cholesterol in man. *Am. J. Clin. Nutr.* 17: 281–295.

Hegsted, D. M., and Nicolosi, R. J. 1987. Individual variation in serum cholesterol levels. *Proc. Natl. Acad. Sci. USA* 84: 6259–6261.

Holme, I. 1990. An analysis of randomized trials evaluating the effect of cholesterol on total mortality and CHD incidence. *Circulation* 82: 1916–1924.

Hopkins, P. N. 1992. Effects of dietary cholesterol on serum cholesterol. A meta analysis and review. *Am. J. Clin. Nutr.* 55: 1060–1070.

Hopkins, P. N., and Williams, R. R. 1981. Survey of 246 suggested coronary risk factors. *Atherosclerosis* 40: 1–52.

Houtsmuller, U. M. T. 1978. Biochemical aspects of fatty acids with trans double bonds. *Fette Seifen Anstrichm.* 80: 162–169.

Imaizumi, K., Abe, K., Kuroiwa, C., and Sugano, M. 1993. Fat containing stearic acid increases fecal neutral steroid excretion and catabolism of low density lipoproteins without affecting plasma cholesterol concentration in hamsters fed a cholesterol containing diet. *J. Nutr.* 123: 1693–1702.

Jacobs, D., Blackburn, H., Higgins, M., Reed, D., Iso, H., McMillan, G., Neaton, J., Nelson, J., Potter, F., Rifkind, B., Rossouw, J., Shekelle, R., and Yusuf, S. 1992. Report of the conference on low blood cholesterol: mortality associations. *Circulations* 86: 1046–1060.

Katan, M., Zock, P. L., and Mensink, R. P. 1994. Effects of fats and fatty acids on blood lipids in humans: An overview. *Am. J. Clin. Nutr.* 60: 1017S–1022S.

Kayden, H. J., Senior, J. R., and Mattson, F. H. 1967. The monoglyceride pathway of fat absorption in men. *J. Clin. Invest.* 46: 1695–1703.

Keys, A., Anderson, J. T., and Grande, F. 1965. Serum cholesterol responses to changes in the diet IV. Particular saturated fatty acids in the diet. *Metabolism* 14: 776–787.

Krauss, R. M., and Burke, J. 1982. Identification of multiple subclasses of plasma low-density lipoproteins in humans. *J. Lipid Res.* 23: 97–104.

Kritchevsky, D. 1985. Variation in serum cholesterol levels. In *Nutrition Update*, Vol. 2, J. Weiniger and G. M. Briggs (Ed), pp. 91–103. John Wiley and Sons, Inc., New York.

Kritchevsky, D. 1988. Cholesterol vehicle in experimental atherosclerosis. A brief review with special reference to peanut oil. *Arch. Pathol. Lab Med.* 112: 1041–1044.

Kritchevsky, D. 1994. Stearic acid metabolism and atherogenesis: history. *Am. J. Clin. Nutr.* 60: 997S–1001S.

Kritchevsky, D., and Baldino, A. R. 1978. Pancreatic cholesteryl ester synthetase: Effects of trans-unsaturated and long chain saturated fatty acids. *Artery* 4: 480–486.

Kritchevsky, D., Davidson, L. M., Weight, M., Kriek, N. J. P., and du Plessis, J. P. 1982. Influence of native and randomized peanut oil on lipid metabolism and aortic sudanophilia in Vervet monkeys. *Atherosclerosis* 42: 53–58.

Kritchevsky, D., Davidson, L. M., Weight, M., Kriek, N. P. J., and du Plessis, J. P. 1984. Effect of trans unsaturated fats on experimental atherosclerosis in Vervet monkeys. *Atherosclerosis* 51: 123–133.

Kritchevsky, D., Moyer, A. W., Tesar, W. G., Logan, J. B., Brown, R. A., Davies,

M. C., and Cox, H. R. 1954. Effect of cholesterol vehicle in experimental atherosclerosis. *Am. J. Physiol.* 178: 30–32.

Kritchevsky, D., and Tepper, S. A. 1967. Cholesterol vehicle in experimental atherosclerosis. X. Influence of specific saturated fatty acids. *Exp. Mol. Pathol.* 6: 394–401.

Kritchevsky, D., Tepper, S. A., Kuksis, A., Eghtedary, K., and Klurfeld, D. M. 1995. Influence of triglyceride structure on experimental atherosclerosis. *FASEB J.* 9: A320.

Kritchevsky, D., Tepper, S. A., Vesselinovitch, D., and Wissler, R. W. 1971. Cholesterol vehicle in experimental atherosclerosis XII. Peanut Oil. *Atherosclerosis* 14: 53–64.

Kritchevsky, D., Tepper, S. A., Vesselinovitch, D., and Wissler, R. W. 1973. Cholesterol vehicle in experimental atherosclerosis XIII. Randomized peanut oil. *Atherosclerosis* 17: 225–243.

Kritchevsky, D., Tepper, S. A., Williams, D. E., and Story, J. A. 1977. Experimental atherosclerosis in rabbits fed cholesterol-free diets. 7. Interaction of animal and vegetable protein with fiber. *Atherosclerosis* 26: 397–403.

Kritchevsky, S. B., and Kritchevsky, D. 1992. Serum cholesterol and cancer risk. An epidemiological perspective. *Annu. Rev. Nutr.* 12: 391–416.

Kummerow, F. A., Kim, Y., Pollard, J., Ilenov, P., Dorossiev, D. L., and Valek, J. 1977. The influence of egg consumption on the serum cholesterol level in human subjects. *Am. J. Clin. Nutr.* 30: 664–673.

La Rosa, J. 1993. Cholesterol lowering, low cholesterol and mortality. *Am. J. Cardiol.* 72: 776–786.

Lichtenstein, A. H., Ausman, L. M., Carrasco, W., Jenner, J. L., Ordovas, J. M., and Schaefer, E. T. 1993. Hydrogenation impairs the hypolipidemic effect of corn oil in humans. Hydrogenation, trans fatty acids and plasma lipids. *Arterioscler. Thromb.* 12: 154–161.

Mattson, F. H., and Grundy, S. M. 1985. Comparison of effects of dietary saturated, monounsaturated and polyunsaturated fatty acids on plasma lipids and lipoproteins in man. *J. Lipid Res.* 26: 194–202.

Mattson, F. H., and Volpenhein, R. A. 1964. The digestion and absorption of triglycerides. *J. Biol. Chem.* 239: 2772–2777.

McGandy, R. B., Hegsted, D. M., and Myers, M. L. 1970. Use of semi synthetic fats in determining effects of specific dietary fatty acids on serum lipids in man. *Am. J. Clin. Nutr.* 23: 1288–1298.

McMillan, G. C., Silver, M. D., and Weigensberg, B. I. 1963. Elaidinized olive oil and cholesterol atherosclerosis. *Arch. Pathol.* 76: 106–112.

McNamara, D. J. 1990. Relationship between blood and dietary cholesterol.

In: *Meat and Health Adv. Meat Res.*, Vol. 6, A. M. Pearson and T. R. Dutson (Ed.), pp. 63–87. Elsevier Applied Science, London.

McNamara, D. J., Kolb, R., Parker, T. S., Batwin, H., Samuel, P., Brown, C. D., and Ahrens, E. H., Jr. 1987. Heterogeneity of cholesterol homeostatasis in man. Response to changes in dietary fat quality and cholesterol quantity. *J. Clin. Invest.* 79: 1729–1739.

Mensink, R. P., and Katan, M. B. 1990. Effect of dietary trans fatty acids on high density and low density lipoprotein cholesterol levels in healthy subjects. *N. Engl. J. Med.* 323: 439–445.

Mensink, R. P., and Katan, M. B. 1992. Effect of dietary fatty acids on serum lipids and lipoproteins—a meta analysis of 27 trials. *Arterioscler. Thromb.* 12: 911–919.

Moore, C. E., Alfin-Slater, R. B., and Aftergood, L. 1980. Incorporation and disappearance of trans fatty acids in rat tissues. *Am. J. Clin. Nutr.* 33: 2318–2323.

Muldoon, M., Manuck, S., and Matthews, K. 1990. Lowering cholesterol concentrations and mortality: A quantitative review of primary prevention trials. *Br. Med. J.* 301: 309–314.

Nestel, P., Noakes, M., Belling, B., McArthur, R., Clifton, P., Janus, E., and Abbey, M. 1992. Plasma lipoprotein lipid and Lp(a) changes with substitution of elaidic for oleic acid in the diet. *J. Lipid Res.* 33: 1029–1036.

Ono, K., and Fredrickson, D. S. 1964. The metabolism of ^{14}C labeled cis and trans isomers of octadecadienoic acids. *J. Biol. Chem.* 239: 2482–2488.

Porter, M. W., Yamanaka, W., Carlson, S. D., and Flynn, M. A. 1977. Effect of dietary egg on serum cholesterol and triglycerides in human males. *Am. J. Clin. Nutr.* 30: 490–495.

Privett, O., Stearns, E. M., Jr., and Nickell, E. C. 1967. Metabolism of the geometric isomers of linoleic acid in the rat. *J. Nutr.* 92: 303–310.

Robinson, D., Bevan, G. A., Hinohara, S., and Takabashi, T. 1992. Seasonal variation in serum cholesterol levels—evidence from the UK and Japan. *Atherosclerosis* 95: 15–24.

Ruttenberg, H., Davidson, L. M., Little, N. A., Klurfeld, D. M., and Kritchevsky, D. 1983. Influence of trans unsaturated fats on experimental atherosclerosis in rabbits. *J. Nutr.* 113: 835–844.

Sgoutas, D. S. 1968. Hydrolysis of synthetic cholesterol esters containing trans fatty acids. *Biochim. Biophys. Acta* 164: 317–326.

Slater, G., Mead, J., Dhopeshwarkar, G. M., Robinson, S., and Alfin-Slater, R. B. 1976. Plasma cholesterol and triglycerides in men with added eggs in the diet. *Nutr. Rep. Int.* 14: 249–260.

Small, D. M. 1991. The effects of glyceride structure on absorption and metabolism. *Annu. Rev. Nutr.* 11: 413–434.

Sommerfeld, M. 1983. Trans unsaturated fatty acids in natural products and processed foods. *Prog. Lipid Res.* 22: 221–233.

Stender, D., and Zilversmit, D. B. 1981. Transfer of plasma lipoprotein components and of plasma proteins in aortas of cholesterol-fed rabbits. Molecular size as a determinant of plasma lipoprotein influx. *Arteriosclerosis* 1: 38–49.

Strong, J. P. 1995. Natural history and risk factors for early human atherogenesis. *Clin. Chem.* 41: 134–138.

Utermann, G., Hees, M., and Steinmetz, A. 1977. Polymorphism of apolipoprotein E and occurrence of dysbetalipoproteinemia in man. *Nature* 269: 604–607.

Vander Wal, R. J. 1955. The triglyceride composition of natural fats. *Prog. Chem. Fats Other Lipids* 1: 327–350.

Vesselinovitch, D., Getz, G. S., Hughes, R. H., and Wissler, R. W. 1974. Atherosclerosis in the rhesus monkey fed three food fats. *Atherosclerosis* 20: 303–321.

Wood, R., Kubena, K., O'Brien, B., Tseng, S., and Martin, G. 1993. Effect of butter, mono- and poly-unsaturated fatty acid enriched butter, trans fatty acid margarine, and zero trans fatty acid margarine on serum lipids and lipoproteins of healthy men. *J. Lipid Res.* 34: 1–11.

3
Dietary Lipids and Cancer: Lessons from the Past, Directions for the Future

Michael W. Pariza

University of Wisconsin—Madison
Madison, Wisconsin

INTRODUCTION

Understanding the relationship between dietary fat and cancer risk is complicated by the effects of energy (calories) and specific fatty acids. The calorie effect (defined below) is general and not limited to fat per se. However, among the components of dietary fat, two structurally related C-18 fatty acids—linoleic acid and conjugated linoleic acid (CLA)—exert direct though opposite effects on carcinogenesis in certain model systems.

The purpose of this presentation is to concisely review the general and specific effects of dietary fat on carcinogenesis.

DIETARY FAT AND THE CALORIE EFFECT

Watson and Mellanby (1930) were the first to report an increase in chemically induced epidermal neoplasms in mice fed diets to which fat had been added (Boutwell, 1995). However, this was not a systematic study of dietary fat effects and was no doubt complicated by differences in caloric intake between control and test animals. Within two decades it was apparent that dietary fat effects on carcinogenesis were tied closely to the "calorie effect." The calorie effect is the observation that, for rodents, reducing calorie intake decreases cancer risk and increases life span. The source of calories—carbohydrate, protein, or fat—is essentially unimportant; it is necessary only that total caloric intake be reduced below that of the ad libitum state (Boutwell, 1988). There is evidence that the calorie effect is effective for humans as well, particularly in reducing the risks of developing breast or colon cancer (Pariza and Simopoulos, 1987).

It is important to recognize that while the calorie effect is arguably the most effective means of reducing cancer risk in rodents, it is only marginally effective in slowing the growth of malignancies (Boutwell, 1995). This is because established cancer is parasitic and does not respond to physiological signals that influence the biochemical behavior of normal cells (LePage et al., 1952).

The mechanism(s) whereby the calorie effect reduces the development of cancer has been extensively studied (Boutwell, 1995). It appears to involve changes in hormonal balance, which in turn influence the promotion of preneoplastic lesions to autonomous cancers cells that no longer respond to normal physiological signals. Calorie intake affects the regulation of numerous hormones. For example, the anti-inflammatory adrenal steroids, which inhibit cell division while promoting cellular differentiation, are enhanced during caloric restriction. Hence the experimental outcome is determined directly by changes in hormone balance, which are in turn influenced by calorie intake.

The interaction between caloric intake and dietary fat consumption in modulating carcinogenesis has been explored in depth. Lavic and Baumann (1943) were the first to study the relationship, showing that the cancer-depressing effect of reduced caloric intake is dominant over cancer enhancement by dietary fat. This finding was confirmed and expanded by Boutwell et al. (1949) and much later by Kritchevsky et al. (1984), Boissonneault et al. (1986), and Welsch et al. (1990), using other experimental carcinogenesis models. In addition, Welsch et al. (1990) reported that dietary fat enhanced mammary carcinogenesis in rats only when the animals were allowed free access to food (ad libitum feeding). Restricting the amount of diet available by just 12% effectively abolished the effect. Evidently the changes in hormone levels induced by even modest caloric restriction are able to override the enhancement of mammary carcinogenesis by dietary fat.

MODULATION OF CARCINOGENESIS BY FATTY ACIDS

Linoleic Acid

Dietary lipid, of course, is not a single substance but rather a diverse collection of biological materials that are soluble to various degrees in organic solvents (e.g., ethanol, ether, hexane). In carcinogenesis research the most studied lipids are triglycerides, referred to as dietary fat. The dietary triglycerides usually used in these investigations are those that are sold commercially as commodities, for example, corn oil, soybean oil, and beef tallow.

It is well documented that for experimental mammary, pancreatic, and colon carcinogenesis, the linoleic acid content of a dietary fat determines the extent of tumor enhancement that will occur when the lipid is fed. Linoleic acid is the only fatty acid shown unequivocally to enhance carcinogenesis in these models under ad libitum feeding conditions (Ip et al., 1985; Welsch et al., 1990). Interestingly, however, induced epidermal carcinogenesis in mice is also inhibited by dietary linoleic acid (Lo et al., 1994). This may be a reflection of the fact that linoleic acid is essential for skin integrity. As such, linoleic acid will stimulate epidermal cell differentiation rather than continued cell growth, which is necessary for tumor development.

The mechanism of carcinogenesis enhancement in some tissues by linoleic acid is not clear but very likely involves effects on prostaglandin synthesis and signal transduction pathways. Oxidation products of fatty acids (including linoleic acid) that may form in vivo are hypothesized to modulate carcinogenesis in various models. However, there is little direct proof for this conjecture (Pariza, 1988). It has been proposed that bile acids may be involved in colon cancer promotion, but the evidence that this occurs in vivo is also equivocal (Boutwell, 1988).

Conjugated Linoleic Acid

There is considerable interest in the possibility that some fatty acids may inhibit carcinogenesis. For example, the inhibition of epidermal carcinogenesis by linoleic acid was discussed above (Lo et al., 1994). The omega-3 fatty acids of fish oil have been postulated to be anticarcinogenic, but the evidence supporting this is not strong (Pariza, 1988). Of all fatty acids studied, only conjugated linoleic acid (CLA) has unequivocally been shown to inhibit carcinogenesis in a number of animal model systems.

CLA was isolated from grilled ground beef extracts that displayed anticarcinogenic activity and was shown to be the active principal (Ha et al., 1987). In addition to inhibiting carcinogenesis in mouse epidermis, CLA has also been shown to inhibit carcinogen-induced neoplasia in the mouse fore-stomach and the rat mammary gland (Ha et al., 1990; Ip et al., 1991). Most recently, Ip and coworkers (1994) established that CLA at 0.1% of the diet significantly reduced DMBA-induced mammary carcinomas in the rat.

We have conducted extensive research aimed at determining the mechanism whereby CLA inhibits carcinogenesis. Our findings lead us to believe that CLA is a previously unrecognized nutrient which has as its primary function the regulation of energy metabolism and retention within the body. The anticancer effect of CLA may be a reflection of more fundamental biochemical activity.

CLA exerts substantial effects on the immune system. Specifically, it modulates the catabolic effects of immune stimulation without adversely affecting immune function—indeed, antibody synthesis is unaffected by CLA feeding, whereas cell-mediated immunity is actually enhanced (Cook et al., 1993; Miller et al., 1994). The catabolic effects induced by immune stimulation are mediated by cytokines and regulated by prostaglandin E_2 synthesis. Through this mechanism immune stimulation induces a spectrum of disease symptoms that range from brief mild episodes of appetite and weight loss, which can result from vaccination (Cook et al., 1993), to the severe wasting that often accompanies chronic illness such as congestive heart failure, cancer, rheumatoid arthritis, and acquired immunodeficiency syndrome (AIDS) (Freeman et al., 1994). The finding that CLA mitigates these effects in animals exposed to immune stimulants is of considerable potential importance, indicating that CLA may have pharmaceutical and medical nutrition applications.

Catabolism induced by immune stimulation partitions energy away from other physiological processes. In young animals this can result in growth retardation (Klasing and Austic, 1984; Klasing et al., 1987). Accordingly we investigated the possibility that CLA might be a previously unrecognized growth factor (Chin et al., 1994). We found that feeding CLA (0.5% of diet) to rat dams during gestation and lactation significantly enhanced pup growth while producing no gross evidence of harm. Continuing the pups after weaning on CLA-fortified diets further extended the body weight gain. Interestingly, the animals reared on CLA-fortified diets exhibited statistically significant improvements in feed efficiency.

In addition to regulating the metabolism and retention of protein, diets containing CLA exert substantial effects on body fat stores. Specifically, we have found that feeding CLA reduces body fat accumulation and increases lean body mass (Park et al., 1995). In a series of experiments to be published elsewhere involving mice, rats, and chickens, CLA was shown to significantly reduce body fat accumulation, often by 50% or more. These results indicate a possible relationship between the inhibition of cancer by CLA and the inhibition of cancer via the calorie effect.

Dietary CLA also appears to alter fat metabolism by affecting the desaturation of saturated fatty acids to monounsaturated fatty acids (Lee et al., 1995). Dietary CLA reduces blood LDL levels and the development of atherosclerosis in rabbits fed on atherogenic diet (Lee et al., 1994).

CONCLUSIONS

Among diet-related factors, the calorie effect is the most effective known means of modulating carcinogenesis in rodents. The calorie effect acts to prevent the development of cancer; it is only marginally effective against established malignancy. There is evidence that the calorie effect is effective for humans as well, particularly in reducing the risks of developing breast or colon cancer. The mechanism of action of the calorie effect appears to involve changes in hormonal balance, which in turn influence the promotion of preneoplastic lesions to autonomous cancer cells that no longer respond to normal physiological signals.

Dietary fat influences the process of carcinogenesis in two ways, the most important of which appears to be its contribution to the energy content of the diet. Additionally, however, linoleic acid and CLA exert specific effects on carcinogenesis that are beyond the calorie effect. It is noteworthy that adding CLA to the diet at just 0.1% produces a statistically significant reduction in chemically induced mammary carcinomas in rats. CLA appears to act, at least in part, by regulating energy metabolism and retention (e.g., fat and protein stores) within the body.

REFERENCES

Boissonneault, G. A., Elson, C. E., and Pariza, M. W. 1986. Net energy effects of dietary fat on chemically induced mammary carcinogenesis in F344 rats. *J. Natl. Cancer Inst.* 76: 355–358.

Boutwell, R. K. 1988. An overview of the role of diet and nutrition in carcinogenesis. In *Nutrition, Growth and Cancer*, G. T. Tryfiates and K. N. Prasad (Ed.), pp. 81–104. Alan R. Liss, Inc., New York.

Boutwell, R. K. 1995. Nutrition and carcinogenesis: Historical highlights and future prospects. *Adv. Exp. Med. Biol.* 369: 111–123.

Boutwell, R. K., Brush, M. K., and Rusch, H. P. 1949. The stimulating effect of dietary fat on carcinogenesis. *Cancer Res.* 9: 741–746.

Chin, S. F., Storkson, J. M., Albright, K. J., Cook, M. E., and Pariza, M. W. 1994. Conjugated linoleic acid is a growth factor for rats as shown by enhanced weight gain and improved feed efficiency. *J. Nutr.* 124: 2344–2349.

Cook, M. E., Miller, C. C., Park, Y., and Pariza, M. W. 1993. Immune modulation by altered nutrient metabolism: Nutritional control of immune-induced growth depression. *Poultry Sci.* 72: 1301–1305.

Freeman, L. M. and Roubenoff, R. 1994. The nutrition implications of cardiac cachexia. *Nutr. Rev.* 52: 340–347.

Ha, Y. L., Grimm, N. K., and Pariza, M. W. 1987. Anticarcinogens from fried ground beef: heat-altered derivatives of linoleic acid. *Carcinogenesis* 8: 1881–1887.

Ha, Y. L., Storkson, J. M., and Pariza, M. W. 1990. Inhibition or benzo[a]-pyrene-induced mouse forestomach neoplasia by conjugated dienoic derivatives of linoleic acid. *Cancer Res.* 50: 1097–1101.

Ip, C., Carter, C. A., and Ip, M. M. 1985. Requirement of essential fatty acid for mammary tumorigenesis in the rat. *Cancer Res.* 45: 1997–2001.

Ip, C., Chin, S. F., Scimeca, J. A., and Pariza, M. W. 1991. Mammary cancer prevention by conjugated dienoic derivative of linoleic acid. *Cancer Res.* 51: 6118–6124.

Ip, C., Singh, M., Thompson, H. J., and Scimeca, J. A. 1994. Conjugated linoleic acid suppresses mammary carcinogenesis and proliferative activity of the mammary gland in the rat. *Cancer Res.* 54: 1212–1215.

Klasing, K. C. and Austic, R. E. 1984. Changes in protein degradation in chickens due to an inflammatory challenge. *Proc. Soc. Exp. Biol. Med.* 176: 292–296.

Klasing, K. C., Laurin, D. E., Peng, R. K., and Fry, D. M. 1987. Immunologically mediated growth depression in chicks: influence of feed intake, corticosterone, and interleukin-1. *J. Nutr.* 117: 1629–1637.

Kritchevsky, D., Webber, M. M., and Klurfeld, D. M. 1984. Dietary fat versus caloric content in initiation and promotion of 7, 12-dimethylbenz[a]anthracene-induced mammary tumorigenesis in rats. *Cancer Res.* 44: 3174–3177.

Lavik, P. S. and Baumann, C. A. 1943. Further studies on the tumor promoting action of fat. *Cancer Res.* 3: 749–756.

Lee, K., Kritchevsky, D., and Pariza, M. W. 1994. Conjugated linoleic acid inhibits atherosclerosis in rabbits. *Atherosclerosis* 108: 19–25.

Lee, K. N., Storkson, J. M., and Pariza, M. W. 1995. Dietary conjugated linoleic acid changes fatty acid composition in different tissues by decreasing monounsaturated fatty acids. 1995 IFT Annual Meeting: *Book of Abstracts*.

LePage, G. A., Potter, V. R., Busch, H., Heidelberger, C., and Hurlbert, R. B. 1952. Growth of carcinoma implants in fasted and fed rats. *Cancer Res.* 12: 153–157.

Lo, H.-H., Locniskar, M. F., Bechtel, D., and Fischer, S. M. 1994. Effects of type and amount of dietary fat on mouse skin tumor promotion. *Nutr. Cancer* 22: 43–56.

Miller, C. C., Park, Y., Pariza, M. W., and Cook, M. E. 1994. Feeding conjugated linoleic acid to animals partially overcomes catabolic response due to endotoxin injection. *Biochem. Biophys. Res. Commun.* 198: 1107–1112.

Pariza, M. W. 1988. Dietary fat and cancer risk: Evidence and research needs. *Annu. Rev. Nutr.* 8: 167–183.

Pariza, M. W. and Simopoulos, A. P. (Eds.). 1987. Calories and energy expenditure in carcinogenesis. *Am. J. Clin. Nutr.* 45(Suppl.): 149–372.

Park, Y., Albright, K. J., Liu, W., Cook, M. E., and Pariza, M. W. 1995. Dietary conjugated linoleic acid (CLA) reduces body fat content and isomers of CLA are incorporated into phospholipid fraction. 1995 IFT Annual Meeting: *Book of Abstracts*.

Watson, A. F. and Mellanby, E. 1930. Tar cancer in mice II: The condition of the skin when modified by external treatment or diet, as a factor in influencing the cancerous reaction. *Br. J. Exp. Pathol.* 11: 311–322.

Welsch, C. W., House, J. L., Herr, B. L., Eliasberg, S. J., and Welsch, M. A. 1990. Enhancement of mammary carcinogenesis by high levels of dietary fat: A phenomenon dependent on *ad libitum* feeding. *J. Natl. Cancer Inst.* 82: 1615–1620.

4
Dietary Lipids and the Immune Response

David M. Klurfeld and Kobra Eghtedary

Wayne State University
Detroit, Michigan

INTRODUCTION: IMMUNE SYSTEM

Although research has been published on food lipids and the immune response since the early part of this century, this subject has never received serious attention from either the nutrition or the immunology communities. The major early interest in this area was due to observations that poor nutrition was a factor in the development of clinically apparent tuberculosis, which was the leading cause of death in the United States during the first several decades of this century. While the majority of individuals were exposed to, and infected with, tuberculosis, most developed only a localized infection; those that were subject to malnutrition or other forms of environmental stress developed pulmonary or disseminated tuberculosis. When antibiotics and vaccines became available, interest in diet as a mediator of this disease waned. Modulation of the immune response by dietary lipids is difficult to characterize primarily because the immune system is the most dispersed of bodily functions. Numerous cell types that are both fixed and mobile and interact with each other are one component of this system; the other major portion is the soluble products of these cells, which can come in contact with foreign substances and every cell in the body. With this in mind, it is easy to understand that not all aspects of the immune system would respond in the same way and with similar magnitude to alterations in dietary fat. This chapter will give a very brief overview of the components of the immune system and then describe the effects of amount and type of dietary fatty acids, cholesterol and antioxidants on various aspects of the immune response. This will be followed by an attempt to explain the mechanisms for these effects and how both over- and undernutrition interact with or independently affect immunological phenomena.

A variety of immunological cells are involved in protecting the host against foreign substances, including microbial pathogens. These include the polymorphonuclear leukocytes (or granulocytes), which consist of neutrophils, basophils, and eosinophils. Neutrophils participate in acute inflammatory reactions against bacteria or foreign bodies; both basophils and eosinophils participate in atopic allergic reactions, and eosinophils are also involved in combating parasitic infections. Viral infections, transplantation of foreign tissues, autoimmunity, and chronic inflammation elicit lymphocytic and monocytic responses.

Cell-Mediated Immunity

It is artificial to divide the functioning of the immune system into cell- and humoral-mediated compartments, and this practice stems, in part, from the original competing hypotheses of how this system functioned. In the mid-1800s Elie Metchnikoff proposed that immunity was due to motile cells, while Robert Koch and others maintained immunity was due to humoral factors (Fudenberg et al., 1978). However, it is easier conceptually to study these parts of the system individually, and this has become standard for discussion of the immune system. Cell-mediated immunity is characterized by events in which the participation of lymphocytes and macrophages is predominant, although these cells elaborate a variety of cytokines that participate in the domain labeled humoral, or antibody-dependent, immunity. Also, there is cooperation between the cells responsible for cell- and antibody-mediated immunity. These cells can be found in solid organs or tissues such as the thymus, spleen, lymph nodes, gut-associated lymphoid tissue, or bone marrow. The last two sources and the circulating blood generally have the highest numbers of these cells. While T (thymus-dependent) lymphocytes are the prototypical cell in this component of the immune response, they are not the only participant; macrophages also play a role. T lymphocytes can be further subdivided into a number of phenotypes, based on cell surface markers and functionality. The scheme used to classify T-lymphocyte subsets is the CD (cluster designation or cluster of differentiation) method, which depends on monoclonal antibodies that identify specific subsets of these cells. Therefore, one can classify T cells by their CD number such as CD4$^+$ or CD8$^+$ cells, but these cells are also described by their effector functions; older but still commonly used terms for these cells are helper cells or suppressor cells. In addition, there are NK (natural killer) cells, LAK (lymphokine-activated killer) cells, and lymphocytes responsible for delayed-type hypersensitivity. NK cells are present in nonimmunized individuals and are capable of attacking tumor cells and other targets, but their activity is increased by cytokines such as interleukin-2. The terms "thymocytes" or "splenocytes" usually refer to a relatively unpurified population of lymphocytes. Finally, mononuclear cells isolated from peripheral blood are primarily lymphocytes but contain a fair number of monocytes. In rodents, lymphocytes are the predominant cell type in the blood, while in humans granulocytes are the most common form of circulating leukocytes.

Macrophage subpopulations include stem cells found in the bone marrow, monocytes circulating in the blood, histiocytes that are fixed phagocytic cells in tissues, reticulum cells in lymphoid organs that process antigen for T cells, and Langerhans cells in the epithelium that also process antigen for T cells. Circulating monocytes migrate into tissues, often in response to some chemotactic signal, and become macrophages. Fixed histiocytes of the reticuloendothelial system include the Kupffer cells lining hepatic sinusoids and specialized phagocytic cells in the lungs, lymph nodes, spleen, and bone marrow.

Cytokines are peptides released by lymphocytes or monocytes and are signals for other cells in the immune system. Some of the better characterized cytokines include the interleukins, the interferons, tumor necrosis factor, and granulocyte/monocyte colony-stimulating factor. These cytokines regulate lymphocyte proliferation, antibody secretion, inflammatory responses, and many other pathophysiological responses.

Humoral Immunity

While this aspect of the immune system is often thought of as distinct from the cell-mediated component, there is some overlap in function. Lymphocytes are responsible for specific immunity; that is, they serve as the "memory" of the immune system. Once exposed to an antigen, these cells persist and upon rechallenge induce rapid proliferation of lymphocytes to produce appropriate antibodies. B (for bursa of Fabricius in birds, which is the immunological equivalent of bone marrow in mammals) cells are the precursors of plasma cells; they synthesize and secrete immunoglobulins but do so assisted by signals from T cells. Circulating antibodies are, therefore, products of B cells but cannot be produced without interaction with T cells. In addition to antibody production, the complement system is part of humoral immunity. Complement is a series of plasma enzymes that participate in antigen-antibody reactions, which have a diverse array of functions ranging from aiding phagocytosis to killing of tumor cells; essentially, complement activates other components of the immune system.

Major regulatory elements of the immune system are the eicosanoids, compounds derived from the metabolism of essential fatty acids. For most mammals, linoleic (18:2, ω-6) and α-linolenic (18:3, ω-3) acids need to be supplied by diet. Through a series of elongations and desaturations, these fatty acids result in the production of arachidonic (20:4, ω-6) or eicosapentaenoic (20:5, ω-3) acids. These 20-carbon fatty acids are significant because they are the immediate precursors for the production of eicosanoids, which are classified into prostaglandins, thromboxanes, and leukotrienes. These compounds will be discussed more fully in the section on mechanisms below.

DIETARY FATTY ACID EFFECTS

Amount

Research in a number of model systems and in human volunteers indicates that the amount of dietary fat affects certain immunological responses. Some of the earliest work in this area showed that animals fed high-fat diets had increased susceptibility to a variety of infections. These diseases included avian tuberculosis (Solotorovsky et al., 1961), parasitic diarrhea in monkeys (Scrimshaw et al., 1968), canine hepatitis (Fiser et al., 1972), and canine distemper (Newberne, 1966). It was found that high levels of polyunsaturated fat (PUFA) prolonged the rejection of skin grafts in mice, improved renal graft survival in humans, and lessened the severity of multiple sclerosis in humans (McHugh et al., 1977; Meade and Mertin, 1978). These studies were followed by rapid growth in understanding of the immune system. Many others showed that high-fat diets altered immune responsiveness, but most studies have only compared different levels of polyunsaturated fats, so it is difficult to differentiate the effect of total fat from an excess of linoleic acid. Another issue is that diets high in saturated fatty acids can induce higher essential fatty acid (EFA) requirements in animals, so there may be relative EFA deficiency in animals fed very high–saturated fat diets. Much of the attention related to high-fat diets and the immune response has centered on the relationship with development of cancer since the 1970s. Erickson and associates have contributed significantly to this field and showed that splenocyte-mediated cytotoxicity against tumor cells was highest when the EFA requirement was just met, but there was a dose-dependent decrease in cytotoxicity that appeared to be mediated via cytotoxic T cells and not through alterations in helper or suppressor cell numbers (Thomas and Erickson, 1985). Erickson and Hubbard (1993) recently reviewed much of this area. Just as excess fat can suppress T-cell responses, EFA deficiency has also been associated with impaired immune response (DeWille et al., 1981). When rats were fed diets containing either 2 or 20% fat by weight, the feeding of high-fat diets (whether saturated, monounsaturated, or polyunsaturated) was associated with significantly decreased proliferation of splenic lymphocytes and a marginal reduction of thymocyte proliferation (Yaqoob et al., 1994a). This study concluded that olive, evening primrose, and menhaden oils were immunosuppressive at high levels in the diet but hydrogenated coconut and safflower oils were not. Reports by Locniskar et al. (1983, 1986) described changes in rats fed either 5% mixed fat or 24% beef tallow, corn oil, or vegetable shortening made of partially hydrogenated soybean oil plus palm oil. They found that there was splenic follicular and germinal center hyperplasia at 2.5 or 5 months, but this was not seen in mesenteric lymph nodes (MLN). There was significant reduction in splenocyte blastogenesis only in the corn oil group at both time points; this finding seems inconsistent with the histological observations but may be explained by enhanced sequestration of lymphocytes in the spleen or increased survival of these cells on high-fat diets. MLN lymphocytes from rats fed tallow or shortening had enhanced responses to mitogen at 5 months. These data indicate that the effect of fat on lymphocytic responses depends on the time of feeding, the type of fat, and the source of the lymphocytes.

In contrast to the relatively large amount of information on T-cell responses to changes in dietary fat, there are only a small number of reports on NK cell activity in animals, and some are contradictory (Leung and Ip, 1986; Erickson and Schumacher, 1989), perhaps because the feeding periods were quite short. Longer feeding studies indicate that high-fat diets significantly suppress the NK cell activity toward a variety of tumor target cells. When mice were fed 5 or 20% soybean oil for 9 months, there was clear reduction of cytotoxicity (Olson et al., 1987); this change was not associated with alterations in splenocyte phospholipids. Olson and Visek (1990) followed up this observation with a study in which mice were fed the same diets for 12 weeks. It was determined that the avidity of NK cells for target cells was unaffected but the rate of cell lysis was significantly reduced. A more recent study found that high-fat diets fed to rats for 10 weeks suppressed NK and LAK activity compared with animals fed low-fat diets (Yaqoob et al., 1994b). One controlled study of the effect of total dietary fat on NK cell activity in humans has been conducted. Barone et al. (1989) reported that reduction in fat as a percent of energy from 32 to 23 for 3 months resulted in a significant enhancement of NK cell activity against tumor cells in vitro among 17 young, healthy male volunteers. In addition to changing the percent energy from fat, these subjects lost a small but significant amount of weight, exercised less, and ate fewer total calories. They did not significantly change their dietary P:S ratio, which was 1.02 at baseline and 0.81 on the low-fat diet. Multivariate analyses revealed that the reduction in percentage of fat calories retained the only significant effect on NK cells.

A recent study (Yaqoob et al., 1995) showed the interactive effect of dietary treatment with the dose of lymphocyte stimulant used. When concanavalin A (ConA) was added to whole blood as a T-cell mitogen, three important points were observed: optimal proliferation was observed at 25 μg/mL of ConA; at 1 or 5 μg/mL there was significant reduction in proliferation with high-fat diets; and at 50 μg/mL there was significant enhancement of T-cell proliferation in blood from rats fed the high-fat diets. This indicates that interaction between dietary fat and strength of the immune stimulation can result in divergent findings. In addition, it is perhaps as important that at the optimal concentration of mitogen there was not a significant influence of dietary fat. B-cell responses are lower in mice fed high amounts (20% of diet) of polyunsaturated fat but significantly higher in animals fed saturated fat when compared with animals fed just enough lipid to satisfy the EFA requirement (Erickson et al., 1986). Another study reported that high-fat feeding decreased the sensitivity of B cells to lipopolysaccharide (LPS) but had no effect on the response to this mitogen (Yaqoob et al., 1995), that is, the amount of LPS needed to induce proliferation was increased with high-fat feeding but there were no significant effects of amount of dietary fat at any individual dose of LPS. This same study also found no effect of amount of dietary fat on the numbers of leukocytes in the peripheral blood including T cells, B cells, CD4[+] cells, CD8[+] cells, monocytes, or NK cells.

A study that compared low- and high-fat diets in volunteers also examined the effect of high and low PUFA in a low-fat diet (Kelley et al., 1992). Seven healthy women in a metabolic unit consumed a basal diet that derived 41% of energy from fat with a P:S ratio of 0.3. They then consumed a diet with 31% of energy from fat with a P:S ratio of 1.0 or a diet containing 26% energy from fat and a P:S ratio of 0.3 for 40 days. Feeding of both lower-fat diets resulted in significant increases in blastogenesis of peripheral blood lymphocytes in response to additions of the mitogens phytohemagglutinin, ConA, protein A, and pokeweed. In addition, the serum concentrations of complement fractions C3 and C4 were significantly increased after either of the low-fat diets. Unaffected were levels of immunoglobulins and interleukin-2 (IL-2). This study indicated that there were no differences in immunological alterations between high- and low-PUFA diets but that low total fat enhanced several responses. Another controlled human study was reported by Meydani et al. (1993), who fed National Cholesterol Education Program (NCEP) Step-2 diets that either contained fish-derived ω-3 fatty acids or excluded fish-derived ω-3 fatty acids and were prepared in a metabolic kitchen. Twenty-two subjects consumed a baseline diet for 6 weeks followed by the experimental diets for 24 weeks. The baseline diet provided 14.1% of energy from SFA, 14.5% MUFA, 6.1% [ω-6] PUFA, 0.8% [ω-3] PUFA, and 147 mg cholesterol per 1000 kcal. The NCEP diets provided 4.3% SFA, 11.3% MUFA, 10.4% PUFA and 61 mg cholesterol per 1000 kcal. The fish-enriched NCEP diet provided 0.54% eicosapentaenoic (EPA) and docosahexaenoic (DHA) acids, while the other diet contained 0.13% EPA and DHA. The low-fat, non–fish-enriched diet resulted in increased lymphocyte mitogenic response to ConA and increased IL-1β and tumor necrosis factor (TNF) production; no effect was seen on delayed hypersensitivity skin response, IL-6, GM-CSF, or prostaglandin E_2 production. In contrast, the low-fat, fish-enriched diet decreased helper T cells and increased suppressor cells. There were significant reductions of lymphocyte mitogenic responses to ConA, delayed hypersensitivity, IL-1β, TNF, and IL-6. These results suggest that low-fat diets can augment lymphocytic responses but low-fat diets enriched in ω-3 fatty acids have clear immunosuppressive effects. While the latter may be beneficial for conditions in which there is hyperactivity of the immune system such as autoimmune diseases or rheumatoid arthritis, low-fat diets enriched in ω-3 fatty acids may have negative effects on immune surveillance against pathogens or tumor cells.

Macrophage tumoricidal activity was decreased significantly when mice were fed 8 or 20% safflower oil but not 8 or 20% coconut oil (Chapkin et al., 1988), therefore it appears that high dietary fat does not intrinsically suppress macrophage function but that only specific fatty acids have this effect.

Type

There is general agreement that polyunsaturated fats are immunosuppressive relative to the effects of saturated or monounsaturated fats. The pioneering work in this area was conducted by Mertin and colleagues (Meade and Mertin, 1978), who reported that linoleic and arachidonic acids inhibited the responses of lymphocytes to antigenic stimuli. A placebo-controlled, double-blind trial of evening primrose versus olive oil supplements was conducted in renal transplant patients. Each oil was administered in doses of 3.6 mL/day in capsules to 44 or 45 patients, who were followed for 6 months. Graft survival was significantly better in the evening primrose

oil group for the first 4 months, but there was no significant benefit thereafter (McHugh et al., 1977). Although the benefit to allograft survival may
have been due to alterations in the immune system, there could also have
been differences due to effects on the coagulation system since polyunsaturated fat reduces platelet aggregation. Since the 1970s, immunosuppressive
medication for organ transplants has improved substantially, and there
seems to be little interest in the additional potential effects of dietary
polyunsaturated fat. There may be effects of dietary lipids on the immune
system that are not accounted for by differences in fatty acid composition.
Acute feeding of 18 g soy phosphatidylcholine (PC) or 15 g soybean or
safflower oils to eight subjects revealed that the oils had no effects, but the
PC increased neutrophil phagocytosis and killing of *Candida albicans* significantly (Jannace et al., 1992); the fatty acid composition of the PC was similar
to the two oils. Nevertheless, most studies in both humans and animals have
concentrated on changes resulting from differences in dietary fatty acids
rather than lipid species.

There are inconsistencies among the studies reported as to whether the
type of fatty acids, ratios between different fatty acids or the quantity of total
dietary fat has greater impact on the immune response. Studies suggest that
high levels of PUFA have the strongest immunosuppressive effect. Some
immune functions can be regulated by dietary fat through an influence on
lymphocytes. Fifteen elderly men who consumed a diet with 28% of energy
from fat and a P:S ratio of 0.7 for 5 weeks had blood drawn for measurement
of NK cell activity. There were significant negative correlations of basal NK
activity with total plasma PUFA, plasma ω-6 fatty acids, and plasma linoleic
acid (Rasmussen et al., 1994). Similar negative correlations were found with
NK activity stimulated by interleukin-2 or interferon-α (IFN-α). Feeding rats
20% fat from menhaden fish oil (MO), evening primrose oil (EPO), or olive
oil decreased proliferation of lymph node lymphocytes in response to ConA
as compared to 20% hydrogenated coconut oil, safflower oil, or a low-fat
(2%) diet (Yaqoob et al., 1994a). There was also a significant reduction of
T-cell proliferation in lymphocytes from the spleen when comparing the
high-fat–fed groups to the low-fat diet, with the highest suppression of cell
proliferation in rats fed the MO and EPO diets. ConA-stimulated lymphocytes from the thymus and spleen had reduced IL-2 receptor expression
from rats fed the MO diet. When the diets of 12 healthy adult females were
supplemented with 2.4 g/day of EPA and DHA for 3 months, there was
decreased interleukin-2 and blood lymphocyte proliferation in response to
phytohemagglutinin and ConA (Meydani et al., 1991). Thomas and Erickson (1985) reported a decrease in lymphocyte-mediated cytotoxicity of
mammary tumor cells in mice fed 8 or 20% of either safflower oil or corn oil
when compared to controls fed 0.5% fat, with a greater reduction in the
higher-fat groups.

Although the results from many animal studies show suppression of the immune response with increased levels of ω-6 fatty acids (Thomas and Erickson, 1985; Erickson, 1986; Dupont et al., 1990), other studies reported a greater reduction of various indices of immune response with ω-3 fatty acids (Somers et al., 1989; Meydani et al., 1993; Hubbard et al., 1994). In a study by Meydani et al. (1993), 22 normolipidemic subjects consumed either a low-fat, high-fish diet or a low-fat, low-fish diet for 24 weeks. The results indicated a significant decrease in delayed-type hypersensitivity, percent helper T cells, and mitogenic response of lymphocytes to ConA with intake of the low-fat, high-fish diet. After 24 weeks consumption of the low-fat, high-fish diet the subjects showed a reduced percentage of CD4$^+$ cells and an increased percentage of CD8$^+$ cells. However, a reduction of the CD8$^+$ cells was observed in subjects fed the low-fat, low-fish diet. Cytokine production was also affected with consumption of the high-fish diet. There was a decrease in production of IL-1β and TNF after stimulation with LPS or *Staphylococcus epidermidis*, and reduced production of IL-6 was observed with intake of the low-fat, high-fish diet. Intake of the low-fat, low-fish diet, which was high in ω-6 PUFA, on the other hand, resulted in enhancement of mitogenic response to ConA, and increased LPS or *S. epidermidis* stimulated production of IL-1β and TNF. Fish oil supplementation has also been associated with reduced cytokine production, mitogen response by lymphocytes, and delayed hypersensitivity in other studies (Yoshino and Ellis, 1987; Endres et al., 1989; Kelley et al., 1991; Meydani et al., 1991). However, Kelley et al. (1992) reported no adverse effect on the immune system in a study of six healthy men consuming a diet supplemented with 500 g of salmon every day for 40 days. Consumption of a high-fish diet for a short period did not affect peripheral blood mononuclear cell blastogenesis in response to ConA, protein A, pokeweed, or phytohemagglutinin (PHA). Kelley and colleagues also looked at the effect of two different concentrations of ω-6 PUFA on the immune response of seven healthy adult women (Kelley et al., 1992). In this study the subjects consumed a diet containing 5.2% energy from ω-6 PUFA and 41.1% energy from total fat for a period of 20 days. For the next 40 days the subjects consumed one of two diets diet providing either 3.2% energy from ω-6 PUFA and 26.1% energy from total fat or 9.1% energy from ω-6 PUFA and 31.1% energy from total fat. There was no difference in lymphocyte blastogenesis to ConA, protein A, PHA, or pokeweed mitogen between the group fed the high or low concentration of ω-6 PUFA.

The same type of inconsistency is also present in studies of immunoglobulin production by B cells. High levels of ω-6 PUFA decreased antibody responses in guinea pigs (Friend et al., 1980) and in mice (Erickson, 1986). A study of immune status in two groups of healthy adult males consuming a diet of about 30% energy from fat was conducted by Kelley et al. (1989). The diets provided either 3.5 or 12.9% energy from PUFA. Comparison between the two experimental diet groups did not show any effect on serum concentrations of IgE, IgG, and IgM in healthy adult males. Similar effects were observed in adult females (Kelley et al., 1992). Healthy adult women consumed a diet of either 3.2% energy from PUFA and 26.1% energy from total fat or 9.1% energy from PUFA and 31.1% energy from total fat. No differences were found in serum concentrations of IgG, IgM, and IgA between the high- and the low-PUFA diet groups. Kelley and colleagues suggested that a moderate increase in the amount of ω-6 PUFA does not have an adverse effect on human immune response when the total fat intake is low.

An in vitro study of the effects of ω-3 PUFAs on the activity of natural killer cells in human peripheral blood lymphocytes was conducted by Yamashita et al. (1991). The results indicated a marked decrease in NK cell activity, which was proportional to the concentration of ω-3 PUFAs in a lipid emulsion added to the incubation medium. In addition, intravenous infusion of 30 mL ω-3 PUFAs emulsion in healthy volunteers was also reported to suppress NK cell activity. Yaqoob et al. (1994b) studied NK cell activity of rat spleen lymphocytes from groups fed different types of fat. Twenty percent hydrogenated coconut, olive, safflower, evening primrose, or menhaden fish oil was fed to each group of rats. There was a reduction of NK cell activity in spleen lymphocytes from rats fed the 20% olive, fish, or evening primrose oils when compared with the 2% fat diet, with the fish oil diet having the strongest suppressive effect. Three hours of stimulation with IFN-α significantly increased the NK cell activity of spleen lymphocytes from the rats fed the different types of fat, except from rats fed the olive oil diet. This suppressive effect of olive oil on NK cells was unexpected and does not agree with most published studies.

The type of dietary fat can also affect the regulation of immunity by influencing various functions of macrophages and neutrophils. To examine tumoricidal activity of macrophages, Chapkin et al. (1988) fed mice diets containing 8 or 20% safflower or coconut oil. A lower level of LPS-stimulated cytotoxicity of macrophages was reported from mice fed the safflower oil diet. ω-3 PUFA from dietary fish oil can also reduce immune response. The diets of 12 healthy adult males were supplemented with 30 ml of cod liver oil for 6 weeks (Schmidt et al., 1989). The results showed a reduction of both neutrophil and monocyte chemotactic responsiveness with daily supplementation of 5.3 g ω-3 PUFA from cod liver oil. The same effect was also reported in hyperlipidemic patients after 6 weeks of daily supplementation with 6 g ω-3 PUFAs (Schmidt et al., 1991). This study also found a dose-dependent reduction of monocyte and neutrophil chemotaxis when the diet of healthy volunteers was supplemented with 1.3, 4, or 9 g ω-3 PUFA for 6 weeks. The reduction in leukocyte functions was noted even at the low dose of 1.3 g.

A number of reports indicate a stronger inhibitory effect of ω-3 PUFAs compared to the ω-6 PUFAs. Somers et al. (1989) reported a significant reduction of macrophage tumoricidal activity in mice fed 10% fish oil compared to 10% safflower or hydrogenated coconut oil. A reduced capacity to kill tumor cells was observed when macrophages from fish oil–fed mice were treated with LPS and IFN-γ. However, linseed oil, a plant source of ω-3 PUFA, did not show the same effect as fish oil with respect to macrophage tumoricidal capacity (Hubbard et al., 1994). In this study mice were fed diets containing 10% linseed, safflower, or menhaden fish oils. Linseed oil is enriched in linolenic acid, whereas fish oil contains high amounts of the longer-chain ω-3 PUFAs, EPA, and DHA. There was reduced production of prostaglandin and leukotriene C_4 in macrophages from mice fed the linseed or fish oil diets compared to macrophages from mice fed safflower oil; this reduction in eicosanoid production was stronger in fish oil–fed mice compared to the linseed oil group. Linseed and safflower oil diets did not reduce tumoricidal capacity of macrophages activated with LPS or IFN-γ and did not alter the production of TNF. However, fish oil did reduce macrophage cytolytic capacity and production of TNF-α as expected. Hubbard et al. (1994) suggested that the type of ω-3 PUFAs may be important in alteration of macrophage function.

The ratio of ω-3 to ω-6 PUFAs may also be responsible for some of the effects on the immune system. Macrophage cytotoxicity was reduced with increasing amounts of ω-3 PUFA and constant dietary fat and ω-6 PUFA in the diets of mice (Black and Kinsella, 1993). In this study, mice were fed diets that contained 1.5% safflower oil and increasing amounts of sardine oil up to 1.5%, with a total fat intake of 10% by weight; the ratios of ω-6 to ω-3 were 1:0, 1:0.1, 1:0.2, and 1:1. When stimulated with LPS the macrophages from mice fed higher amounts of ω-3 PUFA had lower synthesis of prostaglandin E_2, and this reduction was dose-dependent. In addition, increasing the ω-6:ω-3 ratio to 1:0.2 reduced macrophage cytotoxicity toward target L929 cells by 50%. Grimm et al. (1994) used cardiac allograft survival rate to study the influence of different ratios of ω-3 to ω-6 PUFA on immune response. Twenty percent fat emulsions containing safflower, fish, or soybean oil or a 1:1 mixture of safflower and fish oils were used, with ω-3:ω-6 ratios of 1:370, 7.6:1, 1:6.5, and 1:2.1, respectively. Graft survival rate was significantly prolonged with infusion of safflower, fish, and soybean oils. However, soybean oil was found to be less immunosuppressive than either safflower or fish oil, which showed similar responses. The 1:1 mixture of safflower and fish oils with the ω-3:ω-6 ratio of 1:2.1, on the other hand, showed no immunosuppressive effect. The report suggested a stronger immunosuppressive effect when there was a higher ratio of ω-3 to ω-6 fatty acids.

When there is a sufficient amount of essential fatty acids present in the diet, recent studies indicate that high amounts of total fat, ω-3 PUFAs, ω-6 PUFAs, and the ratio between the fatty acids may all have immunosuppressive effects. Both phagocytes (Schmidt et al., 1991; Grimm et al., 1994; Hubbard et al., 1994) and lymphocytes (Meydani et al., 1993; Yaqoob et al., 1994a; Yaqoob et al., 1995) have been reported to be adversely affected by high intake of PUFAs. Dietary fats have been shown to reduce proliferation and activity of different cells of the immune system. Dietary lipids may exert these effects by altering several components of immune function such as TNF (Kelley et al., 1992; Meydani et al., 1993; Engelberts et al., 1993; Hubbard et al., 1994; Utsunomiya et al., 1994), interleukins (Engelberts et al., 1993; Meydani et al., 1993 Yaqoob et al., 1994a), and eicosanoids.

DIETARY CHOLESTEROL

The immunological effects of dietary cholesterol have only been demonstrated among animals in which the serum cholesterol varies over a wider range than that seen in humans. However, serum lipoproteins at physiological levels in humans clearly have the ability to modulate immunological activity. This suggests that however serum cholesterol is elevated, there will be immunological consequences; this has been confirmed in animals that have hypercholesterolemia induced by either dietary cholesterol or high–saturated fat diets. Early work in this area has been reviewed by Klurfeld (1983; 1993). In the first two decades of this century there was so much interest in dietary fat therapy of tuberculosis that there was enough material to publish a review in the 1930s (Levinson, 1931). Hypercholesterolemic patients generally showed reduced responsiveness to antigens that stimulate the proliferation of either B or T cells. Antonaci et al. (1988) reported that synthesis of immunoglobulins was significantly reduced in B cells from type II, but not type IV, hyperlipidemics; that is, hypercholesterolemia but not hypertriglyceridemia was associated with decreased antibody production. Similar results were found in elderly hyperlipidemics except that both elevations of cholesterol and triglycerides were associated with significant reductions in immunological response (Carnazzo et al., 1989). In the normal range of serum cholesterol, there was no correlation with multiple immunological parameters among healthy males (Berry et al., 1987). An intriguing report associated hypocholesterolemia with early, asymptomatic HIV infection (Shor-Posner et al., 1993). Despite greater consumption of saturated fat and cholesterol, HIV-positive men displayed hypocholesterolemia, with 40% having concentrations below 150 mg/dL. This condition was associated with elevated serum levels of β_2-microglobulin, and the authors suggested that decreased serum cholesterol may be a marker for early immunological changes in HIV infection. Peripheral blood monocytes from hypercholesterolemic patients showed increased chemotaxis using autologous serum as the chemoattractant (Schmidt et al., 1991). This would be expected because monocytes play a major role in the development of atherosclerosis, and hypercholesterolemia would be expected to induce monocyte adhesion and extravasation.

When rabbits were fed enough dietary cholesterol to raise their serum concentrations 20-fold, there were increased in vivo responses to the B- and T-cell stimulants, typhoid vaccine, and tuberculin antigen (Klurfeld et al., 1979). While a similar T-cell–dependent response to tuberculin was seen in hypercholesterolemic monkeys, B-cell responsiveness to injected ovalbumin was significantly impaired (Fiser et al., 1973). There do not appear to be any changes in the proportions of B and T cells in the blood of hypercholesterolemic rabbits (Brito et al., 1989) so the functional changes must occur at a cellular level. NK cell activity in cholesterol fed guinea pigs was studied and found to be reduced by 54% when serum cholesterol averaged around 200 mg/dL but the activity of these cells was significantly elevated early in the study when cholesterol rose from the normal concentration of 50 mg/dL to 100 mg/dL (Duwe et al., 1984). This suggests that both low and high serum cholesterol concentrations depress immune responses compared with moderate levels of circulating sterol.

Cholesterol feeding to rats resulted in loading of plasma membranes from monocytes with excess cholesterol (Feo et al., 1976). This was associated with a significant reduction in the phagocytic ability of these cells; latex bead ingestion was reduced by 36% while internalization of larger lipid droplets was 82% lower. The same phenomenon was observed in peritoneal macrophages harvested from cholesterol-fed rabbits (Klurfeld et al., 1979), and these cells had reduced ability to kill bacteria. Along with decreased function, the macrophages showed significant reductions in several enzyme activities to more than 80% below control levels that control energy utilization in the cells. The studies cited above suggest the effect of cholesterol on phagocytosis of markers is partially dependent on size and speed of ingestion. The speed of ingestion is, in turn, related to the microviscosity of the cell membrane, which is controlled by its cholesterol concentration.

In subjects with familial hypercholesterolemia, neutrophils displayed no defects in chemotaxis, chemokinesis, or random movement (Leirisalo-Repo et al., 1990). In markedly hypercholesterolemic rabbits, neutrophils showed reductions in phagocytosis and bactericidal ability (Klurfeld et al., 1979). Neutrophils from guinea pigs fed cholesterol also showed decreases in phagocytosis (Duwe et al., 1981). The influence of hypercholesterolemia on clearance of substances from the bloodstream by Kupffer cells seems to be a function of the marker used and the degree of hypercholesterolemia; it may also have some species specificity, and the amount of hepatic lipid deposition is probably also a factor. Trypan blue clearance was not affected in rabbits (Klurfeld et al., 1979), carbon particle clearance was slightly impaired in rabbits (Neveu et al., 1956), carbon was cleared faster in hypercholesterolemic monkeys (Fiser et al., 1973), and erythrocytes or bacteria were taken up less rapidly in mice (Pereira et al., 1987).

The end result of diet-induced hypercholesterolemia on immune response seems somewhat mixed, but functionally there is increased susceptibility to infections among a variety of animals. For example, normal rabbits are completely resistant to infection with *Bacteroides fragilis*, but cholesterol-fed animals almost all develop infection upon injection with this organism and there is a 25% mortality associated with these infections (Klurfeld et al., 1979). Mice of the A/J strain cannot be infected with mouse hepatitis virus type 3, but those with dietary hypercholesterolemia develop hepatitis with a high mortality rate (Pereira et al., 1987).

MECHANISMS OF EFFECT

A number of potential mechanisms responsible for changes in immune cell functions have been investigated in animals and humans who consumed different amounts or types of food lipids. The dietary changes are probably mediated via the plasma lipoproteins or free fatty acids as these constituents can transfer lipids directly to the cell membranes of various cells of the immune system. Changes in relative concentrations of the lipoprotein classes and in their composition have been associated with alterations in immune cell functions. There are direct changes in membrane sterol, phospholipid fatty acids, and resultant variations in membrane microviscosity that control a wide range of cellular responses. These include alterations in membrane ion channels and differential expression of receptors on the cell membrane surface. Lipoproteins themselves have been shown repeatedly to have immunomodulatory properties. Human lymphocyte proliferation in response to phytohemagglutinin was inhibited significantly by addition of isolated LDL (Cuthbert and Lipsky, 1986). Morse et al. (1977) reported that all classes of lipoproteins inhibited lymphocyte proliferation and that IDL and VLDL were more potent inhibitors than LDL, which was in turn a much stronger inhibitor of these reactions than was HDL. Curtiss et al. (1977) described a subspecies of normal human LDL that they designated LDL-In which was 35–50 times stronger than LDL in inhibiting lymphoproliferation.

Another potential mechanism is via the eicosanoids produced by macrophages. Since several dietary fatty acids are precursors to eicosanoids, it seems reasonable to relate their levels to changes in type and amount of food lipids. Arachidonic acid is the immediate primary precursor of most eicosanoids and is metabolized via cyclooxygenase to a series of prostaglandins and thromboxanes or via lipoxygenase to a variety of leukotrienes and hydroxyeicosatetraenoic (HETE) acids. Both the concentration of arachidonic acid in the phospholipids and its rate of metabolism are controlling factors in the amount of eicosanoids released by cells. Competition with arachidonic acid by ω-3 fatty acids for the enzymes cyclooxygenase and lipoxygenase results in production of different amounts and types of eicosanoids. There is currently much debate about the requirements for ω-3 fatty acids; these lipids seem to be needed for optimal neural and visual development, but it is unclear what the requirement is for other systems in the body. While α-linolenic (18:3) acid is the prototypical fatty acid in the ω-3 series, the effects of 20-carbon or longer fatty acids found predominantly in marine life are far stronger probably because of direct competition with arachidonic acid. A review relating diets with eicosanoid formation and subsequent immune function requires more detail than is possible here (Hummell, 1993). Eicosanoids act, at least in part, by elevating cyclic GMP levels, which then elicit cellular responses. However, these responses can be stimulated by other second messengers.

In addition to the effects of specific fatty acids on eicosanoid production, there are probably indirect effects on signal transduction. The generally accepted metabolic scheme is that phospholipase C activity at the inner plasma membrane results in the release of diacylglycerol (DAG) and inositol triphosphate (IP$_3$). DAG induces the translocation of protein kinase C from the cytosol to the plasma membrane and promotes its activation; IP$_3$ induces the endoplasmic reticulum to release calcium, thereby stimulating the calmodulin-dependent kinase and ion flux through the cell membrane. However, recent work suggests that lipid mediators other than DAG may play regulatory roles, including free fatty acids and lysophosphatidylcholine (Nishizuka, 1995). Activation of these kinases regulates phosphorylation of cellular proteins and signals genes to turn on or off. Modification of the substrate (the fatty acids of the membrane phospholipids) upon which phospholipase C acts can modulate its reaction products and this entire cascade.

Altered levels of cytokines have also been reported in response to changes in dietary fat; these changes may be secondary to some of the other changes induced by dietary fat suggested above or due to changes in signal transduction. Another potential mechanism for mediation of immune responses by dietary fat is via increased entry of lymphocytes into intestinal lymph during lipid absorption. Oleic acid, but not octanoic acid, stimulated a significant increase in lymphocytes found in lymph of cannulated rats

(Miura et al., 1993); in addition, these cells proliferated significantly more in response to phytohemagglutinin.

ANTIOXIDANTS

Both increased dietary total fat and polyunsaturated fat are immunosuppressive; the more double bonds in a fat, the more immunosuppressive it is. One common denominator of these two dietary manipulations is that they increase the need for antioxidants. The more total lipid or the more double bonds in a lipid, the greater the requirement for an antioxidant. Acute administration of 100 mg oxidized methyl linoleate via stomach tube to mice greatly depressed both DNA synthesis and the mitogenic response of splenocytes to ConA; chronic feeding of oxidized soybean oil resulted in reduced DNA synthesis of thymocytes, but the mitogenic response of splenocytes to ConA was increased (Oarada et al., 1989). Immune suppression may also be mediated, in part, by peroxidation of lipoproteins by the generation of reactive oxygen species from peripheral blood mononuclear cells (Kasiske and Keane, 1991); this phenomenon was dependent on the lipid concentration of the lipoprotein fractions. Therefore, both exogenous and endogenous production of lipid peroxides may feed back to suppress immune status. The antioxidant nutrients that have been shown to have beneficial effects on immune status are vitamins C, E, and A, β-carotene, and selenium.

Vitamin C is found in high concentrations in peripheral blood leukocytes; the level is reduced in cigarette smokers who are exposed to strong prooxidants. While it is clear that vitamin C enhances cell-mediated immune function and that the free radical quenching effect of the vitamin is one of its more important activities (Siegel, 1993), it is not clear that the effect is related to the lipid domains of the cells involved. However, vitamin C does regenerate the reduced antioxidant form of vitamin E and therefore leads to inhibition of lipid peroxidation in membranes (Bendich, 1990).

There is an entire body of literature on the effects of vitamin E on the immune response, and this micronutrient is clearly linked to protecting lipid species against oxidation. Much of the work in this area has been reviewed by Bendich (1993). A particularly relevant study showed that human volunteers consuming a controlled diet that supplied 40% of energy from fat supplemented with 15 g/day of fish oil for 10 weeks had significantly reduced peripheral blood lymphocyte mitogenesis after exposure to ConA compared with a group given 15 g/day of a placebo oil composed of lard, tallow, and corn oil, but this effect was reversed by the concurrent administration of 200 mg/day all-rac-α-tocopherol (Kramer et al., 1991). A dosage of 20 times the RDA may no longer have vitaminlike actions but may have other pharmacological properties. The vitamers of vitamin E have a range of biological activity: α-tocopherol, 100; β-tocopherol, 25–50; γ-tocopherol, 10–35; and α-tocotrienol, 30. However, recent work suggests that the tocotrienols, especially the gamma form, are more potent at affecting certain in vitro and in vivo oxidation reactions. Related to this is a recent study that fed 38 volunteers a diet in which up to 70% of their dietary fat was replaced by palm oil for 6 weeks (Engelberts et al., 1993) (palm oil is the richest dietary source of tocotrienols). Although the P:S ratio dropped significantly between control and palm oil diets, the actual ratios were 0.43 and 0.40, respectively. Peripheral lymphocyte stimulation in response to lipopolysaccharide and subsequent measurement in vitro of TNF, IL-6 and IL-8 concentrations were done. While the interleukin levels were unaffected, dietary palm oil resulted in a significant reduction of TNF. Although it is possible that this was in response to the small but significant change in saturated fat, the more likely explanation is that it was due to increased dietary tocotrienol.

Carotenoids also have been shown to have both antioxidant and immunomodulatory roles that may be related. Although β-carotene is converted to vitamin A, the latter is a very weak antioxidant. Carotenoids have been shown to increase the number of circulating lymphocytes, enhance rejection of skin grafts, and increase proliferation of cytotoxic T cells in mice (Seifter et al., 1981, 1982). In 24 volunteers consuming a low-carotenoid diet, exposure to controlled amounts of ultraviolet light for 21 days resulted in significantly reduced delayed-type hypersensitivity (DTH) skin reactions to seven antigens. Supplementation with 30 mg of β-carotene decreased the reductions in DTH reactions (Fuller et al., 1992). This study indicated that plasma β-carotene levels had to be above 1.5 μmol/liter to prevent the significant reductions seen in the DTH reactions but there was no dose response seen with plasma concentrations up to 7.5 μmol/liter, suggesting a threshold effect. Another study of nine healthy women housed in a metabolic ward for 100 days used a low-carotene diet to deplete serum levels over 68 days and then the subjects were repleted with 15 mg/day of β-carotene. Neither depletion nor repletion of β-carotene had any significant impact on peripheral blood mononuclear cell blastogenesis in response to phytohemagglutinin or ConA, in vitro production of soluble IL-2 receptor, or the concentrations of circulating lymphocytes and their subsets (Daudu et al., 1994). It was presumed by the authors that because the subjects were consuming adequate vitamin A, there was no effect of manipulating β-carotene levels in the blood. A dose response to β-carotene was reported in older humans with an average age of 56 years who were given supplements of 30, 45, or 60 mg/day for 60 days; there were significant increases in the level of

NK cells in the blood, total lymphocytes, and IL-2 receptors (Watson et al., 1991).

OVERNUTRITION—OBESITY

Although the subject of this review is dietary lipids and the immune response, an interrelated condition is obesity. While excess calories from any source can induce obesity, calories derived from dietary fat are more efficiently stored as body fat than are calories from protein or carbohydrate. As obesity is a widespread condition in much of the developed world where high-fat diets are consumed, it is difficult to clearly distinguish the effects of high-fat diets from those of excessive body weight. Current estimates of the prevalence of obesity in the United States indicate that approximately one third of the adult population is obese. A condition concomitant with obesity is hyperglycemia, which also interferes with leukocyte function (Kumari and Chandra, 1993). There is general agreement that obesity in animals, whether genetic or diet induced, suppresses a variety of immunological responses that result in increased susceptibility to infections (Newberne, 1966; Chandra, 1980). Similar findings have been reported for humans (Hallberg et al., 1976). Paradoxically, weight loss in obese subjects has been associated with a further depression in some immunological reactions. Fourteen obese women who lost 21 kg were challenged with seven antigens intradermally, and both the number of positive DTH reactions and their size were significantly reduced; the decrease in reaction size was correlated with weight loss (Stallone et al., 1994). Kelly et al. (1994) examined the effect of using high-fat (41% energy) or low-fat (19% energy) diets to induce a 7–9 kg weight loss in 10 obese women over an 84-day period. While there was no effect of the amount of fat in the weight loss diets, weight loss itself was associated with significant decreases in serum concentrations of IgG, IgA, C_3, and the number of circulating NK cells; unaffected by weight loss were lymphocytes other than NK cells, serum IgM, C_4, and DTH skin responses. It is likely that the reduced immune responses associated with weight loss are temporary and that on maintenance of lower body weight, immune function would be closer to normal levels.

UNDERNUTRITION—CALORIC RESTRICTION

As obesity results in reduced immune reactivity, undernutrition might be expected to result in the converse. This is generally the case if nutrient deficiencies are avoided. There is abundant evidence that single or multiple nutrient deficiencies can result in deleterious effects on the immune system

(Beisel, 1981; Kuvibidila et al., 1993). However, restriction of total energy intake that avoids nutrient deficiencies improves most measured parameters of the immune system (Weindruch and Walford, 1988), particularly those functions that change with age. Only a single study has reported the effects of significant chronic energy restriction in humans who were not overweight at the beginning of the study; four males and four females consumed a low-fat (10% of energy) diet that resulted in weight loss of about 14% over 6 months. This was correlated with reductions in serum concentrations of cholesterol, triglycerides, glucose, and total leukocyte count (Walford et al., 1992). As the volunteers were in a closed ecosystem with exposure only to each other, it is impossible to attribute the reduction in circulating leukocytes exclusively to the diet or to the reduced antigenic challenge to which the individuals were exposed.

There is extensive literature on the effects of food restriction modulating the immune system in animals, in particular as it relates to aging (Fernandes and Venkatraman, 1993). While virtually all immunological functions decline with age, some of the better characterized changes that accompany aging are progressive declines in most B, T, and NK cell functions. One exception seems to be the production of prostaglandins, which do not decrease and sometimes increase during aging (Fernandes and Venkatraman, 1993). Both mean and maximal life span of mice are lengthened by food restriction; this is especially true of shorter-lived strains, and more so for those that display immunological dysfunctions such as autoimmunity. Dietary restriction in lymphoma-bearing mice improved the blastogenic response of peripheral blood lymphocytes to phytohemagglutinin, increased the tumoricidal capability of peritoneal macrophages, and raised serum IgG and IgM levels (Mukhopadhyay et al., 1994). An interesting observation in this study was that serum concentrations of vitamins A and E were lower in tumor-bearing mice but were further decreased by dietary restriction, suggesting that food restriction has a stronger immunostimulatory effect than do these antioxidant nutrients.

Although energy restriction has a strong immunomodulatory effect, there is scant evidence to determine if the fat effect is independent. It would be expected that diets containing low amounts of saturated fat and adequate EFA but in restricted amounts would be best for the control of immunological phenomena. One of the basic conceptual issues that this raises is if ad libitum feeding is a proper control. That is, are freely fed rats actually obese? There is some evidence to suggest that this is the case (Klurfeld et al., 1989), although this view is not widely accepted. However, toxicologists are gathering evidence that heavier substrains of rats have higher incidences of various tumors and other diseases associated with aging, shorter life spans, and declining immunity.

CONCLUSION

There is fairly widespread agreement that dietary lipids modulate many aspects of the immune response in both humans and animals. Those components of the immune system associated with chronic inflammatory responses respond more to amount and type of fat. High-fat diets tend to be immunosuppressive, and the more polyunsaturated the fat, the greater the degree of immunosuppression. It appears that the ω-3 fatty acids are more immunosuppressive primarily because of the position of their double bonds and secondarily because they have more double bonds per acyl group. It is somewhat remarkable that the human and animal data coincide so well, in contrast to many other areas of research into dietary effects of health. Dietary cholesterol in very large excess seems to modulate some immune reactions, but some increase, others decrease, and a few are unchanged. Since cholesterol tends to increase cell membrane microviscosity and polyunsaturated fat decreases it, this is a plausible explanation for why cholesterol increases lymphocytic responses and may relate to the mechanism by which polyunsaturated fat suppresses immune function. It is also clear that dietary polyunsaturated fats alter eicosanoid balance, which in turn affects a variety of immunological responses. However, this is almost certainly not the only mechanism by which dietary fat modulates immunological responses. It is possible that the proportion of antioxidant nutrients relative to the number of double bonds in dietary fat may also play a role in controlling many immune reactions. Overnutrition appears to lessen, and undernutrition without deficiency enhances, many immunological functions, but it does appear that there is an independent effect of dietary lipids distinct from that seen with changes in body weight. Relatively small amounts of supplemental polyunsaturated fats (approximately 5 g/day in humans or only a few percent of the daily intake) have the potential to significantly modify immune reactions. It is not clear if the absolute amount of polyunsaturated fat, or the P:S ratio, or the position of double bonds in fatty acids is the key in this situation. An unresolved issue relating modulation of immunity by dietary lipids is whether it is beneficial for immune functions to be at their highest potential. That is, are reductions of some immune responses beneficial? This would certainly seem to be the case for autoimmune diseases but would not be desirable for surveillance against infectious agents or transformed cells. The relationship between the immune system and development of cancer is still unresolved since most tumors are not immunogenic and escape immune surveillance. Since the realization that atherosclerosis exhibits most components of chronic inflammation, dietary modulation of the immune system may also have beneficial effects on this condition. A correlate of aging is a general decline in cell-mediated immunity; low-fat and low-energy diets have the potential to restore some responses to levels seen at younger ages. It is obvious that food lipids have the potential of playing a major role in modulation of many aspects of immunological responses and other related diseases.

REFERENCES

Antonaci, S., Jirillo, E., Garofalo, A. R., Polignano, A., Resta, F., Pugliese, P., Capurso, A., and Bonomo, L. 1988. Cell-mediated immune response in patients with type IIa, type IIb and type IV primary hyperlipoproteinaemia. *Cytobios.* 54: 181–189.

Barone, J., Hebert, J. R., and Reddy, M. M. 1989. Dietary fat and natural-killer-cell activity. *Am. J. Clin. Nutr.* 50: 861–867.

Beisel, W. R., Edelman, R., Nauss, K., and Suskind, R. M. 1981. Single nutrient effects on immunological functions. *J. Am. Med. Assoc.* 254: 52–58.

Bendich, A. 1990. Antioxidant nutrients and immune functions—introduction. *Adv. Exp. Biol. Med.* 262: 1–12.

Bendich, A. 1993. Biological functions of dietary carotenoids. *Ann. NY Acad. Sci.* 691: 61–67.

Berry, E. M., Hirsch, J., Most, J., McNamara, D. J., and Cunningham-Rundles, S. 1987. Dietary fat, plasma lipoproteins, and immune functions in middle-aged American men. *Nutr. Cancer* 9: 129–142.

Black, J. M. and Kinsella, J. E. 1993. Dietary n-3 fatty acids alter murine peritoneal macrophages cytotoxicity. *Ann. Nutr. Metab.* 37: 110–120.

Brito, B., Romano, E., and Soyano, A. 1989. Functional characterization of mononuclear cells of normal and hypercholesterolemic rabbits. *J. Med.* 20: 273–285.

Carnazzo, G., Mirone, G., Turturici, A., Favetta, A., Campo, M. E., Cosenza, C., Chiarenza, G., and Stivala, F. 1989. Pathophysiology of the immune system in elderly subjects with or without diabetes and variations after recombinant interleukin-2. *Arch. Gerontol. Geriatr.* 9: 163–180.

Chandra, R. K. 1980. Cell mediated immunity in obese (c57B1/6Job/ob) mice. *Am. J. Clin. Nutr.* 33: 13–15.

Chapkin, R. S., Somers, S. D., and Erickson, K. L. 1988. Inability of murine peritoneal macrophages to convert linoleic acid into arachidonic acid. *J. Immunol.* 140: 2350–2355.

Curtiss, L. K., DeHeer, D. H., and Edgington, T. S. 1977. In vivo suppression of the primary immune response by a species of low density serum lipoprotein. *Science* 197: 282–285.

Cuthbert, J. A. and Lipsky, P. E. 1986. Low-density lipoprotein (LDL) and lymphocyte responses: Direct suppression by native LDL and indirect inhibition from zinc chelation by contaminating EDTA. *Biochim. Biophys. Acta* 876: 210–219.

Daudu, P. A., Kelley, D. S., Taylor, P. C., Burri, B. J., and Wu, M. M. 1994. Effect of a low beta-carotene diet on the immune functions of adult women. *Am. J. Clin. Nutr.* 60: 969–972.

DeWille, J. W., Fraker, P. J., and Romsos, D. R. 1981. Effects of dietary fatty acids on delayed-type hypersensitivity in mice. *J. Nutr.* 111: 2039–2043.

Dupont, J., White, P. J., Carpenter, M. P., Schaefer, E. J., Meydani, S. N., Elson, C. E., Woods, M., and Gorbach, S. L. 1990. Food uses and health effects of corn oil. *J. Am. Coll. Nutr.* 9: 438–470.

Duwe, A. K., Fitch, M., and Ostwald, R. 1981. Effects of dietary cholesterol on antibody-dependent phagocytosis and cell-mediated lysis in guinea pigs. *J. Nutr.* 111: 1672–1680.

Duwe, A. K., Fitch, M., and Ostwald, R. 1984. Depressed natural killer and lectin-induced cell-mediated cytotoxicity in cholesterol-fed guinea pigs. *J. Natl. Cancer Inst.* 72: 333–338.

Endres, S., Ghorbani, R., Kelley, V. E., Georgilis, K., Lonnemann, G., Van-dermeer, J., Cannon, J. G., Rogers, T. S., Klempner, M. S., Weber, P. C., Schaefer, E. J., Wolf, S. M., and Dinarello, C. A. 1989. The effect of dietary supplementation with n-3 polyunsaturated fatty acids on the synthesis of interleukin-1 and tumor necrosis factor by mononuclear cells. *N. Engl. J. Med.* 320: 265–271.

Engelberts, I., Sundram, K., van Houwelingen, A. C., Hornstra, G., Kester, A. D. M., Ceska, M., Francot, G. J. M., van der Linden, C. J., and Buurman, W. A. 1993. The effect of replacement of dietary fat by palm oil on in vivo cytokine release. *Br. J. Nutr.* 69: 159–167.

Erickson, K. L. 1986. Dietary fat modulation of immune response. *Int. J. Immunopharmacology* 8: 529–543.

Erickson, K. L., Adams, D. A., and Scibienski, R. J. 1986. Dietary fatty acid modulation of murine B-cell responsiveness. *J. Nutr.* 116: 1830–1840.

Erickson, K. L. and Hubbard, N. E. 1993. Dietary fat and immunity. In *Nutrition and Immunology*, D. M. Klurfeld (Ed.), pp. 51–78. Plenum Press, New York.

Erickson, K. L. and Schumacher, L. A. 1989. Lack of an influence of dietary fat in murine natural killer cell activity. *J. Nutr.* 119: 1311–1317.

Feo, F., Canuto, R. A., Torrielli, M. V., Garcea, R., and Dianzani, M. U. 1976. Effect of a cholesterol-rich diet on cholesterol content and phagocytic activity of rat macrophages. *Agents Actions* 6: 135–142.

Fernandes, G. and Venkatraman, J. T. 1993. Dietary restriction: effects on immunological function and aging. In *Nutrition and Immunology*, D. M. Klurfeld (Ed.), pp. 91–120. Plenum Press, New York.

Fiser, R. H., Rollins, J. B., and Beisel, W. R. 1972. Decreased resistance against infectious canine hepatitis in dogs fed a high-fat ration. *Am. J. Vet. Res.* 33: 713–719.

Fiser, R. H., Denniston, J. C., McGann, V. G., Kaplan, J., Adler, W. H. III, Kastello, M. D., and Beisel, W. R. 1973. Altered immune functions in hypercholesterolemic monkeys. *Infect. Immun.* 8: 105–109.

Friend, J. V., Lock, S. O., Gurr, M. I., and Parish, W. E. 1980. Effect of different dietary lipids on the immune responses of Hartley strain guinea pigs. *Int. Arch. Allergy Appl. Immunol.* 62: 292–301.

Fudenberg, H. H., Sites, D. P., Caldwell, J. L., and Wells, J. V. 1978. *Basic & Clinical Immunology*, 2nd ed. Lange Medical Publications, Los Altos, CA.

Fuller, C. J., Faulker, H., Bendich, A., Parker, R. S., and Roe, D. A. 1992. Effect of β-carotene supplementation on photosuppression of delayed-type hypersensitivity in normal young men. *Am. J. Clin. Nutr.* 56: 684–690.

Grimm, H., Tibell, A., Norrlind, B., Blecher, C., Wilker, S., and Schwemmle, K. 1994. Immunoregulation by parenteral lipids: Impact of the n-3 to n-6 fatty acid ratio. *J. Parent. Enter. Nutr.* 18: 417–421.

Hallberg, D., Nilsson, B. S., and Blackman, L. 1976. Immunological functions in patients operated on with small intestinal shunts for morbid obesity. *Scand. J. Gastroenterol.* 11: 41–49.

Hubbard, N. E., Chapkin, R. S., and Erickson, K. L. 1994. Effect of dietary linseed oil on tumoricidal activity and eicosanoid production in murine macrophages. *Lipids* 29: 651–655.

Hummell, D. S. 1993. Dietary lipids and immune function. *Prog. Food Nutr. Sci.* 17: 287–329.

Jannace, P. W., Lerman, R. H., Santos, J. I., and Vitale, J. J. 1992. Effects of oral soy phosphatidylcholine on phagocytosis, arachidonate concentrations, and killing by human polymorphonuclear leukocytes. *Am. J. Clin. Nutr.* 56: 599–603.

Kasiske, B. L. and Keane, W. F. 1991. Role of lipid peroxidation in the inhibition of mononuclear cell proliferation by normal lipoproteins. *J. Lipid Res.* 32: 775–781.

Kelley, D. S., Branch, L. B., and Iacono, J. M. 1989. Nutritional modulation of human immune status. *Nutr. Res.* 9: 965–975.

Kelley, D. S., Branch, L. B., Love, J. E., Taylor, P. C., Rivera, Y. M., and Iacono, J. M. 1991. Dietary α-linolenic acid and immunocompetence in humans. *Am. J. Clin. Nutr.* 53: 40–46.

Kelley, D. S., Daudu, P. A., Branch, L. B., Johnson, H. L., Taylor, P. C., and Mackey, B. 1994. Energy restriction decreases number of circulating natural killer cells and serum levels of immunoglobulins in overweight women. *Eur. J. Clin. Nutr.* 48: 9–18.

Kelley, D. S., Dougherty, R. M., Branch, L. B., Taylor, P. C., and Iacono, J. M. 1992. Concentration of dietary n-6 polyunsaturated fatty acids and the human immune status. *Clin. Immunol. Immunopathol.* 62: 240–244.

Klurfeld, D. M. 1983. Interactions of immune function with lipids and atherosclerosis. *CRC Crit. Rev. Toxicol.* 11: 333–365.

Klurfeld, D. M. 1993. Cholesterol as an immunomodulator. In *Nutrition and Immunology*, D. M. Klurfeld (Ed.), pp. 79–89. Plenum Press, New York.

Klurfeld, D. M., Allison, M. J., Gerszten, E., and Dalton, H. P. 1979. Alterations of host defenses paralleling cholesterol-induced atherogenesis. II. Immunologic studies of rabbits. *J. Med.* 10: 49–64.

Klurfeld, D. M., Welch, C. B., Davis, M. J., and Kritchevsky, D. 1989. Determination of degree of energy restriction necessary to reduce DMBA-induced mammary tumorigenesis in rats during the promotion phase. *J. Nutr.* 119: 286–291.

Kramer, T. R., Schoene, N., Douglas, L. W., Judd, J. T., Ballard-Barbash, R., Taylor, P. R., Bhagavan, H. N., and Nair, P. P. 1991. Increased vitamin E intake restores fish-oil-induced suppressed blastogenesis of mitogen-stimulated T lymphocytes. *Am. J. Clin. Nutr.* 54: 896–902.

Kumari, B. S. and Chandra, R. K. 1993. Overnutrition and immune responses. *Nutr. Res.* 13: S3–S18.

Kuvidibila, S., Yu, L., Ode, D., and Warrier, R. P. 1993. The immune response in protein-energy malnutrition and single nutrient deficiencies. In *Nutrition and Immunology*, D. M. Klurfeld (Ed.), pp. 121–156. Plenum Press, New York.

Leirisalo-Repo, M., Jattela, M., Gylling, H., Miettinen, T. A., and Repo, H. 1990. Phagocyte function in familial hypercholesterolemia: Peripheral blood monocytes exposed to lipopolysaccharide show increased tumour necrosis factor production. *Scand. J. Immunol.* 32: 679–685.

Leung, K. H. and Ip, M. M. 1986. Effect of polyunsaturated fat and 7, 12-dimethylbenz(a)anthracene on rat splenic natural killer cells and prostaglandin E synthesis. *Cancer Immunol. Immunother.* 21: 161–163.

Levinson, S. A. 1931. Fat therapy in experimental tuberculosis of rabbits. *Am. Rev. Tuberc.* 23: 527–541.

Locniskar, M., Nauss, K. M., and Newberne, P. M. 1983. The effect of quality and quantity of dietary fat on the immune system. *J. Nutr.* 113: 951–961.

Locniskar, M., Nauss, K. M., and Newberne, P. M. 1986. Effect of colon tumor development and dietary fat on the immune response of rats treated with DMH. *Nutr. Cancer* 8: 73–84.

McHugh, M. I., Wilkinson, R., Elliott, R. W., Field, E. J., Dewar, P., Hall, R. R., Taylor, R. M. R., and Uldall, P. R. 1977. Immunosuppression with polyunsaturated fatty acids in renal transplantation. *Transplantation* 24: 263–267.

Meade, C. J. and Mertin, J. 1978. Fatty acids and immunity. *Adv. Lipid Res.* 16: 127–165.

Meydani, S. N., Endres, S., Woods, M. M., Goldin, B. R., Soo, C., Labrode, A., Dinarello, C. A., and Gorbach, S. L. 1991. Oral (n-3) fatty acid supplementation suppresses cytokine production and lymphocyte proliferation: Comparison between young and older women. *J. Nutr.* 121: 547–555.

Meydani, S. N., Lichtenstein, A. H., Cornwall, S., Meydani, M., Goldin, B. R., Rasmussen, H., Dinarello, C., and Schaefer, E. J. 1993. Immunologic effects of National Cholesterol Education Panel Step-2 diets with and without fish-derived n-3 fatty acid enrichment. *J. Clin. Invest.* 92: 105–113.

Miura, S., Imaeda, H., Shiozaki, H., Ohkubo, N., Tashiro, H., Serizawa, H., Tsuchiya, M., and Tso, P. 1993. Increased proliferative response of lymphocytes from intestinal lymph during long chain fatty acid absorption. *Immunology* 78: 142–146.

Morse, J. H., Witte, L. D., and Goodman, D. S. 1977. Inhibition of lymphocyte proliferation stimulated by lectins and allogeneic cells by normal plasma lipoproteins. *J. Exp. Med.* 146: 1791–1803.

Mukhopadhyay, P., Gupta, J. D., Senyal, U., and Das, S. 1994. Influence of dietary restriction and soyabean supplementation on the growth of a murine lymphoma and host immune function. *Cancer Lett.* 78: 151–157.

Newberne, P. M. 1966. Overnutrition and resistance of dogs to distemper virus. *Fed. Proc.* 25: 1701–1712.

Neveu, T., Biozzi, G., Benacerraf, B., Stiffel, C., and Halpern, B. N. 1956. Role of reticulo-endothelial system in blood clearance of cholesterol. *Am. J. Physiol.* 187: 269–274.

Nishizuka, T. 1995. Protein kinase C and lipid signaling for sustained cellular responses. *FASEB J.* 9: 484–496.

Oarada, M., Majima, T., Miyazawa, T., Fujimoto, K., and Kaneda, T. 1989. The effect of dietary autoxidized oils on immunocompetent cells in mice. *Biochim. Biophys. Acta* 1012: 156–160.

Olson, L. M., Clinton, S. K., Everitt, J. I., Johnston, P. V., and Visek, W. J. 1987. Lymphocyte activation, cell-mediated cytotoxicity and their relationship to dietary fat-enriched mammary tumorigenesis in C3H/OUJ mice. *J. Nutr.* 117: 955–963.

Olson, L. M. and Visek, W. J. 1990. Kinetics of cell-mediated cytotoxicity in mice fed diets of various fat contents. *J. Nutr.* 120: 619–624.

Pereira, C. A., Steffan, A. M., Koehren, F., Douglas, C. R., and Kirn, A. 1987. Increased susceptibility of mice to MHV 3 infection induced by hypercholesterolemic diet: Impairment of Kupffer cell function. *Immunobiology* 174: 253–265.

Rasmussen, L. B., Kiens, B., Pedersen, B. K., and Richter, E. A. 1994. Effect of diet and plasma fatty acid composition on immune status in elderly men. *Am. J. Clin. Nutr.* 59: 572–577.

Schmidt, E. B., Pedersen, J. O., Varming, K., Ernst, E., Jersild, C., Grunnet, N., and Dyerberg, J. 1991. n-3 Fatty acids and leukocyte chemotaxis. Effects in hyperlipidemia and dose-response studies in healthy men. *Arterioscler. Thromb.* 11: 429–435.

Schmidt, E. B., Pedersen, J. O., Ekelund, S., Grunnet, N., Jersild, C., and Dyerberg, J. 1989. Cod liver oil inhibits neutrophil and monocyte chemotaxis in healthy males. *Atherosclerosis* 77: 53–57.

Scrimshaw, N. S., Taylor, C. E., and Gordon, J. E. 1968. *Interactions of Nutrition and Infection.* Monograph No. 57, World Health Organization, Geneva.

Seifter, E., Rettura, G., and Levenson, S. M. 1981. Carotenoids and cell mediated immune response. In *The Quality of Food and Beverages*, G. Charalambors and G. Inglett (Ed.), pp. 335–342. Academic Press, New York.

Seifter, E., Rettura, G., Padawer, J., and Levenson, S. M. 1982. Moloney murine sarcoma virus tumors in CBA/J mice: Chemopreventive and chemotherapeutic actions of supplemental beta carotene. *J. Natl. Cancer Inst.* 835–840.

Shor-Posner, G., Basit, A., Lu, Y., Carejos, C., Chang, J., Fletcher, M., Mantero-Atienza, E., and Baum, M. K. 1993. Hypocholesterolemia is associated with immune dysfunction in early human immunodeficiency virus-1 infection. *Am. J. Med.* 94: 515–519.

Siegel, B. V. 1993. Vitamin C and the immune response in health and disease. In *Nutrition and Immunology*, D. M. Klurfeld (Ed.), pp. 167–196. Plenum Press, New York.

Solotorovsky, M., Squibb, R. L., and Wogan, G. N. 1961. The effect of dietary fat and vitamin A on avian TB. *Am. Rev. Resp. Dis.* 84: 226–232.

Somers, S. D., Chapkin, R. S., and Erickson, K. L. 1989. Alteration of in vitro murine peritoneal macrophage function by dietary enrichment with eicosapentaenoic and docosahexaenoic acids in menhaden fish oil. *Cell. Immunol.* 123:201–211.

Stallone, D. D., Stunkard, A. J., Zweiman, B., Wadden, T. A., and Foster, G. D. 1994. Decline in delayed-type hypersensitivity response in obese women following weight-reduction. *Clin. Diagnost. Lab. Immunol.* 1: 202–205.

Thomas, I. K. and Erickson, K. L. 1985. Dietary fatty acid modulation of T-cell responses in vivo. *J. Nutr.* 115: 1528–1534.

Utsunomiya, T., Chavali, S. R., Zhong, W. W., and Forse, R. A. 1994. Effect of continuous tube feeding of dietary fat emulsions on eicosanoid production and on fatty acid composition during an acute septic shock in rats. *Biochim. Biophys. Acta* 1214: 333–339.

Walford, R. L., Harris, S. B., and Gunion, M. W. 1992. The calorically restricted low-fat nutrient-dense diet in Biosphere 2 significantly lowers blood glucose, total leukocyte count, cholesterol, and blood pressure in humans. *Proc. Natl. Acad. Sci. USA* 89: 11533–11537.

Watson, R. R., Prabhala, R. H., Plezia, P. M., and Alberts, D. S. 1991. Effects of beta-carotene on lymphocyte subpopulations in elderly humans: Evidence for a dose response relationship. *Am. J. Clin. Nutr.* 53: 90–94.

Weindruch, R. and Walford, R. L. 1988. *The Retardation of Aging and Disease by Dietary Restriction.* C. C. Thomas, Springfield, IL.

Yamashita, N., Maruyama, M., Yamazaki, K., Hamazaki, T., and Yano, S. 1991. Effect of eicosapentaenoic and docosahexaenoic acid on natural killer cell activity in human peripheral blood lymphocytes. *Clin. Immunol. Immunopathol.* 59:335–345.

Yaqoob, P., Newsholme, E. A., and Calder, P. C. 1994a. Inhibition of natural killer cell activity by dietary lipids. *Immunol. Lett.* 41: 241–247.

Yaqoob, P., Newsholme, E. A., and Calder, P. C. 1994b. The effect of dietary lipid manipulation on rat lymphocyte subsets and proliferation. *Immunology* 82: 603–610.

Yaqoob, P., Newsholme, E. A., and Calder, P. C. 1995. The effect of fatty acids on leucocyte subsets and proliferation in rat whole blood. *Nutr. Res.* 15: 279–287.

Yoshino, S. and Ellis, E. F. 1987. Effect of fish-oil-supplemented diet on inflammation and immunological processes in rats. *Int. Arch. Allergy Appl. Immunol.* 84: 233–240.

5
Food Lipids and Bone Health

Bruce A. Watkins

Purdue University
West Lafayette, Indiana

Mark F. Seifert

Indiana University School of Medicine
Indianapolis, Indiana

INTRODUCTION

Long bone growth and modeling are regulated by complex interactions
between an individual's genetic potential, environmental influences, and
nutrition. These interactions produce a bone architecture that balances
functionally appropriate morphology with the skeleton's role in calcium
and phosphorus homeostasis. Long bones of children increase in length
and diameter by a process called modeling. Bone modeling represents an
adaptive process of generalized and continuous growth and reshaping of
bone by the activities of osteoblasts and osteoclasts until the adult bone
structure is attained. This growth requires that bone cells function normally.
Bone modeling is distinct from bone remodeling, which describes the local,
coupled process of bone resorption and formation that maintains skeletal
mass and morphology in the adult. Many of the skeletal pathologies that
afflict the adult are the consequence of abnormal bone remodeling and
metabolism. Data from recent studies suggest the possibility that the onset
and severity of some of these pathologies may be delayed and lessened if the

bone modeling process is enhanced early in life. Because of this, an appreciation of the differences between these two processes is a prerequisite for understanding bone health and disease and for the pursuit of novel approaches to maximize peak bone mass potential.

Numerous cell-derived growth regulatory factors are present within skeletal tissues, e.g., prostaglandins, cytokines, and growth factors. These substances are produced locally by chondrocytes, osteoblasts, monocytes/macrophages, and lymphocytes, and exert powerful effects on skeletal metabolism. These cells are induced to synthesize and secrete these compounds by systemic hormones such as parathyroid hormone, estrogens, and vitamin D_3 metabolites, or by local autocrine/paracrine signaling agents within bone.

Several nutrients influence the development, growth, and modeling of long bones. The effects of calcium, phosphorus, and 1,25-dihydroxyvitamin D_3 on bone growth are well known. Low calcium intake results in reduced serum calcium concentrations, rickets, or osteoporosis. Severe phosphorus deficiency can also lead to rickets. Vitamin D_3, the antirachitic vitamin, affects several aspects of bone metabolism. Since its discovery and chemical synthesis, many foods have been supplemented with this vitamin. The physiologically active, hormonal form of vitamin D, 1,25-dihydroxyvitamin D_3 $[1,25(OH)_2D_3]$, acts on its principle target tissues, intestine, bone, and kidney, to conserve calcium and phosphorus for maintenance of serum mineral levels and for normal skeletal mineralization. New research suggests that dietary lipids and antioxidant nutrients influence bone modeling and the risk for degenerative bone diseases.

The goal of this chapter is to (1) describe the types of cells located in bone, (2) review the basic elements of bone modeling and remodeling, (3) discuss the roles of prostaglandins, cytokines, and growth factors involved in the local regulation of bone metabolism, (4) document the role of lipids in bone biology and the relationship between dietary lipids and factors regulating skeletal metabolism, and (5) discuss the importance of lipids in bone modeling and in degenerative diseases of bone in the elderly.

BONE CELLS AND BONE METABOLISM

Bone is a metabolically active, multifunctional tissue that consists of a structural framework of mineralized matrix and contains heterogeneous populations of chondrocytes, osteoblasts, osteocytes, osteoclasts, endothelial cells, monocytes, macrophages, lymphocytes, and hemopoietic cells. This complex milieu of cells produces a variety of biological regulators that control bone metabolism locally. Systemic calciotropic hormones [parathyroid hormone (PTH), estrogens, and $1,25(OH)_2D_3$] and autocrine and paracrine factors, including prostaglandins, cytokines, and growth factors (insulinlike growth factors I and II) orchestrate the cellular activities of bone modeling to increase the length, diameter, and shape of long bones in children. The activities controlling bone growth include bone matrix formation, matrix mineralization, and bone resorption. Bone matrix is produced and mineralized through the activity of osteoblasts, while bone matrix resorption is accomplished by specialized multinucleated cells called osteoclasts (Baron, 1993). The combined and cooperative activities of osteoblasts and osteoclasts result in a bone architecture that provides mechanical support and maintains normal serum concentrations of mineral (e.g., calcium).

Osteoblasts are mononucleated bone-forming cells that originate locally from mesenchymal stem cells (Baron, 1993). Functionally mature osteoblasts are recruited to a site of bone formation where they actively synthesize and secrete an organic bone matrix called "osteoid," which is composed of type I collagen, proteoglycans, glycoproteins, and other protein components (Malluche and Faugere, 1986a,b). Following its formation, osteoid normally undergoes rapid mineralization with hydroxyapatite. In addition to synthesizing bone matrix, osteoblasts maintain a high alkaline phosphatase activity and produce numerous regulatory factors such as prostaglandins, cytokines, and growth factors (Canalis, 1993; Puzas, 1993). These locally produced compounds are reported to stimulate bone formation as well as bone resorption (Schmid et al., 1992; Baylink et al., 1993; Canalis, 1993; Mundy, 1993; Raisz, 1993).

The osteocyte is an osteoblast that has become surrounded by mineralized bone matrix. Osteocytes are contained within lacunae and maintain cytoplasmic continuity with adjacent osteocytes and with osteoblasts lining the surfaces of trabecular or cortical bone (Heersche, 1993; Puzas, 1993). Osteocytes are the most abundant cell type in mature bone (Parfitt, 1977); however, their role in bone metabolism is poorly understood. At one time it was believed that they could become activated under certain conditions to resorb bone ("osteolytic osteolysis") (Belanger, 1969), but current research suggests that they play a central role in transduction of signals generated during mechanical loading (Cowin et al., 1991).

Osteoclasts are large multinucleated bone-resorbing cells. They form at skeletal sites from the fusion of mononuclear precursors arriving via the vasculature. These precursor cells originate from pluripotent hemopoietic stem cells located within bone marrow; the most likely stem cell is a colony-forming unit of the granulocyte-macrophage series (CFU-GM) (Schneider and Relfson, 1988; Kurihara et al., 1990). During bone resorption, osteoclasts produce and release lysosomal enzymes, hydrogen protons, and free radicals into a confined space or resorptive compartment next to bone, which dissolve the mineral and degrade bone matrix (Blair et al., 1993). Active osteoclasts are in contact with mineralized surfaces and produce distinctive resorptive cavities called Howship's lacunae.

Thus, the bone cells are under the regulatory control of systemic and local factors, which modulate their activities and influence bone modeling and remodeling processes. The effects of dietary lipids on altering the amount of local factors produced in bone will be discussed in subsequent sections of this chapter.

BONE TISSUE AND GROWTH

Bone is a dynamic connective tissue consisting of living cells embedded within or lining surfaces of a mineralized organic matrix. Bone functions to provide mechanical support for the body and, through attachment of muscles, allows for locomotive movement through space. In addition, skeletal tissue protects vital organs and serves as a metabolic reservoir of calcium and phosphate for the body. Anatomically, the bones of the skeleton can be classified according to their individual shapes: flat (bones forming the roof of the skull, scapula, and ilium), short (carpal and tarsal bones), irregular (vertebrae), and long (humerus, radius, ulna, femur, and tibia).

All bone is derived from mesenchymal tissue, however, two different histogenetic processes exist for producing bone: one direct and another indirect through a temporary cartilage model. Intramembranous ossification occurs within presumptive flat bones by direct differentiation of mesenchymal cells into osteogenic cells. These cells deposit organic matrix within their embryonic connective tissue membrane, which becomes mineralized. Long bones are formed by endochondral ossification, a process where embryonic mesenchymal cells differentiate into chondroblasts that secrete hyaline cartilage matrix and produce a cartilage model of the future bone. Diaphyseal and, later, epiphyseal centers of ossification develop following local cartilage mineralization and invasion by the vasculature. Cartilage matrix is removed and replaced with bone by newly arrived osteogenic cells. The location of a plate of cartilage interposed between epiphyseal and metaphyseal regions of a bone provides the means for bones to grow in length (Fig. 5.1). In this process, chondrocyte proliferation, matrix production, mineralization, and vascular invasion is balanced with removal of mineralized trabeculae from the metaphyseal side of the growth plate through osteoclastic activity. These primary trabeculae of mineralized cartilage enclosed by bone are progressively replaced by secondary trabeculae of bone produced by osteoblasts. This trabecular or cancellous bone consti-

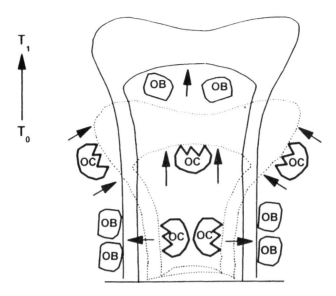

FIG. 5.1   Long bones increase in length over time (T_0 to T_1) by endochondral ossification. The epiphyseal cartilage becomes mineralized followed by vascular invasion. The activities of bone resorption by the osteoclasts (OC) and bone formation by the osteoblasts (OB) result in dissolution of bone and reshaping of the ends.

tutes a meshwork of tissue at the ends of long bones whose surfaces are lined by bone cells and whose intertrabecular spaces are filled with hemopoietic tissue. Trabecular bone is mainly involved with metabolic functions. Dense or cortical bone completely encases bones and is especially thick within the diaphyses or shafts of long bones. The diameters of bones increase via intramembranous ossification through apposition of bone matrix by osteoblasts located within the periosteum (Fig. 5.2). Cortical bone serves primarily mechanical and protective functions.

BONE MODELING

Bone modeling describes the continuous changes in bone shape, length, and width throughout the growth of an individual until skeletal maturity is reached. In contrast to bone remodeling, bone modeling lacks local coupling of resorption with bone formation on modeling bone surfaces (Table 5.1). Resorption and formation in bone modeling occurs on separate sur-

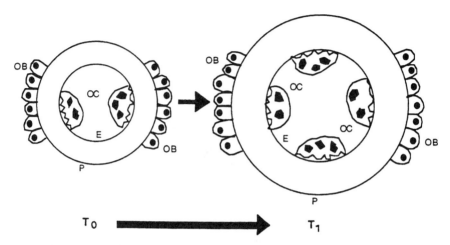

FIG. 5.2   Diagram illustrating intramembranous ossification of bone leading to an increase in long bone diameter over time (T_0 to T_1). Osteoclasts (OC) located on the endosteal surface (E) resorb bone and osteoblasts (OB) on the periosteal surface (P) form new bone matrix.

TABLE 5.1   Comparison of Bone Modeling and Remodeling Activities

	Bone modeling	Bone remodeling
Local coupling	Formation and resorption are *not* coupled	Formation and resorption are coupled
Timing and sequence of activity	F and RS are continuous and occur on separate surfaces	Cyclical: A-RS-RV-F; formation always follows resorption
Extent of surface activity	100% of surfaces are active	20% of surfaces are active
Anatomical objectives	Gain in skeletal mass and change in skeletal morphology	Skeletal maintenance

A = activation; RS = resorption; RV = reversal; F = formation.

faces (periosteal or cortico-endosteal); therefore, surface activation in modeling bone may be followed by either resorption or formation.

BONE REMODELING

The skeletal morphology of the adult represents a sophisticated compromise between structural obligation and metabolic responsibility, serving the individual in support and locomotion while actively participating in the regulation of calcium homeostasis. This compromise is accomplished through the individual's genetic potential for growth and intricate interactions between nutrition, metabolism, and endocrine factors. Hormones and certain nutrients modulate the autocrine and paracrine cellular relationships (actions of prostaglandins, cytokines, and growth factors) responsible for the maintenance of bone mass and architecture. In the adult skeleton, the coordination of bone-resorbing and bone-forming activities is termed the "bone-remodeling cycle."

The regulation of bone remodeling and its corresponding role in the maintenance of adult bone mass is distinctly different from the processes that control skeletal growth and modeling in the young. As the name implies, modeling is responsible for creating bone shape. Modeling of bone is an adaptive process, providing order and specificity to the generalized increase in bone mass that accompanies body growth.

Bone remodeling involves the removal and internal restructuring of previously existing bone and is responsible for the maintenance of tissue mass and architecture in the adult skeleton (Frost, 1973). Chemical and/or electrical stimuli activate local bone cell populations and coordinate their activities in removing and replacing discrete "packets" of bone at skeletal sites. These organized groups of cells are called "basic multicellular units," or BMU (Frost, 1963), which function within a defined remodeling cycle. Osteoblasts and osteoclasts are important members of the BMU.

The cellular interactions occurring within a remodeling cycle are divided into four main events: activation, resorption, reversal, and formation (Parfitt, 1990) (Fig. 5.3). A remodeling cycle begins when a nonremodeling quiescent bone surface becomes "activated." The signals effecting activation are not fully understood, but it is believed that the bone-lining cells covering inactive surfaces initiate this event. It is during this activation event that osteoclasts attach to the bone surface and resorb bone. This marks the resorption phase and results in the release of bone Ca^{2+}. As the period of bone resorption subsides, the reversal phase represents a period of transition when the bone surface is repopulated with newly formed osteoblasts.

The formation phase begins as the osteoblasts commence deposition of

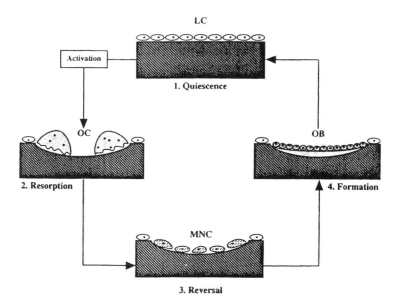

FIG. 5.3   Schematic representation of the bone remodeling cycle. The remodeling cycle is initiated when the lining cells (LC) on a quiescent surface
(1) retract and expose the underlying mineral. Once the remodeling site is
activated, osteoclasts (OC) are recruited and a period of bone resorption
ensues (2). During the reversal phase (3), mononuclear cells (MNC) smooth
the surface of the eroded cavity created by the OC and osteoblasts (OB) are
mobilized to refill the remodeling space during a period of bone formation
(4). After the cavity has been refilled, the bone surface returns to quiescence.

new bone matrix (osteoid), which subsequently becomes mineralized. This
phase, and the bone-remodeling cycle, is complete when the osteoblasts
refill the cavity created during the resorption phase (Fig. 5.3). These events
of resorption and formation are believed to be "coupled" such that resorption is always followed by bone formation (Table 5.1). It is hypothesized that
a reservoir of growth factors and cytokines, previously produced by osteoblasts and incorporated into the bone matrix, becomes available locally as
autocrine/paracrine factors during osteoclastic bone resorption. These factors subsequently direct the proliferation, differentiation, and recruitment
of new osteoblasts to the remodeling site and, thus, regulate the remodeling
cycle (Baylink et al., 1993; Mundy, 1993; Raisz, 1993).

     To summarize the activities of bone cells during modeling (or remodel-
ing), osteoclasts resorb bone while osteoblasts add matrix onto bone sur-

faces. As bones grow, osteoblastic and osteoclastic activities lead to increases in bone size and changes in longitudinal and cross-sectional geometry in accordance with individual genetic, nutritional, and biochemical influences.

LOCAL AND SYSTEMIC FACTORS AFFECTING BONE METABOLISM

Bone formation and bone resorption are regulated by systemic hormones and factors produced locally primarily by osteoblasts (Watrous and Andrews, 1989; Watkins, 1992; Baylink et al., 1993; Mundy, 1993; Raisz, 1993). Systemic hormones involved in stimulating bone formation include insulin (Nilsson et al., 1994), growth hormone (Nilsson et al. 1994), and estrogen (Chow et al., 1992), while those involved in stimulating bone resorption include $1,25(OH)_2D_3$ (Raisz, 1990), PTH (Kream et al., 1990), and thyroid hormone (Klaushofer et al., 1989). In addition, calcitonin (Lin et al., 1991) and glucocorticoids (Lukert and Raisz, 1990) inhibit bone resorption.

Cytokines and local growth factors produced by immunocompetent cells and osteoblasts exert powerful effects on bone. Cytokines, such as interleukin (IL)-1 (Marusic and Raisz, 1991), IL-6 (Ishimi et al., 1990), and tumor necrosis factor (TNF) (Watrous and Andrews, 1989), stimulate bone resorption as do epidermal growth factor (EGF) (Lorenzo et al., 1986), fibroblast growth factor (FGF) (Simmons and Raisz, 1991), and platelet-derived growth factor (PDGF) (Canalis et al., 1989). On the other hand, insulinlike growth factors (IGF-I and IGF-II) (McCarthy et al., 1989) and transforming growth factor-β (TGF-β) (Centrella et al., 1987) enhance bone formation.

In addition to the cytokines and growth factors, which act as local modifiers of bone metabolism, certain eicosanoids [e.g., prostaglandins (PG), leukotrienes (LT)] also exert stimulatory effects on bone formation and resorption. PGE_2 stimulates bone formation at low concentrations but is inhibitory at high concentrations (Raisz and Fall, 1990). In addition, PGE_3 (Raisz et al., 1989a) and the leukotrienes (LTB_4, LTC_4, and LTD_4) (Meghji et al., 1988) have been shown to be potent stimulators of bone resorption.

Prostaglandins

The essential fatty acid, linoleic acid, is metabolically converted to polyunsaturated fatty acids (PUFA) in the liver (Watkins et al., 1996). Linoleic acid [18:2(n-6)] is referred to as an (n-6) PUFA because the terminal double bond nearest the methyl end of the molecule in its carbon chain is located at the 6th position. Enzymatic desaturation (addition of double bonds) and chain elongation (by 2-carbon units) of 18:2(n-6) leads to the formation of arachidonic acid, an (n-6) PUFA (Fig. 5.4). The Δ-6 desaturase is probably the major rate-regulating step in PUFA synthesis. Hormonal and nutritional regulation of the Δ-6 and Δ-5 desaturases controls the rates of conversion of 18:2(n-6) to its respective long-chain (n-6) PUFA (Watkins et al., 1996).

Specific PUFA serve as substrates for the biosynthesis of a variety of oxygenated compounds called eicosanoids (prostacyclins, prostaglandins, thromboxanes, hydroperoxy and hydroxy acids, lipoxins, and leukotrienes). For example, 20:3(n-6), 20:4(n-6), and 20:5(n-3) are substrates for the 1, 2, and 3 series of prostaglandins, respectively. The synthesis of eicosanoids is ubiquitous and these oxygenated C_{20} carboxylic acids affect nearly all physiological systems. In skeletal tissues, their established biological actions include stimulation of chondrocyte and bone cell differentation and mediation of bone formation and resorption.

Prior to the synthesis of PG, substrate must be made available. Activation of phospholipases cleaves substrate from membrane phospholipids (Fig. 5.4). The liberated fatty acid becomes available for oxidative transformation via the cyclooxygenase or lipoxygenase pathways. Various stimuli (physical,

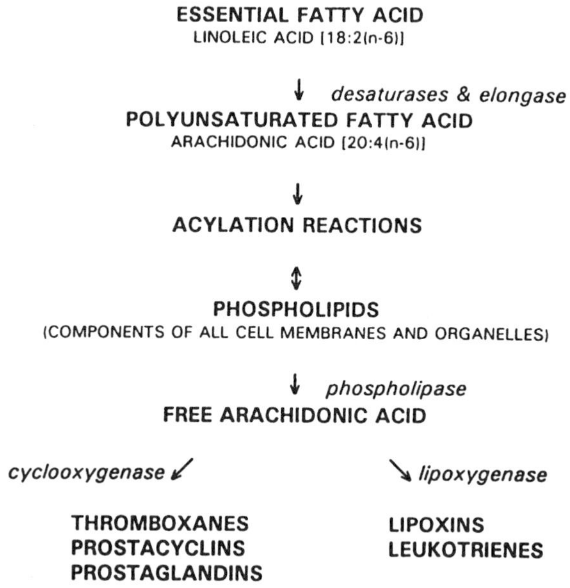

ESSENTIAL FATTY ACID
LINOLEIC ACID [18:2(n-6)]

↓ *desaturases & elongase*
POLYUNSATURATED FATTY ACID
ARACHIDONIC ACID [20:4(n-6)]

↓
ACYLATION REACTIONS

↕
PHOSPHOLIPIDS
(COMPONENTS OF ALL CELL MEMBRANES AND ORGANELLES)

↓ *phospholipase*
FREE ARACHIDONIC ACID

cyclooxygenase ↙   ↘ *lipoxygenase*

THROMBOXANES   **LIPOXINS**
PROSTACYCLINS   **LEUKOTRIENES**
PROSTAGLANDINS

FIG. 5.4   Conversion of the essential fatty acid linoleic acid to arachidonic acid, its incorporation into phospholipids, and subsequent biosynthesis into eicosanoids (see text for details).

hormonal, chemical, and toxic) cause the release of prostaglandins in tissues. Prostaglandins, prostacyclins, and thromboxanes are the major products evolved from the cyclooxygenase pathway, while leukotrienes and lipoxins are produced from the lipoxygenase pathway (Fig. 5.4). Cyclooxygenase is inhibited by aspirin and indomethacin. Arachidonic acid is the primary substrate for most of the eicosanoids produced. Once formed, the eicosanoids exert localized, autocrine, or paracrine effects on cells. The eicosanoids are short-lived biological regulators, which produce immediate cellular responses before being rapidly degraded by enzymes in tissues where they are synthesized.

In 1970, PGE_2 was observed to cause calcium release from bone tissue indicating effects on bone resorption (Klein and Raisz, 1970). Production of PG has been measured in human tissues, bone organ cultures, and osteoblasts (Marks and Miller, 1993; Raisz, 1993). Physical stress (Somjen et al., 1980) and systemic and local bone regulatory factors (PTH, epidermal growth factor, platelet-derived growth factors, transforming growth factors, and interleukin-1) stimulate PG synthesis and release in osteoblasts or bone organ cultures (Mohan and Baylink, 1991; Mundy, 1993).

Cytokines

Cytokines are extracellular signaling proteins, secreted by effector cells, which act on nearby target cells. Cytokines exert their effects at low concentrations in an autocrine or paracrine fashion in cell-to-cell communications. While generally stimulating anabolic processes in cells, cytokines also inhibit cell activity; hence, they could be called biological modifiers. One of the principle cellular responses produced by the action of cytokines is the synthesis and release of PGE_2.

The cytokines involved in bone modeling and remodeling include, epidermal growth factor (EGF), fibroblast growth factor (FGF), interferon-γ (IFN-γ), interleukins (IL-1, IL-6), platelet-derived growth factor (PDGF), transforming growth factors (TGF-α, TGF-β), tumor necrosis factor-α (TNF-α), and insulinlike growth factors (IGF-I, IGF-II) (Canalis et al., 1989, 1991, 1993). Table 5.2 provides a brief summary of effects produced by eicosanoids, cytokines, and regulatory peptides on bone cells and tissues. Whereas most cytokines are potent stimulators of bone resorption, few, in fact, enhance bone formation (Table 5.2). FGF, PDGF, and TGF-β stimulate proliferation and differentiation of collagen-synthesizing cells.

Many of the cytokines exert a positive effect on bone resorption. EGF, IL, PDGF, TGF-α, and TNF-α all stimulate bone resorption in vitro (Table 5.2). IFN-γ inhibits bone resorption previously stimulated in vitro by IL-1, TNF-α, TNF-β, PTH, and $1,25(OH)_2D_3$. The mechanism by which IFN-γ inhibits

TABLE 5.2   Reported Responses of Autocrine and Paracrine
Factors in Bone

Responses observed in bone	Cytokine, eicosanoid, or peptide growth factor
Bone formation or matrix production	FGF, IGF, PGE, TGF-β
Bone resorption	EGF, IL, LT, PDGF, TGF-α, TNF-α
Collagen synthesis	FGF, IGF, TGF-β

FGF = Fibroblast growth factor; IGF = insulinlike growth factor; PGE =
prostaglandin E; TGF = transforming growth factor; EGF = epidermal
growth factor; IL = interleukin; LT = leukotriene; PDGF = platelet-
derived growth factor; TNF = tumor necrosis factor.
Source: Adapted from Norrdin et al., 1990; Canalis et al., 1991; Spencer
et al., 1991; Mundy, 1993; Raisz, 1993.

bone resorption is controversial, but recent investigations suggest that this
cytokine interferes with osteoclast formation (Canalis et al., 1991).

Insulinlike Growth Factors

The insulinlike growth factors (IGF), also called somatomedins, are described as paracrine or autocrine regulatory polypeptides of cells. These
compounds stimulate growth and synthesis of DNA, RNA, and proteins in
cells. IGF are mitogenic and stimulate differentiation in a variety of cell
types. Pituitary growth hormone (GH) controls tissue biosynthesis and
secretion of IGF-I (insulinlike growth factor I or somatomedin C) post-
natally, and it is through IGF-I that the tissue effects of GH are mediated.
Serum concentrations of IGF-I are maintained by liver synthesis under the
influence of GH. Much of the circulating IGF is bound to plasma IGF–
binding proteins (IGFBP). The genes for IGF-I are found in a number of
species, including humans (Rotwein et al., 1986), rats (Shimatsu and Rotwein, 1987), mice (Bell et al., 1986), and chickens (Kajimoto and Rotwein,
1989).

   Both IGF-I and IGF-II are conserved in skeletal tissue of vertebrates,
including chickens and humans (Bautista et al., 1990). The amount of IGF-I
and IGF-II produced by bone cells is species dependent. For example,
humans, neonatal mice and chickens produce more IGF-II than IGF-I in the
skeletal tissues, but adult mice and rats have more IGF-I than IGF-II in
skeletal extracts (Zangger et al., 1987; Bautista et al., 1990). While IGF-II is
generally more abundant than IGF-I (Mohan and Baylink, 1991), IGF-I

appears to be under greater regulatory control in bone (Canalis et al., 1991; McCarthy et al., 1991). For example, PGE_2 (0.01–1 μM) elevated IGF-I mRNA and polypeptide levels 1.9- to 4.7-fold; however, PGE_2 did not increase IGF-II mRNA or polypeptide levels in bone organ cultures of fetal rat calvaria (McCarthy et al., 1991).

ROLE OF LIPIDS IN BONE BIOLOGY

Sources of Dietary Polyunsaturated Fatty Acids

PUFA contain two or more double bonds in their structure. The PUFA are grouped into several families based on the location of the first double bond counting from the methyl or omega end (designated as ω or n, respectively) of the molecule. The PUFA families are (n-3), (n-6), and (n-9), which represent omega-3, omega-6, and omega-9 polyenoic fatty acids, respectively. The essential PUFA include linoleic acid [18:2(n-6)] and α-linolenic acid [18:3(n-3)].

Fatty acids that must be supplied in the diet are called essential fatty acids because the body lacks the enzymes needed to synthesize them de novo (Vergroesen and Crawford, 1989). Two fatty acids are considered essential for humans: linoleic acid and α-linolenic acid (Simopoulos, 1991; Connor et al., 1992). As stated earlier, linoleic acid [18:2(n-6)] belongs to the (n-6) or omega-6 family of PUFA because the terminal double bond is six carbons from the methyl end of the molecule. Likewise, α-linolenic acid [18:3(n-3)] is a member of the (n-3) (omega-3) PUFA family since the double bond is three carbons from the methyl end. Essential fatty acids are crucial for fetal development and growth. The long-chain (n-3) PUFA are important for brain and retinal development (Connor et al., 1992) and appear to be readily digested and absorbed from dietary sources. Learning disabilities and loss of visual acuity have been reported in animals consuming low levels of (n-3) essential fatty acids (Connor et al., 1992).

Formation of PUFA

The essential fatty acids can follow a number of metabolic fates, including β-oxidation in mitochondria to generate ATP (Schulz, 1991), desaturation and chain elongation leading to the formation of long-chain PUFA (Rezanka, 1989), and incorporation into glycerolipids (Tijburg et al., 1989). Total dietary fat intake, type, and amounts of essential fatty acids will influence metabolic use of PUFA. The liver contains desaturases and elongase enzymes to convert linoleic and α-linolenic acids to their respective PUFA (Fig. 5.5). The activities of these enzymes are influenced to some extent by changes in diet and hormones (Vergroesen and Crawford, 1989;

n-6 family
$$\Delta 6 \qquad\qquad E \qquad\qquad \Delta 5$$
18:2(n-6) → 18:3(n-6) → 20:3(n-6) → 20:4(n-6)
(linoleate)   (arachidonate)

n-3 family
$$\Delta 6 \qquad\qquad E \qquad\qquad \Delta 5$$
18:3(n-3) → 18:4(n-3) → 20:4(n-3) → 20:5(n-3)
(linolenate)   (eicosapentaenoate)

n-9 family

$$\Delta 9 \qquad\qquad\qquad \Delta 6 \qquad\qquad E \qquad\qquad \Delta 5$$
18:0 → 18:1(n-9) → 18:2(n-9) → 20:2(n-9) → 20:3(n-9)
(stearate)   (oleate)   (Mead acid)

FIG. 5.5   Formation pathways for the (n-6), (n-3), and (n-9) families of polyunsaturated fatty acids presumed to occur in liver.

Lands, 1991). The rate-limiting step is the delta-6 desaturase (Δ-6), and the preferred substrates are α-linolenic acid > linoleic acid > oleic acid.

The concentrations of 18:3(n-6) and 20:3(n-6) in liver are very low compared to the concentrations of linoleic and arachidonic acids because once 18:3(n-6) is formed it is rapidly elongated to 20:3(n-6), then desaturated to yield 20:4(n-6). Recent studies conducted by Sprecher and coworkers on rat liver suggest that 22:6(n-3) is not produced directly by a putative Δ-4 desaturase (Voss et al., 1991). In the rat, the conversion involves microsomal elongation of 22:5(n-3) to 24:5(n-3) and desaturation to 24:6(n-3) by a Δ-6 desaturase. The 24:6(n-3) is then β-oxidized to 22:6(n-3). Although the major flux through polyene acid formation is towards long-chain PUFA, some retroconversion does occur.

Nonessential fatty acids can be converted to PUFA under certain situations. For example, during essential fatty acid deficiency, oleic acid is converted to Mead acid 20:3(n-9) (Lands, 1991), a PUFA of the (n-9) family (Fig. 5.5). A decrease in the essential fatty acid linoleic acid results in a progressive decrease in arachidonic acid concentration, followed by lowered prostaglandin biosynthesis, thereby compromising normal physiological homeostasis. However, deficiency of essential fatty acids is unlikely to occur in humans.

During essential fatty acid deficiency, stearic acid [18:0] is desaturated and elongated to form Mead acid [20:3(n-9)]. Usually, most organs and tissues contain low concentrations of Mead acid since the essential fatty acid 18:2(n-6) is adequate; however, Adkisson et al. (1991) reported that epiphyseal cartilage in the young animal and human contains 3–4% Mead acid and low levels of (n-6) PUFA compared to other tissues. Xu et al. (1994)

confirmed the presence of Mead acid in epiphyseal cartilage, chondrocytes, and matrix vesicles and reported that dietary linoleate did not affect the concentration of 20:3(n-9) in young chicks.

Lipids in Calcifying Tissues: Bone Mineralization and Bone Growth

Calcifying cartilage in long bones contains chondrocytes, which elaborate matrix vesicles that initiate mineralization (Wuthier, 1988). Wuthier (1988) described the matrix vesicle (MV) structure as a lipid-enclosed microenvironment of acidic phospholipids (e.g., phosphatidylserine) that exhibit high-affinity binding for Ca^{2+}. Indeed, a major proportion of matrix vesicle phosphatidylserine is complexed with Ca^{2+} and inorganic phosphate (Pi) (Wuthier, 1988). Matrix vesicles contain ion-transport proteins for Pi and Ca^{2+} and possess several active phosphatases, especially alkaline phosphatase. The matrix vesicle rapidly accumulates these minerals to yield octacalcium phosphate, which forms apatite crystals (Wuthier, 1988). The developing mineralized crystals eventually rupture the matrix vesicle membrane to facilitate expansion of matrix mineralization by epistaxis.

The PUFA are important (structurally and physiologically) for mineralizing tissues of bone and for the local regulation of bone modeling. Phospholipids in the MV membrane are biosynthesized from PUFA, and PG, which regulate bone formation and resorption, are derived from essential PUFA. Some acidic phospholipids are enriched in the isolated MV, such as phosphatidylserine (PS), phosphatidylinositol, and phosphatidic acid, and PS has been shown to have a strong affinity for ionic calcium (Cotmore et al., 1971; Wuthier and Gore, 1977). The membrane-bound acidic phospholipids located within the MV facilitate mineralization by forming lipid-Ca^{2+}-protein complexes (Genge et al., 1992). These acidic phospholipids may act as non–energy-requiring Ca^{2+} traps for the initial mineralization in MV (Sauer and Wuthier, 1988).

Endochondral mineralization occurs in the extracellular matrix of the hypertrophic cell zone of the growth cartilage (Buckwalter et al., 1986; Hunziker et al., 1987), as illustrated in Fig. 5.6. However, the mechanism of endochondral mineralization remained obscure until the discovery of MVs by Anderson (1967) and Bonucci (1967). Presently, MV are believed to be responsible for initiating de novo mineralization in all calcifying tissues (Anderson, 1989; Wuthier, 1993). MV are chondrocyte-derived cell membrane vesicles (100–200 nm) involved in the process of cartilage mineralization via initial development and maturation of hydroxyapatite crystals along the inner leaflet of the MV membrane (Anderson, 1989). Once initiated, crystals of hydroxyapatite begin to accumulate and grow within the MV eventually rupturing the MV membrane and depositing mineral locally within the matrix (Wuthier, 1988; Anderson, 1989).

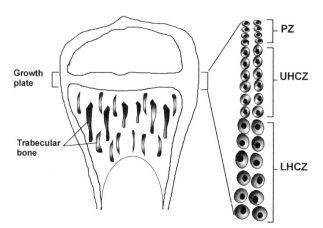

FIG. 5.6   Section of epiphyseal growth plate cartilage in the proximal end of the tibia of a mammal illustrating the location of chondrocytes in the proliferative zone (PZ), upper hypertrophic chondrocyte zone (UHCZ), and the lower hypertrophic chondrocyte zone (LHCZ). Mineralization of cartilage occurs at the interface between the LHCZ and trabecular bone.

High alkaline phosphatase (AP) activity is present in isolated MV (Ali et al., 1970), and the activity is much higher than that found in chondrocytes (McLean et al., 1987; Wuthier, 1988). AP activity has been long associated with bone calcification (Robison, 1923). Early studies revealed that AP is concentrated in calcifying sites and is present in matrix vesicles (Matsuzawa and Anderson, 1971). AP is thought to act upon organic substrates, such as phospholipids present in calcified matrix (Boskey et al., 1980), to yield inorganic phosphate required for nucleation in mineral growth. However, the function of AP in mineral formation is still not clear (Golub et al., 1992).

Biosynthesis of Eicosanoids in Bone

The pathways for the biosynthesis of prostaglandins and leukotrienes are illustrated in Fig. 5.7. As 20:4(n-6) is released from membrane phospholipids of chondrocytes and osteoblasts by the action of phospholipase (PL)A_2, it can undergo oxidative transformation to yield a variety of eicosanoids. For example, PGE_2, prostacyclins (PG)I_2, and thromboxanes (TX)B_2 are produced via the cyclooxygenase (CO) pathway. In contrast, 20:4(n-6) can be converted to other eicosanoid products, i.e., hydroperoxy-eicosatraenoic acid (HPETE), LT, and lipoxins by the lipoxygenase (LO) pathway. Similarly, 20:5(n-3) is the substrate for the biosynthesis of the three

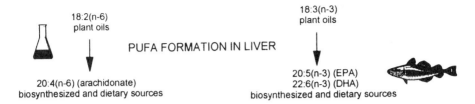

TRANSPORT OF LIPIDS VIA LIPOPROTEINS

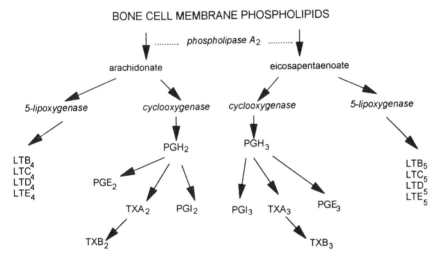

FIG. 5.7   Biosynthesis of eicosanoids in bone from (n-6) and (n-3) PUFA of dietary origin. DHA = docosahexaenoic acid, EPA = eicosapentaenoic acid, PUFA = polyunsaturated fatty acids, LT = leukotrienes (B-E), PG = prostaglandins (H,E), prostacyclins = I, TX = thromboxanes (A-B).

series of prostaglandins (PGE_3, PGI_3, and TXB_3) or the five series products of the LO pathway (Sardesai, 1992).

Eicosanoid Effects on Bone Metabolism

Klein and Raisz (1970) first reported that PGE_1, PGE_2, PGA_1, and $PGF_{1\alpha}$ increased the release of ^{45}Ca into the media from cultured fetal rat bone. Since then, numerous studies have demonstrated that PGE stimulate bone formation as well as bone resorption (Norrdin et al., 1990; Marks and Miller, 1993; Raisz, 1993). For example, PGE_2 stimulated collagen synthesis in cultured rat calvariae (Raisz and Fall, 1990) and in osteoblastic cells

(Hakeda et al., 1985) and also increased the proliferation of osteoblasts in culture (Igarashi et al., 1994). PGE_2 was reported to increase cortical bone mass and intracortical bone remodeling in both intact and ovariectomized rats (Jee et al., 1990). Further, PGE_2 increased proximal tibial metaphyseal bone area in osteopenic ovariectomized rats (Mori et al., 1990). On the other hand, Raisz et al. (1993) reported that infusion of PGE_2 at a high concentration depressed osteogenesis in fetal rat calvariae.

PGE_3 also stimulated bone resorption in cultured fetal rat long bone, and the potency of PGE_3 was nearly equal to that of PGE_2 (Raisz et al., 1989a). Moreover, PGE_2 mediated the effects of $1,25(OH)_2D_3$ (Collins and Chambers, 1992), cytokines [TNF-α (Tashjian et al., 1987), IL-3 (Collins and Chambers, 1992)], and growth factors [TGF-β (Tashjian et al., 1985), PDGF (Tashjian et al., 1982)] in enhancing bone resorption.

Similar to the PG, the LT also play an important role in bone metabolism (Meghji et al., 1988; Ren and Dziak, 1991; Sandy et al., 1991; Gallwitz et al., 1993). Ren and Dziak (1991) demonstrated that LTB_4 inhibited cell proliferation in cultured osteoblasts isolated from rat calvaria in a dose-dependent manner, but LTB_4 may interact with PG to regulate osteoblast activity. Others (Gallwitz et al., 1993) reported that LTC_4, LTD_4, and 5-HETE stimulated isolated avian osteoclasts to resorb bone. Meghji et al. (1988) found that LTB_4, LTC_4, LTD_4, 5-HETE, and 12-HETE stimulated bone resorption in calvariae of mice at picomolar concentrations, whereas PGE_2 produced this stimulatory effect at 10 nM. As a mechanism of action similar to that for PGE_2 and PTH, LTB_4 activated the breakdown of phospholipids in osteoblast membranes and intact osteoblasts to increase bone resorption (Sandy et al., 1991).

Factors Effecting the Concentrations of PUFA and Prostaglandins in Bone

Feeding a semi-purified diet containing 9% of an ethyl ester concentrate of 20:5(n-3) and 22:6(n-3) to male weanling rats enriched the (n-3) PUFA content of phospholipids in alveolar bone compared to those given corn oil (Alam et al., 1993). Watkins et al. (1995a) reported that chicks given a blend of menhaden oil plus safflower oil in a semi-purified diet (45 g menhaden oil/kg diet) had a lower concentration of 20:4(n-6), but higher concentrations of 20:5(n-3) and 22:6(n-3) in cortical bone polar lipids compared to those fed soybean oil. In subsequent studies (Shen et al., 1994; Watkins et al., 1995a), the concentration of 20:4(n-6) was decreased in tibial bone of chicks given dietary sources of (n-3) PUFA, as was the amount of PGE_2 produced ex vivo in bone organ culture. Consumption of (n-3) PUFA readily enriched the (n-3) PUFA fatty acid content of bone (Watkins et al.,

1995a) and cartilage tissue of chicks (Xu et al., 1994). Presumably, altering the concentrations of 20:4(n-6) or 20:5(n-3) in bone with dietary lipids affects bone formation and resorption activities by modulating PGE_2 biosynthesis (Fig. 5.8).

Steroidal and nonsteroidal anti-inflammatory agents are two types of eicosanoid inhibitors. Corticosteroids, which are steroidal anti-inflammatory agents, were reported to inhibit PLA_2 activity, the enzyme responsible for the release of 20:4(n-6) (or other fatty acids) from cell membrane phospholipids. Inhibition of PLA_2 activity would lower the substrate availability for eicosanoid biosynthesis. Acetylsalicylic acid (aspirin), a nonsteroidal anti-inflammatory agent, functions to produce an irreversible acetylation of cyclooxygenase to lower the biosynthesis of PG (Clissold, 1986). Administration of aspirin to immobilized osteoporotic growing dogs decreased bone PGE production, and the reduction in bone PGE was associated with decreased bone loss (Waters et al., 1991). Aspirin stimulated ectopic bone formation induced by demineralized bone matrix in the rat model, suggesting that bone formation may be modulated by the metabo-

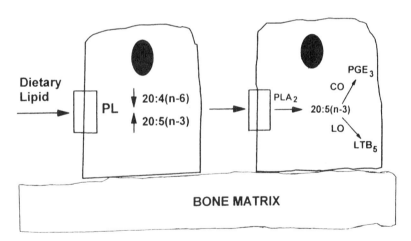

FIG. 5.8 Effect of dietary lipids varying in the amounts of (n-3) and (n-6) polyunsaturated fatty acids on the concentrations of arachidonic acid [20:4(n-6)] and eicosapentaenoic acid [20:5(n-3)] in osteoblast plasma membrane phospholipids (PL). Decreasing the concentration of arachidonic acid in the osteoblast would decrease the production of PGE_2. Likewise, increasing the concentration of 20:5(n-3) would increase the biosynthesis of PGE_3 produced by the cyclooxygenase (CO) pathway and LTB_5 produced by the lipoxygenase (LO) pathway.

lites of arachidonic acid (Yazdi et al., 1992). However, some studies reported that aspirin inhibited bone resorption and formation in rats (Solheim et al., 1986a–d).

Besides aspirin, indomethacin is also reported to inhibit PG biosynthesis in cultured neonatal rat calvariae (Raisz et al., 1989b) and in osteoblasticlike cell cultures (Fujimori et al., 1989). The effects of steroidal and nonsteroidal inhibitors of eicosanoid biosynthesis provide indirect evidence that prostaglandins play an important role in bone metabolism.

IMPORTANCE OF INSULINLIKE GROWTH FACTORS IN BONE HEALTH

Nutritional Regulation of IGF

Nutritional status and diet can regulate IGF-I production (Thissen et al., 1994). Clemmons et al. (1981) reported that fasting in humans reduced plasma IGF-I concentrations. Emler and Schalch (1987) reported that fasted rats had decreased hepatic IGF-I mRNA levels compared to their ad libitum fed controls. Straus and Takemoto (1990) demonstrated that a reduction in the transcriptional level of hepatic IGF-I mRNA was due to a decrease in the GH receptors that mediate the concentration of IGF-I in blood.

Dietary protein restriction (5% vs. 15% dietary protein) in rats lowered IGF-I concentrations in serum (Maes et al., 1984). In contrast to the reduction in GH receptors that occurred during fasting, protein restriction in rats appeared to cause postreceptor resistance to the action of GH (Maiter et al., 1988).

Energy restriction (18–20 kcal/kg ideal body weight/day) for a week lowered IGF-I concentrations in serum of normal-weight human subjects by 38% (Smith et al., 1987) but had no effect on serum IGF-I in obese subjects (Snyder et al., 1988). Energy deprivation in streptozotocin-diabetic rats caused a decrease in hepatic IGF-I mRNA abundance, suggesting that these changes contributed to a reduction of IGF-I in serum (Goldstein et al., 1988).

The effect of energy deprivation on the molecular mechanism of IGF-I regulation, however, remains unclear. Isley et al. (1984) suggested that there was a threshold energy requirement below which optimal protein intake failed to raise the concentration of IGF-I in serum. A highly significant correlation ($r^2 = 0.90$) was reported between the changes in the concentration of IGF-I in serum and changes in nitrogen balance during fasting and refeeding in normal weight human subjects (Isley et al., 1983). Additionally, other studies (Snyder et al., 1989; Vazquez and Adibi, 1992) in obese subjects indicated that when energy intake is restricted, the carbohydrate content of the diet is a major factor for responsiveness of IGF-I to GH compared to a lipid-rich diet. On the other hand, overfeeding (1200–1600 kcal/day) in normal-weight women (20–30 years) for 14 days caused an increase of IGF-I levels in serum (Forbes et al., 1989). However, a negative correlation has been reported between the concentration of IGF-I in serum and the degree of adiposity in obese men (Copeland et al., 1990) and obese women (Crist and Hill, 1990).

Receptors for IGF

The IGF-I receptors on the osteoblasts have been characterized from fetal rat bone by Scatchard plot and chemical cross-link analyses (Centrella et al., 1990). Some studies have demonstrated that IGF-I increases skeletal angiogenesis via an IGF-I type-I receptor in cultured bone cells (Kurose et al., 1989, 1990; Fiorelli et al., 1994). In contrast, Hou et al. (1994) reported that both IGF-I and IGF-II increased bone resorption in mature rabbits via an interaction with type-I receptors. Moreover, $1,25(OH)_2D_3$ increased the numbers of IGF-I receptors for IGF-I on MC3T3-E1 cells (Kurose et al., 1990), and a synergistic effect was demonstrated with IGF-I on alkaline phosphatase activity in these cells (Kurose et al., 1989).

Insulinlike Growth Factor–Binding Proteins

Insulin-like growth factor–binding proteins are circulatory or locally produced proteins, which avidly bind to IGF and transport them from the vascular compartment to their target cell receptors (Shimasaki and Ling, 1991). Currently, six different IGFBP have been identified in bone and are designated IGFBP-1 through IGFBP-6. IGFBP function to modulate the mitogenic and anabolic effects of IGF. Stimulatory or inhibitory effects depend upon the particular IGFBP, the target cell, and the physiological environment (Jones and Clemmons, 1995).

Osteoblastic cells produce both IGF as well as IGFBP in vivo (Schmid et al., 1989; Bautista et al., 1991) and in vitro (McCarthy et al., 1994). IGFBP were reported to regulate the local effects of IGF in bone. For example, coincubation of IGFBP-5 with IGF-I or IGF-II stimulated osteoblastic mitogenesis (Andress and Birnbaum, 1992). $1,25(OH)_2D_3$ was reported to decrease the proliferation of osteoblasts by inhibiting the production of IGF-I. However, $1,25(OH)_2D_3$ stimulated the secretion of IGFBP-2 (Chen et al., 1991), IGFBP-3 (Moriwake et al., 1992), and IGFBP-4 (Scharla et al., 1991) in cultured osteoblastlike cells. Although the production of IGFBP may be regulated by systemic hormones or local factors, few studies have been reported describing the effects of diet on regulation of IGFBP and their effects on bone.

Function of IGF-I in Bone Metabolism

IGF-I stimulates both bone formation and resorption in vivo and in vitro (Baylink et al., 1993; Marks and Miller, 1993; Raisz, 1993). IGF-I has been shown to enhance bone formation in cortical bone (Spencer et al., 1991) as well as in cultured fetal rat calvaria by stimulating DNA (Canalis, 1980) and bone matrix synthesis (Hock et al., 1988). Further, administration of IGF-I to osteopenic rats increased osteoid surface, osteoblastic surface, and total bone formation rate (Mueller et al., 1994).

IGF-I has also been shown to stimulate osteoclastic bone resorption by directly or indirectly activating osteoclasts in cultures of mouse bone cells (Mochizuki et al., 1992). IGF-I appears to be an important regulator of systemic hormones that stimulate bone resorption, including $1,25(OH)_2D_3$ (Battmann et al., 1994), PTH (Goad and Tashjian, 1994), and estrogen (Komm, 1992). Battmann et al. (1994) reported that IGF-I may potentiate the action of $1,25(OH)_2D_3$ by upregulating the receptors for $1,25(OH)_2D_3$ in cultured human bone cells. IGF-I was also shown to downregulate the levels of mRNA for PTH and PTH-related protein receptors in human SAOS-2 osteoblastic cells (Goad and Tashjian, 1994). Moreover, IGF-I increased the transcriptional expression of the estrogen receptor in human osteosarcoma cells, which may be involved in bone remodeling (Komm, 1992).

Romagnoli et al. (1993) reported that the levels of IGF-I in plasma were significantly decreased and were correlated with lower bone mineral density in postmenopausal women. The decreased circulating level of IGF-I and ratio of IGF-I/IGFBP-3 is suggestive that these factors play an important role in bone loss of menopause (Romagnoli et al., 1993, 1994).

Factors Regulating IGF-I Production in Bone

The production of IGF-I in osteoblasts can be modulated by systemic hormones and factors produced locally in bone (Baylink et al., 1993; Marks and Miller, 1993; Raisz, 1993). The stimulatory effect of thyroid hormone (T_3 and T_4) on bone formation may involve an increase in IGF-I production as observed in cultured osteoblastic cells (Schmid et al., 1992). Both PTH and $1,25(OH)_2D_3$ stimulated the production of IGF-I and IGF-II in cultured neonatal mouse calvaria (Linkhart and Keffer, 1991). Injecting PTH into 60-day-old male rats increased the concentration of IGF-I but had no effect on the concentration of IGF-II in bone (Pfeilschifter et al., 1994). Estrogen stimulated the transcriptional levels of IGF-I genes in cultured osteoblasts

(Ernst and Rodan, 1991) and increased skeletal and hepatic IGF-I gene expression in mice (Liu and Richardson, 1991). Growth hormone increased IGF-I mRNA in the growth plate of rat (Isgaard et al., 1988) and enhanced IGFBP-3 mRNA levels (Schmid et al., 1989) and IGFBP-3 production (Ernst and Rodan, 1990) in osteoblastic cells.

PGE$_2$ was reported to stimulate the synthesis of IGF-I in cultured bone cells (McCarthy et al., 1991, 1994; Schmid et al., 1992; Raisz et al., 1993). PGE$_2$ increased the intracellular levels of cAMP, a second messenger, in rat osteoblast cultures (McCarthy et al., 1991), and the increased level of cAMP presumably stimulated the biosynthesis of IGF-I in cultured osteoblasts. Thus, PGE$_2$ may be responsible for stimulating an increase in transcripts and polypeptide levels of IGF-I. Bichell et al. (1993) confirmed that PGE$_2$ rapidly induced production of the precursor of IGF-I mRNA and stimulated gene expression for IGF-I in osteoblasts. Others (Pash et al., 1994) reported that the IGF-I exon 1 promoter had a region (within -1123 to $+358$) on the gene that was activated by PGE$_2$ to increase transcriptional levels of IGF-I mRNA in rat calvarial osteoblasts.

Recent investigations with dietary lipids suggest that (n-3) PUFA raise the concentration of IGF-I in plasma, liver, and cortical bone of chicks compared with those given (n-6) PUFA (Watkins et al., 1995a). In other studies (Shen et al., 1994), the (n-3) PUFA in menhaden oil appeared to upregulate the level of IGF-I in plasma and other tissues of chicks. To our knowledge, no reports have been published describing the effects of PUFA on the levels or production of IGF in tissues.

Although PGE$_2$ modifies the production of IGF-I, it also affects the biosynthesis of IGFBP in skeletal tissues (Schmid et al., 1992; Raisz et al., 1993; McCarthy et al., 1994). PGE$_2$ enhanced the binding affinity of IGFBP-3 and gene expression for IGF-I and IGFBP-3 in osteoblastlike cells (Schmid et al., 1992). McCarthy et al. (1994) demonstrated that PGE$_2$ increased the transcriptional levels for IGFBP-3, IGFBP-4, and IGFBP-5, but had no effect on IGFBP-2 or IGFBP-6 transcription in primary osteoblast-enriched cultures. When they were added to cultured fetal rat calvariae, IGFBP-2 and IGFBP-3 completely blocked the stimulatory effects of exogenous IGF-I on collagen synthesis (Raisz et al., 1993). However, the stimulatory effect of PGE$_2$ on collagen synthesis was not effected by IGFBP-3, indicating that the anabolic effects of PGE$_2$ on collagen synthesis may involve an IGF-I–independent pathway (Raisz et al., 1993).

When bone cultures were treated with indomethacin for 24 hours, IGF-I concentrations were decreased by 50% compared to control cultures not treated with indomethacin (Raisz et al., 1993). In the presence of indomethacin, the addition of exogenous PGE$_2$ to bone cultures elevated IGF-I suggesting that the reduced IGF-I production was due to a lack of endogenous PGE_2 production in bone organ cultures. Moreover, the addition of exogenous PGE_2 exhibited a greater stimulatory effect on IGF-I production compared to endogenously produced PGE_2 in bone organ cultures.

The cytokine IL-1 increased the production of IGF-I in neonatal mouse calvaria by stimulating PGE_2 production (Linkhart and MacCharles, 1992). Some growth factors (e.g., basic FGF, TGF-β_1, and PDGF) were reported to lower IGF-I transcript and polypeptide levels and to decrease the synthesis of IGF-I in cultured osteoblastic cells (Canalis et al., 1993). For example, Gabbitas et al. (1994) demonstrated that basic FGF, TGF-β, and PDGF inhibited osteoblastic differentiation, which correlated with the decreased biosynthesis of IGF-I and IGF-II in osteoblast cell cultures. These data indicate that the production and action of IGF are controlled by complex interactions between systemic and local factors. Further, the production of PGE_2 appears to exert a positive control on the synthesis of IGF and on its regulatory proteins (IGFBP).

Relationships Between Dietary PUFA and IGF-I in Bone

That the concentration of PGE_2 in bone can be manipulated by dietary (n-6) and (n-3) PUFA (Watkins et al., 1995a; Shen et al., 1994) and that changes in ex vivo PGE_2 biosynthesis in bone may regulate IGF-I production to influence bone formation (Watkins et al., 1995a) suggest that dietary lipids could impact bone modeling by separate mechanisms. For example, consumption of dietary PUFA presumably alters the concentrations of (n-6) PUFA, i.e., 20:4(n-6), in the cell membrane phospholipids of osteoblasts to directly affect the production of PGE_2. Once formed, PGE_2 elevates the intracellular level of cAMP in osteoblasts and cAMP acts as a second messenger to stimulate the production of IGFBP and IGF in osteoblasts. The production of IGF-I stimulates the proliferation of osteoblasts and synthesis of bone matrix and, thus, increases bone formation (Fig. 5.9). These responses are of special importance to bone remodeling since a lack of local skeletal growth factors (e.g., IGF) are hypothesized to be, in part, responsible for the development of osteoporosis (Baylink et al., 1993).

Likewise, consumption of menhaden oil increased the concentrations of (n-3) PUFA [i.e., 20:5(n-3) and 22:6(n-3)] but lowered the concentration of 20:4(n-6) in the cell membrane phospholipids of osteoblasts (see Fig. 5.8). The 20:5(n-3) released from membrane phospholipids by PLA_2 could be converted to PGE_3 in osteoblasts by the CO pathway or to LTB_5 by the LO pathway (Fig. 5.10). Similar to the stimulatory effect of PGE_2 on IGF-I production, PGE_3 (or LTB_5) may potentially increase the biosynthesis (or action) of IGF-I in osteoblasts. Thus, the changes in IGF-I production could enhance bone formation by increasing osteoblastic proliferation and bone matrix synthesis.

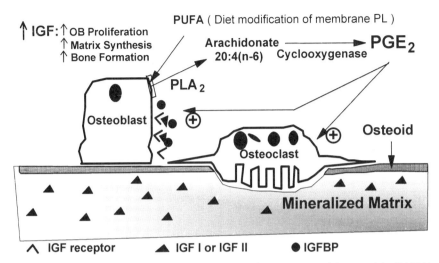

FIG. 5.9   Relationships between dietary polyunsaturated fatty acids (PUFA) and IGF in bone metabolism. IGF = insulinlike growth factor I and II, IGFBP = insulinlike growth factor binding protein, OB = osteoblast, PGE_2 = prostaglandin E_2, PL = phospholipids, PLA_2 = phospholipase A_2.

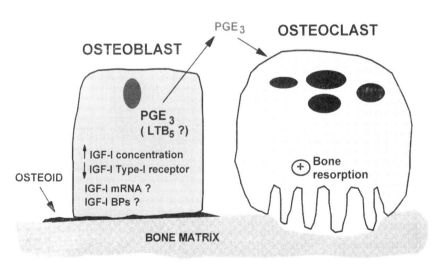

FIG. 5.10   Observed and potential responses of osteoblasts enriched with 20:5(n-3). Formation of prostaglandin E_3 (PGE_3) or leukotriene B_5 (LTB_5) in the osteoblast would stimulate osteoclastic bone resorption and modulate the concentration of insulinlike growth factor-I (IGF-I), IGF-I type-I receptors, and possibly influence the levels of mRNA for IGF and IGF-binding proteins (IGFBP).

Modulation of Cellular Membrane Structure in Bone by Dietary PUFA

The fluidity of cell membranes (e.g., plasma and liver microsomes) is known to be altered by dietary lipids (Bruneau et al., 1987; Muriana and Ruiz-Gutierrez, 1992). Varying the PUFA composition of plasma membrane phospholipids can influence the binding capacity of insulin to cell membrane receptors in vivo (Field et al., 1989, 1990). Based on these observations, one could hypothesize that dietary (n-6) and (n-3) PUFA manipulate the fatty acid composition of membrane-bound phospholipids of osteoblasts. These changes could modify membrane fluidity or receptor binding on the osteoblasts to indirectly influence the action of IGF-I in bone metabolism.

THE ROLE OF LIPIDS IN BONE MODELING AND DEGENERATIVE BONE DISEASES

Oxidative Stress in Bone and Cartilage Tissues

There appears to be a close relationship between lipid peroxidation and degenerative diseases associated with aging (Ames et al., 1993; Halliwell, 1994a,b). Lipid peroxidation is a free radical–mediated chain reaction initiated by the action of the highly active hydroxyl radical (OH·) or by certain metal radicals, such as ferryl or perferryl radicals (Halliwell and Chirico, 1993). These abstract a labile hydrogen from a methylene group adjacent to a double bond of an unsaturated fatty acid (RH). The resulting allyl radical (R·) can further react with O_2 to form a peroxyl radical (ROO·), which can react with another unsaturated fatty acid (RH) to form a lipid hydroperoxide (ROOH).

Lipid hydroperoxides formed in the propagation reaction can further serve as substrates to react with Fe^{2+} to yield ROO· and the alkoxyl radical (RO·). Reducing agents (e.g., ascorbate) convert Fe^{3+} to the more reactive Fe^{2+} (Kappus, 1991). The reduced metal is required for the Fenton reaction (Kalyanaraman et al., 1991), and Fe^{2+} can actively cleave ROOH to produce an alkoxyl radical (RO·). The RO· can initiate additional chain reactions to form R· (Buettner, 1993). The R·, in turn, can react with O_2 to form ROO· to perpetuate oxidation reactions (Halliwell, 1994b).

Lipid peroxidation can also produce mutagenic lipid epoxides, lipid hydroperoxides, lipid alkoxyls, peroxyl radicals, and enals (Ames et al., 1993). Furthermore, these peroxidation products can cause damage to DNA, proteins, and other macromolecules, leading to the development of degenerative diseases associated with aging (Ames et al., 1993; Halliwell,

1994b). The onset of peroxidative reactions within biological membranes could impair the behavior and function of the cell. Oarada and Terao (1992) reported that when mouse thymic lymphocytes were incubated with methyl linoleate hydroperoxide, DNA, RNA, and protein synthesis were greatly decreased, while thiobarbituric acid–reactive substances (indicative of lipid peroxidation) increased.

Oxidative stress occurs when the balance between prooxidants and anti-oxidants favors the prooxidants (Sies, 1991). Garrett et al. (1990) recently reported that oxygen-derived free radicals stimulated bone resorption in vitro and in vivo, and Matsumoto et al. (1991) found that the activities of superoxide dismutase (SOD) and catalase were higher in the premineralized zone of growth cartilage but were lower in the mineralized zone. This research suggests that the mineralized region of growth cartilage may have a limited capacity for handling oxidized lipid species since SOD and catalase activities are low in this region. Both SOD and catalase function as vital antioxidant protective enzyme systems. SOD converts superoxide ($O_2^{\bullet-}$ to hydrogen peroxide (H_2O_2), and catalase degrades hydrogen peroxide to H_2O (Halliwell, 1994b).

Rathakrishnan et al. (1992) reported that normal articular chondrocytes produce reactive oxygen radicals and reactive oxygen intermediates. An excess production of reactive oxygen radicals may be associated with cartilage pathology. Oxygen free radical damage has been reported to exert a pathogenic role in chronic rheumatic diseases (Torrielli and Dianzani, 1984; Harris, 1990; Peretz et al., 1991). Recently, Watkins et al. (1995a) reported that chicks fed butter oil high in saturated fat showed an increase in cortical bone formation rates compared to chicks fed soybean oil. These findings suggest that dietary lipids and oxidation products from fatty acids may affect cartilage mineralization and bone modeling. Dietary lipids and antioxidant nutrients may influence oxidative stress in bone tissues in a manner similar to that observed in other tissues (Ames et al., 1993; Gutteridge, 1993; Halliwell, 1994b).

Potential Antioxidant Role of Vitamin E in Bone Modeling

The antioxidant function of vitamin E has received much attention recently (Ames et al., 1993; Halliwell, 1994a). The function of vitamin E as a primary cellular antioxidant has been well documented (for review, see Meydani, 1995). α-Tocopherol is an important cellular antioxidant that prevents peroxidation in membrane-bound lipids (Burton and Traber, 1990). The antioxidant reaction of vitamin E involves a peroxyl radical and the phenolic hydroxyl group of tocopherol to generate the hydroxide and the tocopherol radical (Meydani, 1995). Therefore, tocopherol breaks the chain reaction peroxidation by decreasing peroxyl radicals, which may react with other lipids during the propagation step.

Ebina et al. (1991) reported that the Fe-induced impairment of bone formation in rats was prevented by dietary vitamin E supplementation compared to rats fed a vitamin E–deficient diet. This response suggests that vitamin E may be important for maintaining normal bone development.

Recently, the effects of dietary vitamin E and lipids on tissue lipid peroxidation, epiphyseal growth plate cartilage development, and trabecular bone formation were evaluated in chicks (Xu et al., 1995). The level of α-tocopherol in plasma was higher, and thiobarbituric acid reactive substances (TBARS) were less in plasma and liver of animals supplemented with additional vitamin E, and the thickness of the entire growth plate cartilage and the lower hypertrophic chondrocyte zone was significantly greater compared to those given a lower level of vitamin E. Kinetic histomorphometric parameters indicated that mineral apposition rate was higher in those given supplemental vitamin E above the requirement.

Watkins et al. (1995b) reported that vitamin E protected primary cultures of avian epiphyseal chondrocytes from the effects of iron-induced oxidative stress when supplemented with 18:2(n-6). Further, vitamin E lowered lactate dehydrogenase activity and partially restored collagen synthesis in the chondrocytes enriched with 18:2(n-6). The data suggest that linoleic acid caused cellular injury and impaired chondrocyte cell function. Vitamin E appears to be important in chondrocyte biology and beneficial to growth cartilage development during early growth. Figure 5.11 illustrates the unusual pattern of PUFA formation in epiphyseal chondrocytes in the young animal and human and the effects of dietary fat on modifying PUFA formation.

Dietary Lipids and Bone Modeling

Watkins et al. (1995a) reported that cortical bone modeling in the tibia of chicks given saturated fat increased compared to those given vegetable oil. Higher values for periosteal bone formation rates (mm^2/day), total new bone formation rates (mm^2/day), and intracortical porosity (mm^2) were observed in animals fed the diet containing butter and corn oil as the lipid sources. In contrast, the values for total bone area (mm^2) and cortical bone area (mm^2) were lowest in animals given a diet containing vegetable oil as the only source of fat. The concentrations of IGF-I in bone increased from 21 to 42 days in animals given vegetable oil or butter plus corn oil. Alterations in fatty acid profiles and histomorphometric data, and the quantitative differences in tissue IGF-I concentrations, indicate that dietary lipids

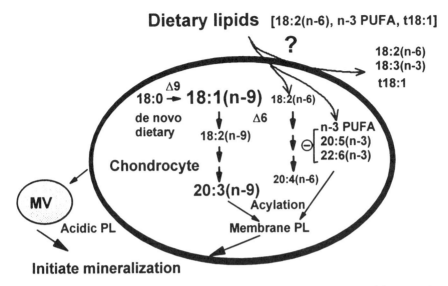

FIG. 5.11   Diagram illustrating the formation of polyunsaturated fatty acids (PUFA) in chondrocytes in the young. (Based on Adkisson et al., 1991; Xu et al., 1994.)

modulate the fatty acid composition of bone and that these changes impact bone modeling. Other studies (Shen et al., 1994) report that dietary PUFA modulate the ex vivo production of PGE_2 in bone organ culture to alter bone formation rate and bone modeling in the young.

A study in caucasian boys and girls (children 8–11 years and adolescents 11–17 years) indicated that bone mineral density in the forearm was predicted by dietary saturated fat intake (Gunnes and Lehmann, 1995). The study also found a positive association with forearm bone mineral density with the intake of calcium, saturated fat, fiber, and vitamin C; however, the associations depended on age and bone type.

Dietary lipids appear to exert important effects on bone modeling. Figure 5.12 demonstrates the relationship between dietary fat (unsaturated vs. saturated fat) and PGE_2 production in bone to influence bone modeling in the young. Dietary fat appears to mediate effects through modulation of PGE_2 production and perhaps through IGF-I action on bone.

Degenerative Bone Diseases in the Elderly

Osteoporosis is a significant health problem in the United States costing $10 billion a year to treat and covalesce adult patients. While dietary supplementation of calcium is currently used as a therapeutic adjunct to slow the loss of

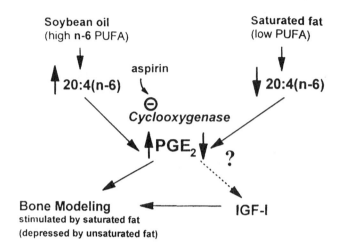

FIG. 5.12   Effects of a diet containing primarily unsaturated fat compared to a diet containing a balance between saturated and unsaturated fat on the production of prostaglandin E_2 (PGE_2) and its subsequent impact on bone modeling. Although the effect of dietary fat on IGF-I is not yet clear, PGE_2 can modulate IGF-I action on bone.

bone mineral, calcium is likely to have its greatest effect on maximizing bone mass accretion, which peaks between 30–35 years and progressively declines thereafter. Fat constitutes 30–40% of the daily total caloric intake of individuals in the United States. The amounts and types of fatty acids consumed in the diet exert profound effects on metabolism and physiology. Notably, dietary fatty acids alter lipoprotein and cholesterol metabolism, affect blood pressure, impact the risk for cardiovascular disease, modulate eicosanoid biosynthesis, and influence immune responses. To a great extent, dietary fat impacts several physiological systems in the body by altering tissue PUFA composition to modulate eicosanoid biosynthesis, influence membrane-ligand interactions, and affect cell permeability and cell-to-cell communications. Dietary lipids likely play a role in optimizing skeletal mass, as described earlier, by their ability to modulate the local production of prostaglandins and growth factors vitally important to skeletal growth, development, and maintenance.

Osteoporosis and osteoarthritis are two extremely important diseases afflicting the aging population. Osteoporosis is a condition of decreased bone mass, which is prevalent in women and places them at risk for fractures. Although dietary calcium is believed to reduce bone mineral loss, calcium is not a singular treatment for osteoporosis. In addition, calcium intake above a daily requirement does not stimulate bone formation. Two theories have emerged recently to explain the pathogenesis of osteoporosis. These theories focus on impaired coupling between bone formation and resorption (Raisz, 1993; Baylink et al., 1993) and a decline in the amount of bone growth factors deposited into bone matrix leading to decreased bone formation. A lack of control of PGE_2 production (Raisz, 1993) or decreased storage of IGF-I or other growth factors in bone (Baylink et al., 1993) may play roles in the etiology of osteoporosis. On the other hand, excessive lipid metabolism and oxidative stress may contribute to osteoarthritis. Over-production of PGE_2 has been linked to joint pathology and is known to exacerbate inflammatory responses (Lippiello et al., 1990). The information presented in this chapter suggests that dietary lipids modulate the skeletal production of PGE_2 and perhaps IGF-I to influence bone modeling in the young as a deterrent to osteoporosis. Because dietary fat constitutes 30–40% of the food calories in Western diets, the type of fat consumed can significantly influence the metabolic and physiological processes controlling bone modeling in children and adults.

NUTRITIONAL RECOMMENDATION FOR DIETARY FAT INTAKES DURING BONE MODELING AND RISK FOR OSTEOPOROSIS AND ARTHRITIS

Current research supports the recommendation that a healthy diet should contain a balance between the amounts of unsaturated fats and saturated fats. For example, animals given a diet containing an unsaturated–to–saturated fat (UNSAT/SAT) ratio of 1.1 had higher bone formation rates compared to those given a diet containing only vegetable oil, which had an UNSAT/SAT ratio of 5.4 (Watkins et al., 1995a). Diets containing meat, poultry, and dairy products, which are sources of saturated fats, are beneficial to a growing child since moderate levels of saturated fats stimulated early bone growth and bone modeling in young animals (Watkins et al., 1995a), and saturated fat intake was significantly correlated with bone mineral density in children (Gunnes and Lehmann, 1995). Research in animals also indicated that a diet high in PUFA depressed bone formation rates and may result in excessive prostaglandin production that would not be conducive to healthy bone modeling in the young.

Additionally, besides the benefits of menhaden oil on reducing the risk of heart disease, clinical trials indicate that menhaden oil may play an important role in joint diseases and inflammatory responses in the elderly (Lippiello et al., 1990; Geusens et al., 1994). The production of PGE_2 in bone was significantly decreased in animals consuming menhaden oil compared to the amount in those given soybean oil (Shen et al., 1994). Since excessive production of PGE_2 is associated with rheumatoid arthritis, (n-3) PUFA may be helpful in reducing the symptoms of this disease.

REFERENCES

Adkisson, H. D., IV, Risener, F. S., Jr., Zarrinkar, P. P., Walla, M. D., Christie, W. W., and Wuthier, R. E. 1991. Unique fatty acid composition of normal cartilage: Discovery of high levels of n-9 eicosatrienoic acid and low levels of n-6 polyunsaturated fatty acids. *FASEB J.* 5: 344–353.

Alam, S. Q., Kokkinos, P. P., and Alam, B. S. 1993. Fatty acid composition and arachidonic acid concentrations in alveolar bone of rats fed diets with different lipids. *Calcif. Tissue Int.* 53: 330–332.

Ali, S. Y., Sajdera, S. W., and Anderson, H. C. 1970. Isolation and characterization of calcifying matrix vesicles from epiphyseal cartilage. *Proc. Natl. Acad. Sci. USA* 67: 1513–1520.

Ames, B. N., Shigenaga, M. K., and Hagen, T. M. 1993. Oxidants, antioxidants, and the degenerative diseases of aging. *Proc. Natl. Acad. Sci. USA* 90: 7915–7922.

Anderson, H. C. 1967. Electron microscopic studies of induced cartilage development and calcification. *J. Cell Biol.* 35: 81–101.

Anderson, H. C. 1989. Biology of disease: Mechanism of mineral formation in bone. *Lab. Invest.* 60: 320–330.

Andress, D. L. and Birnbaum, R. S. 1992. Human osteoblast-derived insulin-like growth factor (IGF) binding protein-5 stimulates osteoblast mitogenesis and potentiates IGF action. *J. Biol. Chem.* 267: 22467–22472.

Baron, R. 1993. Anatomy and ultrastructure of bone. In *Primer on the Metabolic Bone Diseases and Disorders of Mineral Metabolism,* M. J. Favus (Ed.), 2nd ed., pp. 3–9. Raven Press, New York.

Battmann, A., Mohan, S., Tuohimaa, P., Chevalley, T., Schulz, A., and Baylink, D. J. 1994. Evidence that insulin-like growth factors upregulate vitamin D receptor function in human bone cells in vitro. *J. Bone Miner. Res.* 9(Suppl. 1): S345.

Bautista, C. M., Baylink, D. J., and Mohan, S. 1991. Isolation of a novel insulin-like growth factor (IGF) binding protein from human bone: a potential candidate for fixing IGF-II in human bone. *Biochem. Biophys. Res. Commun.* 176: 756–763.

Bautista, C. M., Mohan, S., and Baylink, D. J. 1990. Insulin-like growth factors I and II are present in the skeletal tissues of ten vertebrates. *Metabolism* 39: 96–100.

Baylink, D. J., Finkelman, R. D., and Mohan, S. 1993. Growth factors to stimulate bone formation. *J. Bone Miner. Res.* 8 (Suppl. 2): S565–S572.

Belanger, L. F. 1969. Osteocytic osteolysis. *Calcif. Tissue Res.* 4: 1–12.

Bell, G. I., Stempien, M. M., Fong, N. M., and Rall, L. B. 1986. Sequences of liver cDNAs encoding two different mouse insulin-like growth factor I precursors. *Nucleic Acids Res.* 14: 7873–7882.

Bichell, D. P., Rotwein, P., and McCarthy, T. L. 1993. Prostaglandin E$_2$ rapidly stimulates insulin-like growth factor-I gene expression in primary rat osteoblast cultures: Evidence for transcriptional control. *Endocrinology* 133: 1020–1028.

Blair, H. C., Schlesinger, P. H., Ross, F. P., and Teitelbaum, S. L. 1993. Recent advances toward understanding osteoclast physiology. *Clin. Orthop.* 294: 7–22.

Bonucci, E. 1967. Fine structure of early calcification. *J. Ultrastruct. Res.* 20: 33–50.

Boskey, A. L., Posner, A. S., Lane, J. M., Goldberg, M. R., and Cordella, D. M. 1980. Distribution of lipids associated with mineralization in the bovine epiphyseal growth plate. *Arch. Biochem. Biophys.* 199: 305–311.

Bruneau, C., Staedel-Flaig, C., Cremel, G., Leray, C., Beck, J. P., and Hubert, P. 1987. Influence of lipid environment on insulin binding in cultured hepatoma cells. *Biochim. Biophys. Acta* 928: 287–296.

Buckwalter, J. A., Mower, D., Ungar, R., Schaeffer, J., and Ginsberg, B. 1986. Morphometric analysis of chondrocyte hypertrophy. *J. Bone Jt. Surg.* 68A: 243–255.

Buettner, G. R. 1993. The pecking order of free radicals and antioxidants: lipid peroxidation, α- tocopherol, and ascorbate. *Arch. Biochem. Biophys.* 300: 535–543.

Burton, G. W. and Traber, M. G. 1990. Vitamin E: Antioxidant activity, biokinetics, and bioavailability. *Annu. Rev. Nutr.* 10: 357–382.

Canalis, E. 1980. Effect of insulinlike growth factor I on DNA and protein synthesis in cultured rat calvaria. *J. Clin. Invest.* 66: 709–719.

Canalis, E. 1993. Regulation of bone remodeling. In *Primer on the Metabolic Bone Diseases and Disorders of Mineral Metabolism*, M. J. Favus (Ed.), 2nd ed., pp. 33–37. Raven Press, New York.

Canalis, E., Centrella, M., and McCarthy, T. L. 1991. Regulation of the insulin-like growth factor-II production in bone cultures. *Endocrinology* 129: 2457–2462.

Canalis, E., McCarthy, T. L., and Centrella, M. 1989. Effects of platelet-derived growth factor on bone formation in vitro. *J. Cell. Physiol.* 140: 530–537.

Canalis, E., Pash, J., Gabbitas, B., Rydziel, S., and Varghese, S. 1993. Growth factors regulate the synthesis of insulin-like growth factor-I in bone cell cultures. *Endocrinology* 133: 33–38.

Centrella, M., McCarthy, T. L., and Canalis, E. 1990. Receptors for insulin-like growth factor-I and -II in osteoblast-enriched cultures from fetal rat bone. *Endocrinology* 126: 39–44.

Centrella, M., McCarthy, T. L., and Canalis, E. 1987. Transforming growth factor beta is a bifunctional regulator of replication and collagen synthesis in osteoblast-enriched cell cultures from fetal rat bone. *J. Biol. Chem.* 262: 2869–2874.

Chen, T. L., Chang, L. Y., Bates, R. L., and Perlman, A. J. 1991. Dexamethasone and 1,25-dihydroxyvitamin D_3 modulation of insulin-like growth factor-binding proteins in rat osteoblast-like cell cultures. *Endocrinology* 128: 73–80.

Chow, J., Tobias, J. H., Colston, K. W., and Chambers, T. J. 1992. Estrogen maintains trabecular bone volume in rats not only by suppression of bone resorption but also by stimulation of bone formation. *J. Clin. Invest.* 89: 74–78.

Clemmons, D. R., Klibanski, A., Underwood, L. E., McArthur, J. W., Ridgway, E. C., Beitins, I. Z., and Van Wyk, J. J. 1981. Reduction of plasma immunoreactive somatomedin-C during fasting in humans. *J. Clin. Endocrinol. Metab.* 53: 1247–1250.

Clissold, S. P. 1986. Aspirin and related derivatives of salicylic acid. *Drugs* 32(Suppl. 4): 8–26.

Collins, D. A. and Chambers, T. J. 1992. Prostaglandin E_2 promotes osteoclast formation in murine hematopoietic cultures through an action on hematopoietic cells. *J. Bone Miner. Res.* 5: 555–561.

Connor, W. E., Neuringer, M., and Reisbick, S. 1992. Essential fatty acids: The importance of n-3 fatty acids in the retina and brain. *Nutr. Rev.* 50: 21–29.

Copeland, K. C., Colletti, R. B., Devlin, J. T., and McAuliffe, T. L. 1990. The relationship between insulin-like growth factor-I, adiposity, and aging. *Metabolism* 39: 584–587.

Cotmore, J. M., Nichols, G. Jr., and Wuthier, R. E. 1971. Phospholipid-calcium phosphate complex: Enhanced calcium migration in the presence of phosphate. *Science* 172: 1339–1341.

Cowin, S. C., Moss-Salentijn, L., and Moss, M. L. 1991. Candidates for the mechanosensory system in bone. *J. Biomech. Eng.* 113: 191–197.

Crist, D. M. and Hill, J. M. 1990. Diet and insulin-like growth factor I in relation to body composition in women with exercise-induced hypothalamic amenorrhea. *J. Am. Coll. Nutr.* 9: 200–204.

Ebina, Y., Okada, S., Hamazaki, S., Toda, Y., and Midorikawa, O. 1991. Impairment of bone formation with aluminum and ferric nitrilotriacetate complexes. *Calcif. Tissue Int.* 48: 28–36.

Emler, C. A. and Schalch, D. S. 1987. Nutritionally induced changes in hepatic insulin-like growth factor I (IGF-I) gene expression in rats. *Endocrinology* 120: 832–834.

Ernst, M. and Rodan, G. A. 1991. Estradiol regulation of insulin-like growth factor-I expression in osteoblastic cells: Evidence for transcriptional control. *Mol. Endocrinol.* 5: 1081–1089.

Ernst, M. and Rodan, G. A. 1990. Increased activity of insulin-like growth factor (IGF) in osteoblastic cells in the presence of growth hormone (GH): Positive correlation with the presence of the GH-induced IGF-binding protein BP-3. *Endocrinology* 127: 807–814.

Field, C. J., Ryan, E. A., Thomson, A. B., and Clandinin, M. T. 1990. Diet fat composition alters membrane phospholipid composition, insulin binding, and glucose metabolism in adipocytes from control and diabetic animals. *J. Biol. Chem.* 265: 11143–11150.

Field, C. J., Toyomizu, M., and Clandinin, M. T. 1989. Relationship between dietary fat, adipocyte membrane composition and insulin binding in the rat. *J. Nutr.* 119: 1483–1489.

Fiorelli, G., Orlando, C., Benvenuti, S., Fransceschelli, F., Bianchi, S., Pioli, P., Tanini, A., Serio, M., Bartucci, F., and Brandi, M. L. 1994. Characterization, regulation, and function of specific cell membrane receptors for insulin-like growth factor I on bone endothelial cells. *J. Bone Miner. Res.* 9: 329–337.

Forbes, G. B., Brown, M. R., Welle, S. L., and Underwood, L. E. 1989. Hormonal response to overfeeding. *Am. J. Clin. Nutr.* 49: 608–611.

Frost, H. M. 1973. *Bone Remodeling and Its Relationship to Metabolic Bone Disease*, pp. 28–53. Charles C. Thomas, Springfield, IL.

Frost, H. M. 1963. *Bone Remodeling Dynamics*. Charles C. Thomas, Springfield, IL.

Fujimori, A., Tsutsumi, M., Fukase, M., and Fujita, T. 1989. Cyclooxygenase inhibitors enhance cell growth in an osteoblastic cell line, MC3T3-E1. *J. Bone Miner. Res.* 4: 697–704.

Gabbitas, B., Dong, Y., and Canalis, E. 1994. Skeletal growth factors cause a coordinated inhibition of insulin-like growth factors (IGF) I and II and IGF binding protein (IGFBP) 5 in osteoblasts. *J. Bone Miner. Res.* 9(Suppl. 1): S298.

Gallwitz, W. E., Mundy, G. R., Lee, C. H., Qiao, M., Roodman, G. D., Raftery, M., Gaskell, S. J., and Bonewald, L. F. 1993. 5-Lipoxygenase metabolites of arachidonic acid stimulate isolated osteoclasts to resorb calcified matrices. *J. Biol. Chem.* 268: 10087–10094.

Garrett, I. R., Boyce, B. F., Oreffo, R. O., Bonewald, L., Poser, J., and Mundy, G. R. 1990. Oxygen-derived free radicals stimulate osteoclastic bone resorption in rodent bone in vitro and in vivo. *J. Clin. Invest.* 85: 632–639.

Genge, B. R., Cao, X., Wu, L. N., Buzzi, W. R., Showman, R. W., Arsenault, A. L., Ishikawa, Y., and Wuthier, R. E. 1992. Establishment of the primary structure of the major lipid-dependent Ca^{2+} binding proteins of chicken growth plate cartilage matrix vesicles: Identity with anchorin CII (annexin V) and annexin II. *J. Bone Miner. Res.* 7: 807–819.

Geusens, P., Wouters, C., Nijs, J., Jiang, Y., and Dequeker, J. 1994. Long-term effect of omega-3 fatty acid supplementation in active rheumatoid arthritis. *Arthritis Rheum.* 37: 824–829.

Goad, D. L. and Tashjian, A. H., Jr. 1994. Insulin-like growth factor-I (IGF-I) down-regulates mRNA for the parathyroid hormone/parathyroid hormone-related protein (PTH/PTHrP) receptor in human SAOS-2 osteoblastic cells. *J. Bone Miner. Res.* 9(Suppl. 1): S306.

Goldstein, S., Sertich, G. J., Levan, K. R., and Phillips, L. S. 1988. Nutrition and somatomedin. XIX. Molecular regulation of insulin-like growth factor-I in streptozotocin-diabetic rats. *Mol. Endocrinol.* 2: 1093–1100.

Golub, E. E., Harrison, G., Taylor, A. G., Camper, S., and Shapiro, I. M. 1992. The role of alkaline phosphatase in cartilage mineralization. *Bone Miner.* 17: 273–278.

Gunnes, M. and Lehmann, E. H. 1995. Dietary calcium, saturated fat, fiber and vitamin C as predictors of forearm cortical and trabecular bone mineral density in healthy children and adolescents. *Acta Paediatr.* 84: 388–392.

Gutteridge, J. M. C. 1993. Free radicals in disease processes: A compilation of cause and consequence. *Free Radic. Res. Commun.* 19: 141–158.

Hakeda, Y., Nakatani, Y., Kurihara, N., Ikeda, E., Maeda, N., and Kumegawa, M. 1985. Prostaglandin E_2 stimulates collagen and non-collagen protein synthesis and prolyl hydroxylase activity in osteoblastic clone MC3T3-E1 cells. *Biochem. Biophys. Res. Commun.* 126: 340–345.

Halliwell, B. 1994a. Free radicals and antioxidants: A personal view. *Nutr. Rev.* 52: 253–265.

Halliwell, B. 1994b. Free radicals, antioxidants, and human disease: curiosity, cause, or consequence? *Lancet* 344: 721–724.

Halliwell, B. and Chirico, S. 1993. Lipid peroxidation: Its mechanism, measurement, and significance. *Am. J. Clin. Nutr.* 57: 715S–725S.

Harris, E. D., Jr. 1990. Rheumatoid arthritis. Pathophysiology and implications for therapy. *N. Engl. J. Med.* 322: 1277–1289.

Heersche, J. N. M. 1993. Bone cells and bone turnover. In *Metabolic Bone Disease: Cellular and Tissue Mechanisms*, C. S. Tam, J. N. M. Heersche, and T. M. Murray (Ed.), pp. 1–18. CRC Press, Inc., Boca Raton, FL.

Hock, J. M., Centrella, M., and Canalis, E. 1988. Insulin-like growth factor I has independent effects on bone matrix formation and cell replication. *Endocrinology* 122: 254–260.

Hou, P., Schöller, J., Heegaard, A. M., and Foged, N. T. 1994. Insulin-like growth factor I and II stimulate osteoclastic bone resorption and release of collagen fragments in vitro. *J. Bone Miner. Res.* 9(Suppl. 1): S244.

Hunziker, E. B., Schenk, R. K., and Crus-Orive, L. M. 1987. Quantification of chondrocyte performance in growth-plate cartilage during longitudinal bone growth. *J. Bone Jt. Surg.* 69: 162–173.

Igarashi, K., Hirafuji, M., Adachi, H., Shinoda, H., and Mitani, H. 1994. Role of endogenous PGE_2 in osteoblastic functions of a clonal osteoblast-like cell, MC3T3-E1. *Prostaglandins Leukot. Essent. Fatty Acids* 50: 169–172.

Isgaard, J., Möller, C., Isaksson, O. G., Nilsson, A., Mathews, L. S., and Norstedt, G. 1988. Regulation of insulin-like growth factor messenger ribonucleic acid in rat growth plate by growth hormone. *Endocrinology* 122: 1515–1520.

Ishimi, Y., Miyaura, C., Jin, C. H., Akatsu, T., Abe, T., Nakamura, Y., Yamaguchi, A., Yoshiki, S., Matsuda, T., Hirano, T., Kishimoto, T., and Suda, T. 1990. IL-6 is produced by osteoblasts and induces bone resorption. *J. Immunol.* 145: 3297–3303.

Isley, W. L., Underwood, L. E., and Clemmons, D. R. 1984. Changes in plasma somatomedin-C in response to ingestion of diets with variable protein and energy content. *J. Parenter. Enteral. Nutr.* 8: 407–411.

Isley, W. L., Underwood, L. E., and Clemmons, D. R. 1983. Dietary components that regulate serum somatomedin-C concentrations in humans. *J. Clin. Invest.* 71: 175–182.

Jee, W. S., Mori, S., Li, X. J., and Chan, S. 1990. Prostaglandin E_2 enhances cortical bone mass and activates intracortical bone remodeling in intact and ovariectomized female rats. *Bone* 11: 253–266.

Jones, J. I. and Clemmons, D. R. 1995. Insulin-like growth factors and their binding proteins: Biological actions. *Endocrine Rev.* 16: 3–34.

Kajimoto, Y. and Rotwein, P. 1989. Structure and expression of a chicken insulin-like growth factor I precursor. *Mol. Endocrinol.* 3: 1907–1913.

Kalyanaraman, B., Morehouse, K. M., and Mason, R. P. 1991. An electron paramagnetic resonance study of the interactions between the adriamycin semiquinone, hydrogen peroxide, iron chelators, and radical scavengers. *Arch. Biochem. Biophys.* 286: 164–170.

Kappus, H. 1991. Lipid peroxidation: Mechanism and biological significance. In *Free Radicals and Food Additives*, O. I. Arouma and B. Halliwell (Ed.), pp. 59–75. Taylor and Francis, London, England.

Klaushofer, K., Hoffmann, O., Gleispach, H., Leis, H.-J., Czerwenka, E., Koller, K., and Peterlik, M. 1989. Bone-resorbing activity of thyroid hormones is related to prostaglandin production in cultured neonatal mouse calvaria. *J. Bone Miner. Res.* 4: 305–312.

Klein, D. C. and Raisz, L. G. 1970. Prostaglandins: Stimulation of bone resorption in tissue culture. *Endocrinology* 86: 1436–1440.

Komm, B. S. 1992. Retinoic acid and IGF-I regulate the steady state expression of estrogen receptor mRNA in osteoblast-like cells. *J. Bone Miner. Res.* 7(Suppl. 1): S97.

Kream, B. E., Petersen, D. N., and Raisz, L. G. 1990. Parathyroid hormone blocks the stimulatory effect of insulin-like growth factor-I on collagen synthesis in cultured 21-day fetal rat calvariae. *Bone* 11: 411–415.

Kurihara, N., Gluck, S., and Roodman, G. D. 1990. Sequential expression of phenotype markers for osteoclasts during differentiation of precursors for multinucleated cells formed in long term human marrow cultures. *Endocrinology* 127: 3215–3221.

Kurose, S., Seino, Y., Yamaoka, K., Tanaka, H., Shima, M., and Yabuuchi, H. 1989. Cooperation of synthetic insulin-like growth factor I/somatomedin C and 1,25-dihydroxyvitamin D_3 on regulation of function in clonal osteoblastic cells. *Bone Miner.* 5: 335–345.

Kurose, S., Yamaoka, K., Okada, S., Nakajima, S., and Seino, Y. 1990. 1,25-Dihydroxyvitamin D_3 ($1,25(OH)_2D_3$) increases insulin-like growth factor-I (IGF-I) receptors in clonal osteoblastic cells. Study on interaction of IGF-I and $1,25(OH)_2D_3$. *Endocrinology* 126: 2088–2094.

Lands, W. E. M. 1991. Biosynthesis of prostaglandins. *Annu. Rev. Nutr.* 11: 41–60.

Lin, H. Y., Harris, T. L., Flannery, M. S., Aruffo, A., Kaji, E. H., Gorn, A., Kolakowski, L. F., Jr., Lodish, H. F., and Goldring, S. R. 1991. Expression cloning of an adenylate cyclase-coupled calcitonin receptor. *Science* 254: 1022–1024.

Linkhart, T. A. and Keffer, M. J. 1991. Differential regulation of insulin-like growth factor-I (IGF-I) and IGF-II release from cultured neonatal mouse calvaria by parathyroid hormone, transforming growth factor-β, and 1,25-dihydroxyvitamin D_3. *Endocrinology* 128: 1511–1518.

Linkhart, T. A. and MacCharles, D. C. 1992. Interleukin-1 stimulates release of insulin-like growth factor-I in neonatal mouse calvaria by a prostaglandin synthesis-dependent mechanism. *Endocrinology* 131: 2297–2305.

Lippiello, L., Fienhold, M., and Grandjean, C. 1990. Metabolic and ultrastructural changes in articular cartilage of rats fed dietary supplements of omega-3 fatty acids. *Arthritis Rheum.* 33: 1029–1036.

Liu, C. C. and Richardson, G. D. 1991. Estrogen increases skeletal and hepatic IGF-I gene expression in mice. *J. Bone Miner. Res.* 6(Suppl. 1): S210.

Lorenzo, J. A., Quinton, J., Sousa, S., and Raisz, L. G. 1986. Effects of DNA and prostaglandin synthesis inhibitors on the stimulation of bone resorption by epidermal growth factor in fetal rat long-bone cultures. *J. Clin. Invest.* 77: 1897–1902.

Lukert, B. P. and Raisz, L. G. 1990. Glucocorticoid-induced osteoporosis: Pathogenesis and management. *Ann. Intern. Med.* 112: 352–364.

Maes, M., Underwood, L. E., and Ketelslegers, J. M. 1984. Low serum somatomedin-C in protein deficiency: Relationship with changes in liver somatogenic and lactogenic binding sites. *Mol. Cell. Endocrinol.* 37: 301–309.

Maiter, D., Maes, M., Underwood, L. E., Fliesen, T., Gerard, G., and Ketelslegers, J. M. 1988. Early changes in serum concentrations of somatomedin-C induced by dietary protein deprivation: Contributions of growth hormone receptor and post-receptor defects. *J. Endocrinol.* 118: 113–120.

Malluche, H. H. and Faugere, M.-C. 1986a. Functional and structural organization of bone. In *Atlas of Mineralized Bone Histology*, H. H. Malluche and M.-C. Faugere (Ed.), pp. 1–10. Karger, New York.

Malluche, H. H. and Faugere, M.-C. 1986b. Evaluation of mineralized bone histology. In *Atlas of Mineralized Bone Histology*, H. H. Malluche and M.-C. Faugere (Ed.), pp. 37–48. Karger, New York.

Marks, S. C. Jr. and Miller, S. C. 1993. Prostaglandins and the skeleton: The legacy and challenges of two decades of research. *Endocrine J.* 1: 337–344.

Marusic, Z. and Raisz, L. G. 1991. Cortisol modulates the actions of interleukin-1α on bone formation, resorption, and prostaglandin production in cultured mouse parietal bones. *Endocrinology* 129: 2699–2706.

Matsumoto, H., Silverton, S. F., Debolt, K., and Shapiro, I. M. 1991. Superoxide dismutase and catalase activities in growth cartilage: Relationship between oxidoreductase activity and chondrocyte maturation. *J. Bone Miner. Res.* 6: 569–574.

Matsuzawa, T. and Anderson, H. C. 1971. Phosphatases of epiphyseal cartilage studied by electron microscopic cytochemical methods. *J. Histochem. Cytochem.* 19: 801–808.

McCarthy, T. L., Casinghino, S., Centrella, M., and Canalis, E. 1994. Complex pattern of insulin-like growth factor binding protein expression in primary rat osteoblast enriched cultures: Regulation by prostaglandin E_2, growth hormone, and the insulin-like growth factors. *J. Cell. Physiol.* 160: 163–175.

McCarthy, T. L., Centrella, M., and Canalis, E. 1989. Regulatory effects of insulin-like growth factors I and II on bone collagen synthesis in rat calvarial cultures. *Endocrinology* 124: 301–309.

McCarthy, T. L., Centrella, M., Raisz, L. G., and Canalis, E. 1991. Prostaglandin E_2 stimulates insulin-like growth factor I synthesis in osteoblast-enriched cultures from fetal rat bone. *Endocrinology* 128: 2895–2900.

McLean, F. M., Keller, P. J., Genge, B. R., Walters, S. A., and Wuthier, R. E. 1987. Disposition of preformed mineral in matrix vesicles. Internal localization and association with alkaline phosphatase. *J. Biol. Chem.* 262: 10481–10488.

Meghji, S., Sandy, J. R., Scutt, A. M., Harvey, W., and Harris, M. 1988. Stimulation of bone resorption by lipoxygenase metabolites of arachidonic acid. *Prostaglandins* 36: 139–149.

Meydani, M. 1995. Vitamin E. *Lancet* 345: 170–175.

Mochizuki, H., Hakeda, Y., Wakatsuki, N., Usui, N., Akashi, S., Sato, T., Tanaka, K., and Kumegawa, M. 1992. Insulin-like growth factor-I supports formation and activation of osteoclasts. *Endocrinology* 131: 1075–1080.

Mohan, S. and Baylink, D. J. 1991. Bone growth factors. *Clin. Orthop.* 263: 30–48.

Mori, S., Jee, W. S., Li, X. J., Chan, S., and Kimmel, D. B. 1990. Effects of prostaglandin E_2 on production of new cancellous bone in the axial skeleton of ovariectomized rats. *Bone* 11: 103–113.

Moriwake, T., Tanaka, H., Kanzaki, S., Higuchi, J., and Seino, Y. 1992. 1,25-Dihydroxyvitamin D_3 stimulates the secretion of insulin-like growth factor binding protein 3(IGFBP-3) by cultured osteosarcoma cells. *Endocrinology* 130: 1071–1073.

Mueller, K., Cortesi, R., Modrowski, D., and Marie, P. J. 1994. Stimulation of trabecular bone formation by insulin-like growth factor I in adult ovariectomized rats. *Am. J. Physiol.* 267: E1–E6.

Mundy, G. R. 1993. Cytokines and growth factors in the regulation of bone remodeling. *J. Bone Miner. Res.* 8(Suppl. 2): S505–S510.

Muriana, F. J. G. and Ruiz-Gutierrez, V. 1992. Effect of n-6 and n-3 polyunsaturated fatty acids ingestion on rat liver membrane-associated enzymes and fluidity. *J. Nutr. Biochem.* 3: 659–663.

Nilsson, A., Ohlsson, C., Isaksson, O. G., Lindahl, A., and Isgaard, J. 1994. Hormonal regulation of longitudinal bone growth. *Eur. J. Clin. Nutr.* 48(Suppl. 1): S150–S160.

Norrdin, R. W., Jee, W. S., and High, W. B. 1990. The role of prostaglandins in bone in vivo. *Prostaglandins Leukot. Essent. Fatty Acids* 41: 139–149.

Oarada, M. and Terao, K. 1992. Injury of mouse lymphocytes caused by exogenous methyl linoleate hydroperoxides in vitro. *Biochim. Biophys. Acta* 1165: 135–140.

Parfitt, A. M. 1990. In *Progress in Basic and Clinical Pharmacology*, J. A. Kanis (Ed.), pp. 1–27. S. Karger AG, Basel.

Parfitt, A. M. 1977. The cellular basis of bone turnover and bone loss: A rebuttal of the osteocytic resorption—bone flow theory. *Clin. Orthop.* 127: 236–247.

Pash, J. M., Delany, A. M., and Canalis, E. 1994. Transcriptional regulation of insulin-like growth factor-I (IGF-I) by prostaglandin E_2 (PGE_2) in osteoblasts. *J. Bone Miner. Res.* 9(Suppl. 1): S124.

Peretz, A. M., Neve, J. D., and Famaey, J. P. 1991. Selenium in rheumatic disease. *Semin. Arthritis Rheum.* 20: 305–316.

Pfeilschifter, J., Laukhuf, F., Müller-Beckmann, B., Blum, W., Pfister, T., and Ziegler, R. 1994. Parathyroid hormone selectively increases the concentration of insulin-like growth factor-I in bone. *J. Bone Miner. Res.* 9(Suppl. 1): S415.

Puzas, J. E. 1993. The osteoblasts. In *Primer on the Metabolic Bone Diseases and Disorders of Mineral Metabolism*, M. J. Favus (Ed.), 2nd ed., pp. 15–21. Raven Press, New York.

Raisz, L. G. 1993. Bone cell biology: New approaches and unanswered questions. *J. Bone Miner. Res.* 8(Suppl. 2): S457–S465.

Raisz, L. G. 1990. Recent advances in bone cell biology: Interactions of vitamin D with other local and systemic factors. *Bone Miner.* 9: 191–197.

Raisz, L. G., Alander, C. B., and Simmons, H. A. 1989a. Effects of prostaglandin E_3 and eicosapentaenoic acid on rat bone in organ culture. *Prostaglandins* 37: 615–625.

Raisz, L. G. and Fall, P. M. 1990. Biphasic effects of prostaglandin E_2 on bone formation in cultured fetal rat calvariae: Interaction with cortisol. *Endocrinology* 126: 1654–1659.

Raisz, L. G., Fall, P. M., Gabbitas, B. Y., McCarthy, T. L., Kream, B. E., and Canalis, E. 1993. Effects of prostaglandin E_2 on bone formation in cultured fetal rat calvariae: Role of insulin-like growth factor-I. *Endocrinology* 133: 1504–1510.

Raisz, L. G., Simmons, H. A., and Fall, P. M. 1989b. Biphasic effects of nonsteroidal anti-inflammatory drugs on prostaglandin production by cultured rat calvariae. *Prostaglandins* 37: 559–565.

Rathakrishnan, C., Tiku, K., Raghavan, A., and Tiku, M. L. 1992. Release of oxygen radicals by articular chondrocytes: A study of luminol-dependent chemiluminescence and hydrogen peroxide secretion. *J. Bone Miner. Res.* 7: 1139–1148.

Ren, W. and Dziak, R. 1991. Effects of leukotrienes on osteoblastic cell proliferation. *Calcif. Tissue Int.* 49: 197–201.

Rezanka, T. 1989. Very-long chain fatty acids from the animal and plant kingdoms. *Prog. Lipid Res.* 28: 147–187.

Robison, R. 1923. The possible significance of hexose phosphoric esters in ossification. *Biochem. J.* 17: 286–293.

Romagnoli, E., Minisola, S., Carnevale, V., Rosso, R., Pacitti, M. T., Sarda, A., Scarnecchia, L., and Mazzuoli, G. 1994. Circulating levels of insulin-like growth factor binding protein 3 (IGFBP-3) and insulin-like growth factor I (IGF-I) in perimenopausal women. *Osteoporosis Int.* 4: 305–308.

Romagnoli, E., Minisola, S., Carnevale, V., Sarda, A., Rosso, R., Scarnecchia, L., Pacitti, M. T., and Mazzuoli, G. 1993. Effect of estrogen deficiency on IGF-I plasma levels: Relationship with bone mineral density in perimenopausal women. *Calcif. Tissue Int.* 53: 1–6.

Rotwein, P., Pollock, K. M., Didier, D. K., and Krivi, G. G. 1986. Organization and sequence of the human insulin-like growth factor I gene. Alternative RNA processing produces two insulin-like growth factor I precursor peptides. *J. Biol. Chem.* 261: 4828–4832.

Sandy, J. R., Meikle, M. C., Martin, B. R., and Farndale, R. W. 1991. Leukotriene B_4 increases intracellular calcium concentration and phosphoinositide metabolism in mouse osteoblasts via cyclic adenosine 3',5'-monophosphate-independent pathways. *Endocrinology* 129: 582–590.

Sardesai, V. M. 1992. Biochemical and nutritional aspects of eicosanoids. *J. Nutr. Biochem.* 3: 562–579.

Sauer, G. R. and Wuthier, R. E. 1988. Fourier-transform infrared characterization of mineral phases formed during induction of mineralization by collagenase-released matrix vesicles in vitro. *J. Biol. Chem.* 263: 13718–13724.

Scharla, S. H., Strong, D. D., Mohan, S., Baylink, D. J., and Linkhart, T. A. 1991. 1,25-Dihydroxyvitamin D_3 differentially regulates the production of insulin-like growth factor-I (IGF-1) and IGF-binding protein-4 in mouse osteoblasts. *Endocrinology* 129: 3139–3146.

Schmid, C., Schläpfer, I., Waldvogel, M., Zapf, J., and Froesch, E. R. 1992.

Prostaglandin E_3 stimulates synthesis of insulin-like growth factor binding protein-3 in rat bone cells in vitro. *J. Bone Miner. Res.* 7: 1157–1163.

Schmid, C., Zapf, J., and Froesch, E. R. 1989. Production of carrier proteins for insulin-like growth factors (IGFs) by rat osteoblastic cells. Regulation by IGF I and cortisol. *FEBS Lett.* 244: 328–332.

Schneider, G. B. and Relfson, M. 1988. The effects of transplantation of granulocyte-macrophage progenitors on bone resorption in osteopetrotic rats. *J. Bone Miner. Res.* 3: 225–232.

Schulz, H. 1991. Beta oxidation of fatty acids. *Biochim. Biophys. Acta* 1081: 109–120.

Shen, C-L., Watkins, B. A., Lim, S. S., and McFarland, D. C. 1994. Dietary lipid modulation of fatty acid composition of tibiotarsal bone and IGF-I responses in chicks. *FASEB J.* 8(5): A929.

Shimasaki, S. and Ling, N. 1991. Identification and molecular characterization of insulin-like growth factor binding proteins (IGFBP-1, -2, -3, -4, -5, and -6). *Prog. Growth Factor Res.* 3: 243–266.

Shimatsu, A. and Rotwein, P. 1987. Sequence of two rat insulin-like growth factor I mRNAs differing within the 5′ untranslated region. *Nucleic Acids Res.* 15: 7196.

Sies, H. 1991. Oxidative stress: From basic research to clinical application. *Am. J. Med.* 91(3C): 31S–37S.

Simmons, H. A. and Raisz, L. G. 1991. Effects of acid and basic fibroblast growth factor and heparin on resorption of cultured fetal rat long bones. *J. Bone Miner. Res.* 6: 1301–1305.

Simopoulos, A. P. 1991. Omega-3 fatty acids in health and disease and in growth and development. *Am. J. Clin. Nutr.* 54: 438–463.

Smith, A. T., Clemmons, D. R., Underwood, L. E., Ben-Ezra, V., and McMurray, R. 1987. The effect of exercise on plasma somatomedin-C/insulin-like growth factor I concentrations. *Metabolism* 36: 533–537.

Snyder, D. K., Clemmons, D. R., and Underwood, L. E. 1989. Dietary carbohydrate content determines responsiveness to growth hormone in energy-restricted humans. *J. Clin. Endocrinol. Metab.* 69: 745–752.

Snyder, D. K., Clemmons, D. R., and Underwood, L. E. 1988. Treatment of obese, diet-restricted subjects with growth hormone for 11 weeks: effects of anabolism, lipolysis, and body composition. *J. Clin. Endocrinol. Metab.* 67: 54–61.

Solheim, L. F., Ronningen, H., and Langeland, N. 1986a. Effects of acetylsalicylic acid on heterotopic bone resorption and formation in rats. *Arch. Orthop. Trauma Surg.* 105: 142–145.

Solheim, L. F., Ronningen, H., and Langeland, N. 1986b. Effects of acetyl-salicylic acid and naproxen on bone resorption and formation in rats. *Arch. Orthop. Trauma Surg.* 105: 137–141.

Solheim, L. F., Ronningen, H., and Langeland, N. 1986c. Effects of acetyl-salicylic acid and naproxen on the mechanical properties of intact femora in rats. *Arch. Orthop. Trauma Surg.* 105: 5–10.

Solheim, L. F., Ronningen, H., and Langeland, N. 1986d. Effects of acetyl-salicylic acid and naproxen on the synthesis and mineralization of collagen in the rat femur. *Arch. Orthop. Trauma Surg.* 105: 1–4.

Somjen, D., Binderman, I., Berger, E., and Harell, A. 1980. Bone remodelling induced by physical stress is prostaglandin E_2 mediated. *Biochim. Biophys. Acta* 627: 91–100.

Spencer, E. M., Liu, C. C., Si, E. C., and Howard, G. A. 1991. In vivo actions of insulin-like growth factor-I (IGF-I) on bone formation and resorption in rats. *Bone* 12: 21–26.

Straus, D. S. and Takemoto, C. D. 1990. Effect of fasting on insulin-like growth factor-I (IGF-I) and growth hormone receptor mRNA levels and IGF-I gene transcription in rat liver. *Mol. Endocrinol.* 4: 91–100.

Tashjian, A. H., Jr., Hohmann, E. L., Antoniades, H. N., and Levine, L. 1982. Platelet-derived growth factor stimulates bone resorption via a prostaglandin-mediated mechanism. *Endocrinology* 111: 118–124.

Tashjian, A. H., Jr., Voelkel, E. F., Lazzaro, M., Goad, D., Bosma, T., and Levine, L. 1987. Tumor necrosis factor-α (cachectin) stimulates bone resorption in mouse calvaria via a prostaglandin-mediated mechanism. *Endocrinology* 120: 2029–2036.

Tashjian, A. H., Jr., Voelkel, E. F., Lazzaro, M., Singer, F. R., Roberts, A. B., Derynck, R., Winkler, M. E., and Levine, L. 1985. Alpha and beta human transforming growth factors stimulate prostaglandin production and bone resorption in cultured mouse calvaria. *Proc. Natl. Acad. Sci. USA* 82: 4535–4538.

Thissen, J. P., Ketelslegers, J. M., and Underwood, L. E. 1994. Nutritional regulation of the insulin-like growth factors. *Endocr. Rev.* 15: 80–101.

Tijburg, L. B. M., Geelen, M. J. H., and van Golde, L. M. G. 1989. Regulation of the biosynthesis of triacylglycerol, phosphatidylcholine and phosphatidylethanolamine in the liver. *Biochim. Biophys. Acta* 1004: 1–19.

Torrielli, M. V. and Dianzani, M. V. 1984. Free radicals in inflammatory disease. In *Free Radicals in Molecular Biology, Aging and Disease*, D. Armstrong, R. S. Sohal, and R. E. Culter (Ed.), pp. 355–379. Raven Press, New York.

Vazquez, J. A. and Adibi, S. A. 1992. Protein sparing during treatment of obesity: Ketogenic versus nonketogenic very low calorie diet. *Metabolism* 41: 406–414.

Vergroesen, A. J. and Crawford, M. 1989. In *The Role of Fats in Human Nutrition*. Academic Press, New York.

Voss, A., Reinhart, M., Sankarappa, S., and Sprecher, H. 1991. The metabolism of 7,10,13,16,19-docosapentaenoic acid to 4,7,10,13,16,19-docosahexaenoic acid in rat liver is independent of a 4-desaturase. *J. Biol. Chem.* 266: 19995–20000.

Waters, D. J., Caywood, D. D., Trachte, G. J., Turner, R. T., and Hodgson, S. F. 1991. Immobilization increases bone prostaglandin E. Effect of acetylsalicylic acid on disuse osteoporosis studied in dogs. *Acta Orthop. Scand.* 62: 238–243.

Watkins, B. A. 1992. Factors involved in the local regulation of bone growth. In *Bone Biology and Skeletal Disorders in Poultry*, C. C. Whitehead (Ed.), pp. 67–86. Carfax Publishing Company, Abingdon, England.

Watkins, B. A., Hennig, H., and Toborek, M. 1996. Dietary fat and health. In *Bailey's Industrial Oil and Fat Products*, Vol. I, 5th ed., pp. 159–214. John Wiley & Sons, Inc., New York.

Watkins, B. A., Shen, C.-L., Seifert, M. F., McFarland, D. C., and Allen, K. G. D. 1994. Dietary lipid modulates fatty acid composition, PGE_2 biosynthesis and IGF-I in chick tibia. *J. Bone Miner. Res.* 9(Suppl. 1): A256.

Watkins, B. A., Shen, C.-L., McMurtry, J. P., Xu, H., and Bain, S. D. 1995a. Dietary lipids alter histomorphometry and concentrations of fatty acids and insulin-like growth factor-I in tibiotarsal bone. *J. Nutr.* (submitted).

Watkins, B. A., Xu, H. and Turek, J. J., 1995b. Linoleate impairs collagen synthesis in primary cultures of avian chondrocytes. *P.S.E.B.M.* (accepted.)

Watrous, D. A. and Andrews, B. S. 1989. The metabolism and immunology of bone. *Semin. Arthritis Rheum.* 19: 45–65.

Wuthier, R. E. 1993. Involvement of cellular metabolism of calcium and phosphate in calcification of avian growth plate cartilage. *J. Nutr.* 123: 301–309.

Wuthier, R. E. 1988. Mechanism of matrix vesicle-mediated mineralization of cartilage. *ISI Atlas Sci. Biochem.* 1: 231–241.

Wuthier, R. E. and Gore, S. T. 1977. Partition of inorganic ions and phospholipids in isolated cell, membrane and matrix vesicle fractions: Evidence for Ca-Pi-acidic phospholipid complexes. *Calcif. Tissue Res.* 24: 163–171.

Xu, H., Watkins, B. A., and Adkisson, H. D. 1994. Dietary lipids modify the fatty acid composition of cartilage, isolated chondrocytes and matrix vesicles. *Lipids* 29: 619–625.

Xu, H., Watkins, B. A., and Seifert, M. F. 1995. Vitamin E stimulates trabecular bone formation and alters epiphyseal cartilage morphometry. *Calcif. Tissue Int.* 57: 293–300.

Yazdi, M., Cheung, D. T., Cobble, S., Nimni, M. E., and Schonfeld, S. E. 1992. Effects of non-steroidal anti-inflammatory drugs on demineralized bone-induced bone formation. *J. Periodontal Res.* 27: 28–33.

Zangger, I., Zapf, J., and Froesch, E. R. 1987. Insulin-like growth factor I and II in 14 animal species and man as determined by three radioligand assays and two bioassays. *Acta Endocrinol.* 114: 107–112.

6
Enzymatic Modification of Lipids

Casimir C. Akoh

The University of Georgia
Athens, Georgia

INTRODUCTION

Lipases are currently used as biocatalysts for the modification of existing lipids, to synthesize new lipids, to add value or improve the functionality of lipids in foods, or to improve their use in nutrition and therapeutics as "medical lipids, pharmafoods or nutraceuticals." Enzymes can be used to produce lipids that may benefit persons with coronary heart disease, obesity, cancer, lipid malabsorption disorders, and for the improvement of general health. Because enzymes are specific as to the nature of their substrates and operate at mild reaction conditions, they are preferred over chemical catalysts for the modification of lipids intended for modern consumers who demand more natural and less synthetic food products and additives.

Lipases (triacylglycerol acylhydrolase, EC 3.1.1.3) previously known to catalyze essentially hydrolytic reactions are now known to also catalyze reverse reactions of hydrolysis in organic solvents and near anhydrous conditions. This unique phenomenon is being exploited by lipid biotechnologists to modify existing fats and oils or to synthesize novel ester products with potential applications in the food, cosmetics, nutritional, and pharmaceutical industries. Enzymes are of particular interest in lipid modifications because of their ability to select the type of reactions catalyzed. For example, enzymes can discriminate based on the position of the bond to be cleaved (regioselectivity), optical activity (enantioselectivity), and functional group (chemoselectivity) in the substrate molecule. Phospholipases primarily catalyze the hydrolysis of glycerophospholipids with strict position or regiospecificity. For example, phospholipase A_1 and A_2 will catalyze reactions at the sn-1 and sn-2 positions of the glycerophospholipids. Phospholipase C will cleave the phosphoryl bond next to the phosphate group. These phospholipases can be used to hydrolyze or modify glycerophospholipids to introduce unique fatty acids with unique functions. Lysolecithin, which is an excellent emulsifier, can be produced by phospholipase A_2–catalyzed hydrolysis of glycerophosphocholine. Lipases catalyze exchange of acyl radicals between a triacylglycerol and a fatty acid (acidolysis), an alcohol (alcoholysis), or an ester (transesterification) to produce a new triacylglycerol.

ADVANTAGES OF ENZYMES OVER CHEMICAL CATALYSTS

Advantages of enzymes over chemical catalysts include ease of product recovery from low-boiling organic solvents, formation of very few side products favoring of synthesis over hydrolysis, ability to recover enzymes by simple filtration since they are not soluble in organic solvents, and increased solubility of the nonpolar lipid substrates. In order to drive the reaction towards synthesis, the enzymatic reaction must be conducted in a low water environment. Compared to chemical catalysts, enzymes are specific, selective, have high turnover numbers, and function under mild conditions of temperature, pH, and pressure, making them energy efficient. Enzymes are well-suited catalysts for the production of chiral compounds important to the pharmaceutical industry. They can be economically produced in large quantities through recombinant DNA technology and fermentation techniques.

IMMOBILIZATION TECHNIQUES

Most synthetic and hydrolysis reactions can be carried out with powdered nonimmobilized enzymes. However, if costs are to be considered, it may be advantageous to immobilize the enzyme in some form of support to confer rigidity to the enzyme. It has been shown that immobilized enzymes are cost-effective because they can be recovered and reused several times. Immobilized enzymes are more thermostable and can be stored over a longer period of time than nonimmobilized enzymes. Immobilization support should have the following properties: (1) high porosity to allow good flow while retaining the enzyme, (2) high surface area to allow maximum contact, (3) high physical strength, (4) solvent resistant, (5) high flow properties, and (6) chemically and microbiologically inert (West, 1988a, b). Enzymes can be immobilized in various ways.

Immobilization by Adsorption

Lipases can be physically adsorbed onto solid matrices such as glass beads, alumina, silica gel, and duolite. The lipase is dissolved in a proper buffer of known pH and ionic strength or deionized water and added to a prewashed support material with agitation. The enzyme is dried to a known water activity or moisture content and is ready for use. Alternatively, the enzyme can be packed in a column, bed, or membrane. Problems such as weak adsorption can lead to low recovery of the enzyme and low activity. It is important to take into consideration the particle size and surface-to-volume ratio of the matrix.

Immobilization Through Covalent Bonding

The enzyme is covalently attached to a water-insoluble matrix via a functional group in the enzyme, which is not responsible for catalysis. A typical example is nylon, and typical functional groups include NH_2, OH, and COOH. The only requirement is that the support material must be activated. A classical example is the cyanogen bromide (CNBr) activation of sephadex or sepharose.

Immobilization Through Cross-Linking

This technique involves the formation of a covalent bond between two or more enzyme molecules with the aid of a bi- or multifunctional reagent such as aliphatic diamines, carbodiimide, or glutaraldehyde.

TYPICAL EXAMPLES AND APPLICATIONS OF LIPASE-CATALYZED MODIFICATION REACTIONS

Hydrolysis (Fat Splitting)

Hydrolysis is currently used for the industrial production of fatty acids and glycerols ("fat splitting"). Lipases catalyze the hydrolysis of fats and oils to give free fatty acids, partial acylglycerols, and glycerol depending on the position specificity of the lipase. They also catalyze the hydrolysis of a wide range of fatty acid esters, although triacylglycerols are their preferred sub-strates. Generally, the hydrolysis of water-soluble carboxylic acid esters by lipases is very slow (Macrae, 1983). Equation (1) in Figure 6.1 illustrates a typical hydrolysis reaction catalyzed by lipases.

Various techniques have been used to increase the rate of lipase-catalyzed hydrolysis. One method involves the use of two lipases (Park et al., 1988) to affect complete hydrolysis. The use of organic solvents sometimes increases the rate of hydrolysis. Lipase-catalyzed hydrolysis is carried out in biphasic medium, and various types of membrane reactors have been used in this process (Mukherjee, 1990). Food flavors have been enhanced by partial hydrolysis of triacylglycerols. Well-known examples include the manufac-ture of various cheeses (Italian, American, cheddar) and lipolyzed milk fat products such as butter flavors and cultured cream flavors (Malcata et al., 1990).

Direct Esterification

Direct esterification reaction is the exact reverse of hydrolysis. The equilib-rium between the forward reaction (hydrolysis) and the reverse reaction (direct esterification) is controlled by the water content of the reaction mixture. Iwai et al. (1964) demonstrated that water activity plays a crucial role in the synthetic capability of lipases. Since then, lipase-catalyzed direct esterification reactions have been performed in biphasic aqueous systems (Okumura et al., 1979; Iwai et al., 1980; Lazar et al., 1986) and especially in organic media (Marlot et al., 1985; Gillies et al., 1987; Akoh et al., 1992; de Castro, 1992; Claon and Akoh, 1993; Janssen et al., 1993). Equation (2) in Figure 6.1 illustrates a typical direct esterification reaction.

Solvent-free lipase-catalyzed esterification (Ergan et al., 1988; Akoh, 1993) as well as the use of supercritical fluid as a reaction medium (Ham-mond et al., 1985; Marty et al., 1992) have been successfully conducted. The major advantage of supercritical fluid is that they can be vented to the atmosphere, allowing products to be recovered without a trace of solvent. This aspect is very important in the food industry (Dordick, 1989). Exam-ples of high-value chemicals obtained via the use of lipases as biocatalysts for esterification reactions include partial acylglycerols and triacylglycerols (Iwai et al., 1964; Akoh et al., 1992; Akoh, 1993), short chain esters (Gillies et al., 1987; Langrand et al., 1990; de Castro et al., 1992), and terpene esters (Okumura et al., 1979; Iwai et al., 1980; Marlot et al., 1987; Langrand et al., 1990; Claon and Akoh, 1993, 1994a, b, c, d; Yee et al., 1995). Another possible application of lipase-catalyzed esterification reactions is the syn-thesis of sugar esters, which can be used as emulsifiers or fat substitutes depending on the degree of acyl group incorporation into the sugar mole-

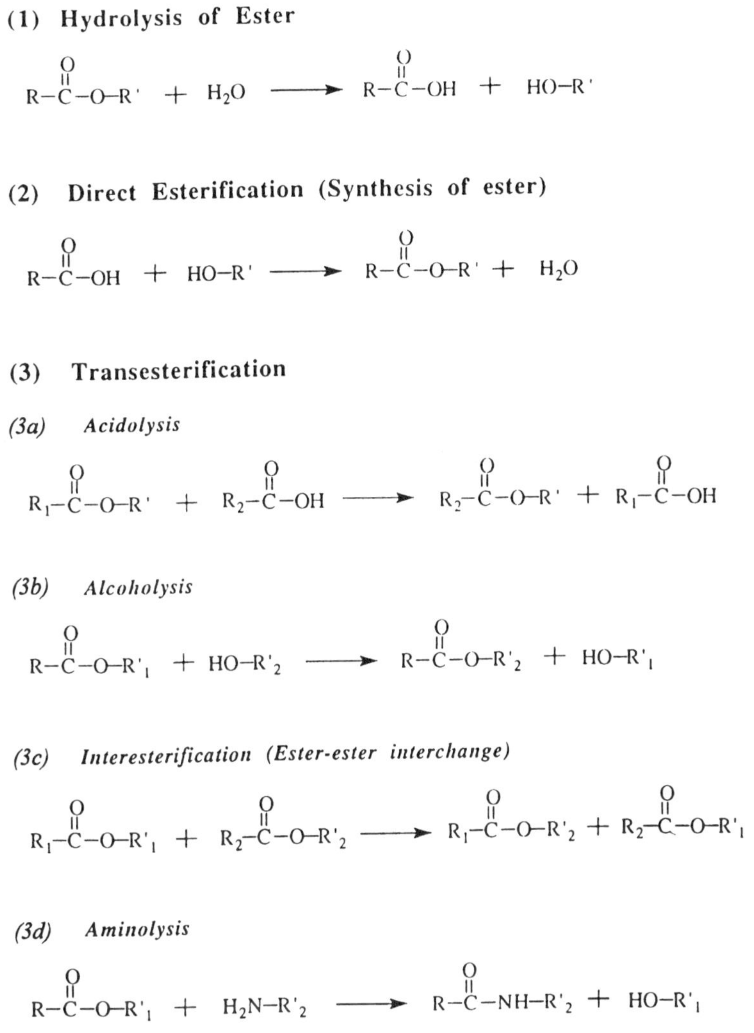

(1) Hydrolysis of Ester

$$R-\overset{O}{\overset{\|}{C}}-O-R' \ + \ H_2O \ \longrightarrow \ R-\overset{O}{\overset{\|}{C}}-OH \ + \ HO-R'$$

(2) Direct Esterification (Synthesis of ester)

$$R-\overset{O}{\overset{\|}{C}}-OH \ + \ HO-R' \ \longrightarrow \ R-\overset{O}{\overset{\|}{C}}-O-R' \ + \ H_2O$$

(3) Transesterification

(3a) Acidolysis

$$R_1-\overset{O}{\overset{\|}{C}}-O-R' \ + \ R_2-\overset{O}{\overset{\|}{C}}-OH \ \longrightarrow \ R_2-\overset{O}{\overset{\|}{C}}-O-R' \ + \ R_1-\overset{O}{\overset{\|}{C}}-OH$$

(3b) Alcoholysis

$$R-\overset{O}{\overset{\|}{C}}-O-R'_1 \ + \ HO-R'_2 \ \longrightarrow \ R-\overset{O}{\overset{\|}{C}}-O-R'_2 \ + \ HO-R'_1$$

(3c) Interesterification (Ester-ester interchange)

$$R_1-\overset{O}{\overset{\|}{C}}-O-R'_1 \ + \ R_2-\overset{O}{\overset{\|}{C}}-O-R'_2 \ \longrightarrow \ R_1-\overset{O}{\overset{\|}{C}}-O-R'_2 \ + \ R_2-\overset{O}{\overset{\|}{C}}-O-R'_1$$

(3d) Aminolysis

$$R-\overset{O}{\overset{\|}{C}}-O-R'_1 \ + \ H_2N-R'_2 \ \longrightarrow \ R-\overset{O}{\overset{\|}{C}}-NH-R'_2 \ + \ HO-R'_1$$

FIG. 6.1 Types of reactions catalyzed by lipases. (Adapted from Yamane, 1987.)

cule. Esters of glucose, fructose, sorbitol, sucrose, alkyl glycosides, etc. were synthesized with lipases (Seino et al., 1984; Lazar et al., 1986; Mutua and Akoh, 1993a; Akoh and Mutua, 1994; Akoh, 1994).

The accumulation of water during direct esterification is a concern because it may inhibit the activity of the lipase or enhance hydrolysis of the formed ester (Klibanov, 1989). Formed water should be continuously removed by carrying the reaction at high temperature (60–75°C) in open test tubes or under reduced pressure (0.01–0.05 mmHg) or in the presence of molecular sieves (Ergan et al., 1988; Novo, 1992; Claon and Akoh, 1993; Akoh, 1994).

Transesterification

The problem caused by water in direct esterification reactions can also be circumvented by using transesterification reactions. Transesterification refers to the exchange of acyl group or radicals between an ester and an acid (acidolysis), an ester and an alcohol (alcoholysis), an ester and another ester (interesterification or ester-ester interchange), or an ester and an amine (aminolysis, less commonly studied) [Fig. 6.1, Eqs. (3a), (3b), (3c), and (3d), respectively] (Yamane, 1987). Transesterification reactions can be accomplished industrially by heating a mixture of anhydrous ester and another reactant at relatively high temperatures for a long time (Malcata et al., 1990). In transesterification reactions, generally, hydrolysis precedes esterification.

Acidolysis and interesterification have been extensively used for the production of partial acylglycerols and sugar esters (Chopineau and Mc-Cafferty, 1988; Akoh et al., 1992; Akoh, 1993, 1994; Mutua and Akoh, 1993a) and designer fats such as cocoa butter (Macrae, 1983; Bloomer et al., 1990; Kanasawud et al., 1992; Marangoni et al., 1993).

Alcoholysis reactions have been performed using nonspecific lipases from *Candida cylindraceae* to produce menthyl acetate and butyrate from menthol, triacetin, and tributyrin (Gray et al., 1990). Acetic acid inhibits lipase activity in direct esterification reactions (Iwai et al., 1980). To minimize this inhibitory effect, Chulalaksananukul et al. (1992, 1993) proposed an alcoholysis reaction to synthesize geranyl acetate from geraniol and propyl acetate using lipozyme IM20, a *Mucor miehei* lipase.

Lipase-catalyzed aminolysis has been used for peptide synthesis in solvents having up to 50% water. Since amino acids are rather hydrophilic, they are derivatized to make them more soluble in the organic solvent used. Ways to maintain lipase esterification activity in these relatively high-water-content media are still being studied (Dordick, 1989).

OTHER LIPASE APPLICATIONS

Glycerophospholipid Modification

Not much work has been done on the modification of glycerophospholipids, either chemically and enzymatically. Glycerophospholipids from natural sources contain several fatty acids, and their proportion depends on the source. For some practical applications it is desirable to have glycerophospholipids that contain specific fatty acids. Glycerophospholipids with specific fatty acid composition can sometimes be obtained by fractionation of natural glycerophospholipids, but the most common approach is to synthesize the desired compounds.

One promising synthetic approach is to use natural glycerophospholipids as starting material and to replace the existing fatty acids with the desired ones (Mukherjee, 1990; Svensson et al., 1990; Mutua and Akoh, 1993b). High selectivity of the lipases or phospholipases make them desirable for the production of modified glycerophospholipids. Phospholipase A_1 and A_2 are specific for the hydrolysis of the fatty acids in the sn-1 and sn-2 positions, respectively. Figure 6.2 shows the scheme for the enzymatic hydrolysis and transesterification of glycerophospholipids. Other lipases, which in general are either nonspecific or specific for the sn-1 and sn-3 positions of triacylglycerols may also be used in glycerophospholipid modifications (Mutua and Akoh, 1993b).

Mutua and Akoh (1993b) used lipozyme from *Mucor miehei* and phospholipase A_1 and A_2 to catalyze the incorporation of eicosapentaenoic acid EPA, 20:5n-3 into glycerophosphocholine (GPC), glycerophosphoinositol (GPI), glycerophosphoethanolamine (GPE), and glycerophosphoserine (GPS) by acidolysis reaction. Na et al. (1990) reported that GPC esterified with docosahexaenoic acid, 22:6n-3 DHA, or EPA at the sn-2 position could be more easily digested in the body and might be of value in nutritional and medical applications.

Mono- and Diacylglycerols

Mono- and diacylglycerols (MAG and DAG) are widely used in food and pharmaceutical industries as emulsifiers. Monoacylglycerols can be synthesized chemically at temperatures in excess of 200°C, leading to unwanted side products. Enzymatically, there are several ways of preparing MAG: direct esterification of glycerol with free fatty acid (Akoh et al., 1992), hydrolysis of triacylglycerol (TAG) with a 1,3-specific lipase forming monoacylglycerol with the fatty acid at sn-2 position, glycerolysis of triacylglycerols in organic solvent (McNeill et al., 1990, 1991) or microemulsions (Singh et al., 1994) to produce a mixture of mono- and diacylglycerols, use of isopropylidene derivatives of glycerol (Pecnik and Knez, 1992; Akoh, 1993), and using vinyl fatty acid esters (Bornsheuer et al., 1994; Bornsheuer and Yamane, 1995). Nutritionally beneficial fatty acids such as eicosapentaenic acid (EPA) and DHA have been incorporated with both 1,3-specific and nonspecific lipases.

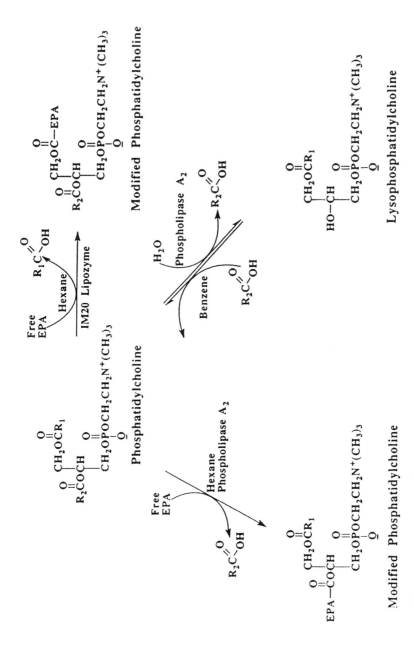

FIG. 6.2   Scheme for hydrolysis and transesterification of glycerophospholipids. (From Akoh, 1995.)

Sugar and Alkyl Glycoside Esters

Sugar and alkyl glycoside fatty acid esters are emulsifiers or biosurfactants, which reduce surface tension and stabilize emulsions. Because of the greater number of free hydroxyl groups in sugar esters, they are more hydrophilic than acylglycerols [i.e., they have wider hydrophilic-lipophilic balance (HLB)]. Biosurfactants have applications in foods, beverages, cosmetics, and pharmaceutical preparations. Chemical synthesis of these molecules is well documented. Their enzymatic synthesis has received recent attention (Seino et al., 1984; Lazar et al., 1986; Mutua and Akoh, 1993a; Akoh and Mutua, 1994; Akoh, 1994; Fregapane et al., 1994; Sarney et al., 1994). Starting substrates include free sugars, sugar acetates, alkyl glycosides, sugar alcohols, and isopropylidene derivatives of the sugars. Figure 6.3 shows the structure of an alkyl glucoside ester (methyl glucoside fatty acid ester) synthesized by Mutua and Akoh (1993a). The only difference between glucose ester and alkyl glycoside ester is that the C-1 anomeric center of the sugar is alkylated (Akoh and Mutua, 1994). Oleic acid, EPA, and DHA have been successfully incorporated into these molecules with *Candida* lipases for potential health reasons.

Vegetable Oil Modifications

There are several functional, health, and nutritional reasons to modify the fatty acid composition of vegetable oils. It has been suggested that the structure of the triacylglycerol as well as the fatty acid content play a role in atherogenicity. These modifications or randomizations can be brought about with chemical catalysts and nonspecific lipases. In order to maintain the balance for n-3, n-6, and n-9 fatty acids in the diet, enzyme-catalyzed vegetable oil modification will play a key role. For example, vegetable oils

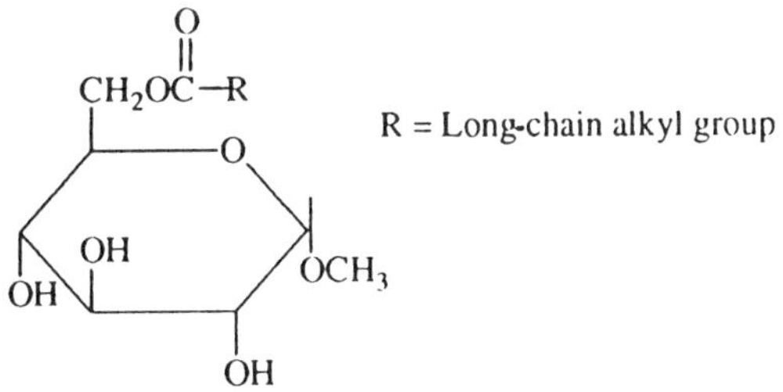

FIG. 6.3 Structure of methyl glucoside fatty acid ester. (Source: Akoh, 1995.)

and melon seed oils containing EPA and DHA have been produced by transesterification with *Mucor miehei* and *Candida antarctica* lipases as biocatalysts (Li and Ward, 1993; Huang and Akoh, 1994; Huang et al., 1994). Tables 6.1 and 6.2 show the fatty acid composition of melon seed oil and soybean oil before and after modification.

Specialty/Structured Lipids

Structured lipids (SL) are triacylglycerols containing both medium-chain fatty acids (MCFA) and long-chain fatty acids (LCFA) in the same molecule and are produced by chemical and enzymatic synthesis/interesterification, but not by physical mixing/blending (Babayan, 1987; Kennedy, 1991; Megremis, 1991). The present commercial manufacturing approach is by chemical interesterification or by physical blending. Enzyme-catalyzed interesterification is a viable alternative to chemical synthesis, and the products may be considered "natural." Very few by-products are formed in enzyme-catalyzed reactions since they are specific. Lipids can be structured

TABLE 6.1   Fatty Acid Composition (Mol%) of Melon Seed
Oil Triacylglycerol Before and After Modification

Fatty acids	IM60		SP435		Before modification
	EPA	EEPA	EPA	EEPA	
16:0	8.1	7.7	10.0	7.6	11.1
16:1 n-7	5.5	7.4	2.4	0.2	0.1
18:0	8.0	0.2	9.5	6.5	9.4
18:1 n-9	12.4	11.2	14.2	9.9	14.2
18:2 n-6	53.4	48.7	56.2	43.9	64.3
18:3 n-6	0.3	0.2	ND	0.4	ND
18:3 n-3	0.3	0.1	0.2	0.1	0.1
20:5 n-3	8.7	24.0	5.2	31.2	ND
22:5 n-3	0.5	ND	0.5	ND	ND
Others	2.8	0.5	1.8	0.2	0.8
Total n-3	9.5	24.1	5.9	31.3	0.1
n-6	53.7	48.9	56.2	44.3	64.3
Saturated	16.1	7.9	19.5	14.1	20.5

ND: not detectable; EEPA: eicosapentaenoic acid ethyl ester; EPA: eicosapentaenoic acid.
Source: Huang et al., 1994.

TABLE 6.2 Fatty Acid Composition of Soybean Oil Before and After Transesterification with Various Acyl Donors by *Mucor miehei* Lipase (IM 60)

Fatty acids	Mol% EPA[a] before transesterification	Mol% EPA after transesterification with		
		EPA45	EPA ethyl ester	DHA ethyl ester
14:0	0.2	0.9	0.6	0.7
14:1	0.1	1.4	1.1	1.3
16:0	11.6	11.8	9.6	12.1
16: n-7	0.1	5.4	0.4	0.2
18:0	3.5	2.5	2.1	2.9
18:1 n-9	21.9	19.1	15.5	19.0
18:2 n-6	53.9	41.8	36.8	43.5
18:3 n-6	0.3			
18:3 n-3	8.4	5.6	5.1	5.8
20:5 n-3		10.5	29.2	
22:5 n-3		0.4		
22:6 n-3				14.6

[a](EPA mol/Total fatty acid mol) × 100%
Source: Huang and Akoh, 1994.

to satisfy essential fatty acid requirements or to incorporate specific fatty acids of interest. These lipids have modified absorption rates because medium-chain triacyglycerols (MCT) are rapidly oxidized for energy, and long-chain triacylglycerols (LCT) are oxidized very slowly (Bell et al., 1991; Kennedy, 1991). MCT were introduced in the 1950s for the treatment of lipid-absorption disorders. Because they are not incorporated into chylomicrons and are not carnitine dependent for transport, they are less likely to be stored in adipose tissue. Pure MCT may be toxic in large doses, and they do not contain essential polyunsaturated fatty acids (PUFA). A combination of MCT and LCT may have theoretical advantages compared to LCT solutions. Simple mixing results in the retention of the original absorption rates of the individual triacylglycerols. Structured triacylglycerols are expected to be less toxic than the physical mixtures, and the tendency to induce metabolic acidosis is also expected to be less. SL may serve as fat substitutes, as in the case of caprenin® (Procter & Gamble Co.) with a defined structure of caprocaprylobehenin (C6:0, C8:0, C22:0), or salatrim® (Nabisco Foods

Group), which is a mixture of stearic acid and short-chain fatty acids such as propionic and/or butyric acid. Behenic and stearic acid are less readily absorbed. The caloric content of caprenin and salatrim is about 5 kcal/g compared to 9 kcal/g for regular triacylglycerols. Again the ability to design lipids (triacylglycerols and glycerophospholipids) with defined structures to target specific diseases or improve general health and well-being has tremendous implications in nutrition and medicine. For example, lipids can be designed to contain the right proportions of the essential fatty acids, MCT, n-3, n-6, and n-9 fatty acids to improve immune function, reduce cholesterol and total fat, prevent thrombosis, atherosclerosis, and cancer, improve nitrogen balance, and reduce the risk of coronary heart disease (Latta, 1990; Bell et al., 1991; Kennedy, 1991; Megremis, 1991). Linoleic acid is required for the formation of arachidonic acid, which is a precursor for the series- 2 prostaglandins and series-4 leukotrienes. Eicosapentaenoic acid (EPA; 20:5 n-3) is an antagonist of the arachidonic acid–derived eicosanoids and may be used to prevent cancer, reduce risk of coronary heart disease, and improve the immune system. Babayan (1987) developed a structured lipid with MCT backbone and containing linoleic acid, 18:2 n-6, which was suitable for critically ill patients. Latta (1990) reviewed current research projects on structuring lipids for nutrition and function and the future of structured lipids.

Designer fats, structured lipids, or "nutraceuticals" can be produced from the MCT and LCT through biotechnology by lipase-catalyzed interesterification reactions with desirable LCFA (Huang, 1995; Shieh et al., 1995), such as oleic, linoleic, and/or EPA with the potential to promote health and nutrition and create new uses in snack foods, foods for obese patients and pediatric patients—particularly immature neonates—and foods for the elderly. Data on the enzymatic synthesis of structured lipids are not extensive. There is a great need for the enzymatic production of these specialty lipids. Indeed, unpublished research from our laboratory indicates that lipids with specific fatty acids can be enzymatically structured for varying specialty uses (Table 6.3). Mucor miehei (IM 60) in the presence of hexane was able to synthesize structured lipid of defined structure containing one or two MCFA (C8-C18:1-C8 and C8-C18:1-C18:1) and very little triolein (Table 6.3) In another study (Huang and Akoh, 1994), it was shown that IM 60 is capable of incorporating up to 10.5% 20:5n-3 (EPA) onto soybean oil with EPA free acid as acyl donor and 29.2% with EPA ethyl ester as acyl donor. Higher incorporation of EPA (34.7%) was obtained with nonspecific Candida antarctica (SP435) lipase and EPA ethyl ester as acyl donor compared to IM 60. Shieh et al. (1995) used four-factor response surface optimization for the enzymatic synthesis of structured triolein. Table 6.4 shows the commercial sources of some of these structured lipids

TABLE 6.3 Synthesis of Structured Lipids Catalyzed by Immobilized *Mucor miehei* (IM 60) Lipase in Hexane

Temperature (°C)	Number of C8:0 attached (%)		Medium-chain	
	1	2	%Incorporation	%Triolein
25	51.7	11.0	62.7	37.3
35	56.9	36.9	93.8	6.2
45	59.1	37.8	96.9	3.1
55	60.6	35.7	96.3	3.7
65	56.2	32.4	88.6	11.4

Condition: IM 60 at 10% by weight of total reactants, molar ratio of C8:0 to triolein of 4, incubation at 200 rpm. Analysis was by HPLC.
Source: Huang and Akoh, 1995.

produced by chemical interesterification reactions. In the future, it is hoped that enzyme-catalyzed synthesis of structured lipids will be the preferred route because of its specificity and natural appeal.

Flavor and Fragrances

The first lipase-catalyzed synthesis of terpene esters was reported by Okumura et al. (1979). Using lipases from *Penicillium cyclopium, Aspergillus niger, Rhizopus delemar,* and *Geotrichum candidum* in a biphasic medium and casein to enhance the stability of the enzyme preparations, they were able to incorporate oleyl group into primary (geraniol and citronellol) and secondary (*l*-menthol) terpene alcohols. Esterification yields were greater than 90% geranyl and citronellyl oleate when lipases from *G. candidum* and *P. cyclopium* were used. With the exception of *G. candidum* lipase, all lipases failed to synthesize the ester of the secondary terpene alcohol, menthol.

TABLE 6.4 [13]Some Commercial Sources of Chemically Synthesized Structured Lipids

Product	Composition	Company
Caprenin	C6:0, C8:0, C22:0	Procter & Gamble, Cincinnati, OH
Salatrim	C3:0, C4:0, C18:0	Nabisco Foods Group, East Hanover, NJ
Captex	C8:0, C10:0, C18:2	ABITEC, Columbus, OH
Neobee	C8:0, C10:0, LCFA	Stepan Co, Maywood, NJ

Recent data from our laboratory indicate that methyl esters can be prepared in organic solvent with acid anhydrides and vinyl esters as acyl donors (unpublished data, Akoh, 1995). No synthesis was observed for the tertiary terpene alcohols (linalool and terpineol). Although the fragrance and flavor properties of terpinyl oleate are unclear, this study nevertheless did establish the feasibility of lipase-catalyzed synthesis of terpene esters.

The first attempt to incorporate short-chain fatty acyl groups (i.e., acetyl, propionyl, butyryl, valeryl, and caproyl) was reported by the same investigators (Iwai et al., 1980) using the same lipase preparations. Lipase from *P. cyclopium* gave the highest yields, 63 and 69%, of geranyl and farnesyl caproate, respectively. No synthesis of terpenyl acetates or of secondary and tertiary terpene alcohol esters was observed. It was concluded that the potent acidity of acetic acid probably inhibited the esterification activity of lipases (Iwai et al., 1980).

Marlot et al. (1985) reported the synthesis of geraniol and menthol esters of butyric and lauric acids by various lipases. The highest yield (74%) was obtained in the synthesis of geranyl laurate by *Candida cylindraceae* lipase immobilized on porous glass beads. This study was the first demonstration of lipase-catalyzed direct esterification in organic solvents, which was thought unsurmountable.

Several authors have addressed lipase-catalyzed terpene ester synthesis in organic media (Langrand et al., 1988, 1990; Claon and Akoh, 1993; 1994a, b, c, d; Yee et al., 1995) and biphasic media (Nishio et al., 1988) Langrand et al. (1988) studied the ability of 13 commercial lipases to incorporate acetyl, propionyl, and butyryl groups into geraniol. While the yield of geranyl propionate and butyrate was greater than 90%, the highest yield of geranyl acetate was 14%. Most lipases gave yields of less than 0.5% geranyl acetate. The results were no better for Nishio et al. (1988). Further attempts by Langrand et al. (1990) did not yield better results. Claon and Akoh (1993, 1994a, b, c, d) and Yee et al. (1995) subsequently reported greatly improved yields (96–100%) of terpene esters with *Candida antarctica* lipase, SP435 (Novo Nordisk Bioindustrial, Inc., Danbury, CT), and lipase AY from *Candida rugosa* (Amano International Enzyme Co., Troy, VA).

Transesterification reactions have been performed to produce terpene esters. Gray et al. (1990) transesterified menthol using triacetin and tributyrin and *C. cylindraceae* lipase. The relative yields reported were 20 and 54% of menthyl acetate and menthyl butyrate after 24 and 48 hours, respectively. To improve the yield of lipase-catalyzed synthesis of geranyl acetate using *Mucor miehei* lipase (Lipozyme™ IM20), Chulalaksananukul et al. (1992, 1993) transesterified geraniol using propyl acetate in hexane and supercritical CO_2. They found that hexane was a better medium for the type of synthesis investigated. Yield of 85% geranyl acetate was obtained after 3 days incubation.

Unlike chemical catalysts, immobilized lipases can be reused. The ability of lipases to be reused is an essential aspect in the cost-effectiveness of biocatalysis. Figure 6.4 shows the conversion obtained after using SP435 10 times in a direct esterification of citronellol reaction.

Others

Lipases are currently being used for the production of optically active compounds for the fine chemicals and pharmaceutical industries. This is important because in some chiral compounds, only one of the enantiomers is biologically active or potent or exhibits more activity than the other enantiomer. Lipases can be used in asymmetrical hydrolysis of an ester or esterification of a carboxylic acid or asymmetrical transesterification reactions (for a recent review, see Santaniello et al., 1993). For example, Patel et al. (1992) used lipase PS-30 for the stereoselective acetylation of a chiral alcohol in organic solvent to produce a hydroxymethyl glutaryl coenzyme A (HMG CoA) reductase inhibitor, which is a potential anticholesterol drug. In order to improve the optical purity it may be necessary to use vinyl esters,

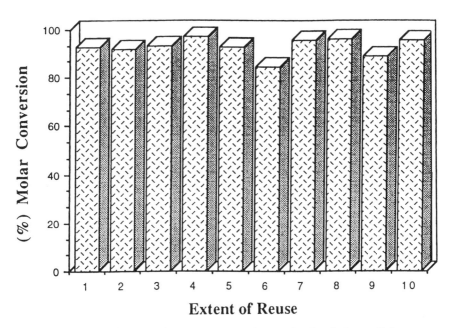

FIG. 6.4   Effect of SP435 lipase reuse on the synthesis of citronellyl acetate by transesterification in n-hexane. (Source: Claon and Akoh, 1994c.)

acid anhydrides, enol, and oxime esters as acyl donors. Shaw and Lo (1994) reported the enzymatic production of propylene glycol fatty acid mono-esters in organic solvent. These esters can be used as emulsifiers in water-in-oil emulsions. They have low HLB values and can be used in cakes, cake mixes, bread, etc.

CONCLUSIONS

The field of nonaqueous enzymology is a reality. Enzymes can be used to catalyze both forward and reverse reactions with the stipulation of controlling the water activity, water content, or formed water during the reaction, which in turn shifts the equilibrium towards the desired product. Immobilization and reuse of immobilized enzymes make this bioprocess commercially and economically feasible. Obvious advantages of using lipases in the modification of lipids include production of value-added lipid, synthesis of novel products, incorporation of desirable fatty acids at specific positions of the lipid to improve functionality and nutrition and for medicinal purposes, and synthesis of specialty lipids, structured lipids, and flavor and fragrances. More research is definitely needed in this growing field, especially in the study of the physical and functional properties as well the metabolism and health benefits, if any, of enzymatically modified lipids.

REFERENCES

Akoh, C. C. 1993. Lipase-catalyzed synthesis of partial glyceride. *Biotechnol. Lett.* 15: 949–954.

Akoh, C. C. 1994. Enzymatic synthesis of acetylated glucose fatty acid ester in organic solvent. *J. Am. Oil Chem. Soc.* 71: 319–323.

Akoh, C. C. 1995. Unpublished data. Department of Food Science & Technology, University of Georgia, Athens.

Akoh, C. C., Cooper, C., and Nwosu, C. V. 1992. Lipase G catalyzed synthesis of monoglycerides in organic solvent and analysis by HPLC. *J. Am. Oil Chem. Soc.* 69: 275–260.

Akoh, C. C. and Mutua, L. N. 1994. Synthesis of alkyl glycoside fatty acid esters: Effect of reaction parameters and the incorporation of n-3 polyunsaturated fatty acids. *Enzyme Microb. Technol.* 16: 115–119.

Akoh, C. C. and Nwosu, C. V. 1992. Fatty acid composition of melon seed oil lipids and phospholipids. *J. Am. Oil Chem. Soc.* 69: 314–316.

Babayan, V. K. 1987. Specialty lipids and their biofunctionality. *Lipids* 22: 417–420.

Bell, S. J., Mascioli, E. A., Bistrain, B. R., Babayan, V. K., and Blackburn, G. L. 1991. Alternative lipid sources for enteral and parenteral nutrition: Long- and medium-chain triacylglycerols, structured triacylglycerols, and fish oils. *J. Am. Diet. Assoc.* 91: 74–78.

Bloomer, S., Aldercreutz, P., and Mattiasson, B. 1990. Triglyceride inter-esterification by lipases. 1. Cocoa butter equivalents from a fraction of palm oil. *J. Am. Oil Chem. Soc.* 67: 519–524.

Bornscheuer, U., Stamatis, H., Xenakis, A., Yamane, T., and Kolisis, F. N. 1994. A comparison of different strategies for lipase-catalyzed synthesis of partial glycerides. *Biotechnol. Lett.* 16: 697–702.

Bornscheuer, U. and Yamane, T. 1995. Fatty acid vinyl esters as acylating agents: A new method for the enzymatic synthesis of monoacylglycerols. *J. Am. Oil. Chem. Soc.* 72: 193–197.

Chopineau, J. and McCafferty, C. C. 1988. Synthesis of alkyl glycoside fatty acid esters in non-aqueous media by *Candida* sp. lipase. *J. Am. Oil Chem. Soc.* 70: 43–46.

Chulalaksananukul, W., Condoret, J. S., and Combes, D. 1992. Kinetics of geranyl acetate synthesis by lipase-catalyzed transesterification in n-hexane. *Enzyme Microb. Technol.* 14: 293–298.

Chulalaksananukul, W., Condoret, J. S., and Combes, D. 1993. Geranyl acetate synthesis by lipase-catalyzed transesterification in supercritical carbon dioxide. *Enzyme Microb. Technol.* 5: 691–698.

Claon, P. A. and Akoh, C. C. 1993. Enzymatic synthesis of geraniol and citronellol esters by direct esterification in n-hexane. *Biotechnol. Lett.* 15: 1211–1216.

Claon, P. A. and Akoh, C. C. 1994a. Lipase-catalyzed synthesis of terpene esters by tranesterification in n-hexane. *Biotechnol. Lett.* 16: 235–240.

Claon, P. A. and Akoh, C. C. 1994b. Enzymatic synthesis of geranyl acetate in n-hexane with *Candida antarctica* lipases. *J. Am. Oil. Chem. Soc.* 71: 575–578.

Claon, P. A. and Akoh, C. C. 1994c. Effect of reaction parameters on SP435 lipase-catalyzed synthesis of citronellyl acetate in organic solvent. *Enzyme Microb. Technol.* 16: 835–838.

Claon, P. A. and Akoh, C. C. 1994d. Lipase-catalyzed synthesis of primary terpenyl acetates by transesterification: Study of reaction parameters. *J. Agric. Food Chem.* 42: 2349–2352.

de Castro, H. F., Anderson, W. A., Moo-Young, M., and Legge, R. L. 1992. Partitioning of water during the production of terpene esters using immobilized lipase. In *Biocatalysis in Non-Conventional Media*, J. Tramper,

M. H. Vermue, H. H. Beeftink, and U. von Stockar (Ed.), Vol. 8, p. 475. Elsevier Science Publishers B. V., New York.

Dordick, J. S. 1989. Enzymatic catalysis in monophasic organic solvents. *Enzyme Microb. Technol.* 11: 194–211.

Ergan, R., Trani, M., and Andre, G. 1988. Solvent-free triacylglycerol synthesis using Lipozyme IM-20. *Biotechnol. Lett.* 10: 629–634.

Fonteyn, F., Blecker, C., Lognay, G., Marlier, M., and Severin, M. 1994. Optimization of lipase-catalyzed synthesis of citronellyl acetate in solvent-free medium. *Biotechnol. Lett.* 16: 693–696.

Fregapane, G., Sarney, D. B., Greenberg, S. G., Knight, D. J., and Vulfson, E. N. 1994. Enzymatic synthesis of monosaccharide fatty acid esters and their comparison with conventional products. *J. Am. Oil Chem. Soc.* 71: 87–91.

Gillies, B., Yamazaki, H., and Armstrong, D. W. 1987. Production of flavor esters by immobilized lipase. *Biotechnol. Lett.* 9: 709–714.

Goh, S. H., Yeong, S. K., and Wang, C. W. 1993. Transesterification of cocoa butter by fungal lipases: effect of solvent on 1,3-specificity. *J. Am. Oil Chem. Soc.* 70: 567–570.

Goto, M., Goto, M., Kamiya, N., and Nakashio, F. 1995. Enzymatic interesterification of triglyceride with surfactant-coated lipase in organic media. *Biotechnol. Bioeng.* 45: 27–32.

Gray, C. J., Narang, J. S., and Barker, S. A. 1990. Immobilization of lipase from *Candida cylindraceae* and its use in the synthesis of menthol esters by transesterification. *Enzyme Micro. Technol.* 12: 800–807.

Hammond, D. A., Karel, M., and Klibanov, A. M. 1985. Enzymatic reactions in supercritical gases. *Appl. Biochem. Biotechnol.* 11: 393–399.

Huang, K-H. 1995. Enzymatic synthesis of structured lipids. M.S. thesis, University of Georgia, Athens.

Huang, K-H. and Akoh, C. C. 1994. Lipase-catalyzed incorporation of n-3 PUFAs into vegetable oils. *J. Am. Oil Chem. Soc.* 71: 1277–1280.

Huang, K-H. and Akoh, C. C. 1995. Unpublished data. Department of Food Science & Technology, University of Georgia, Athens.

Huang, K-H., Akoh, C. C., and Erickson, M. C. 1994. Enzymatic modification of melon seed oil: Incorporation of eicosapentaenoic acid. *J. Agric. Food Chem.* 42: 2646–2648.

Iwai, M., Okumura, S., and Tsujisaka, Y. 1980. Synthesis of terpene alcohol esters by lipase. *Agric. Biol. Chem.* 44: 2731–2732.

Iwai, M., Tsujisaka, Y., and Fukumoto, J. 1964. Studies on lipase II. Hydrolytic and esterifying actions of crystalline lipase of *Aspergillus niger*. *J. Gen. Appl. Microbiol.* 10:13–22.

Janssen, A. E. M., Van der Padt, A., and Vant Riet, K. 1993. Solvent effects on lipase-catalyzed esterification of glycerol and fatty acids. *Biotechnol. Bioeng.* 42: 953–962.

Kanasawud, P., Phutrakul, S., Bloomer, S., Aldercreutz, P., and Mattiasson, B. 1992. Triglyceride interesterification by lipases. 3. Alcoholysis of pure acylglycerols. *Enzyme Microb. Technol.* 14: 959–965.

Kennedy, J. P. 1991. Structured lipids: Fats of the future. *Food Technol.* 45: 78–83.

Klibanov, A. M. 1989. Enzymatic catalysis in anhydrous organic solvents. *Trends Biochem. Sci.* 14: 141–149.

Langrand, G., Rondot, N., Triantaphylides, C., and Baratti, J. 1990. Short chain ester synthesis by microbial lipases. *Biotechnol. Lett.* 12: 581–586.

Latta, S. 1990. "Natural" may be the niche for structured lipids. *Inform* 1: 970–974.

Lazar, A., Wiess, A., and Schmid, R. D. 1986. Synthesis of ester by lipases. In *Proceedings of the World Conference on Emerging Technologies in the Fats and Oil Industry*, A. R. Baldwin (Ed.), pp. 346–354. *American Oil Chemists Society*, Champaign, IL.

Li, Z-Y. and Ward, O. P. 1993. Enzyme catalyzed production of vegetable oils containing omega-3 polyunsaturated fatty acid. *Biotechnol. Lett.* 15: 185–188.

Macrae, A. R. J. 1983. Lipase-catalyzed interesterification of oils and fats. *J. Am. Oil Chem. Soc.* 60: 243A–246A.

Malcata, F. X., Reyes, H. R., Garcia, H. S., Hill, C. G., Jr., and Amundson, C. H. 1990. Immobilized lipase reactors for modification of fats and oils—a review. *J. Am. Oil Chem. Soc.* 12: 890–910.

Marangoni, A. G. 1994. *Candida* and *Pseudomonas* lipase-catalyzed hydrolysis of butter oil in the absence of organic solvents. *J. Food Sci.* 59: 1096–1099.

Marangoni, A. G., McCurdy, R. D., and Brown, E. D. 1993. Enzymatic interesterification of triolein with tripalmitin in canola lecithin-hexane reverse micelles. *J. Am. Oil Chem. Soc.* 70: 103–110.

Marlot, C., Langrand, G., Triantaphylides, C., and Baratti, J. 1985. Ester synthesis in organic solvent catalyzed by lipases immobilized on hydrophilic supports. *Biotechnol. Lett.* 9: 647–650.

Marty, A., Chulalaksananukul, W., Willemot, R. M., and Condoret, J. S. 1992. Kinetics of lipase-catalyzed esterification in supercritical CO_2. *Biotechnol. Bioeng.* 39: 273–280.

McNeill, G. P., Shimizu, S., and Yamane, T. 1990. Solid phase enzymatic glycerolysis of beef tallow resulting in a high yield of monoglyceride. *J. Am. Oil Chem. Soc.* 67: 779–783.

McNeill, G. P., Shimizu, S., and Yamane, T. 1991. High yield enzymatic glycerolysis of fats and oils. *J. Am. Oil Chem. Soc.* 68: 1–5.

McNeill, G. P. and Sonnet, P. E. 1995. Isolation of erucic acid from rapeseed oil by lipase-catalyzed hydrolysis. *J. Am. Oil Chem. Soc.* 72: 213–218.

Megremis, C. J. 1991. Medium-chain triacylglycerols: A nonconventional fat. *Food Technol.* 45: 108–114.

Mojovic, L. and Shiler-Marinkovic, S. 1992. Interesterification of palm oil mid fraction by immobilized lipase in N-hexane: Effect of lecithin addition. In *Food Science and Human Nutrition*, G. Charalambous (Ed.), pp. 585–593. Elsevier Science Publishers B. V.

Mukherjee, K. D. 1990. Lipase-catalyzed reactions for modification of fats and other lipids. *Biocatalysis* 3: 277–293.

Mustranta, A., Suortti, T., and Poutanen, K. 1994. Transesterification of phospholipid in different reaction conditions. *J. Am. Oil Chem. Soc.* 71: 1415–1419.

Mutua, L. N. and Akoh, C. C. 1993a. Synthesis of alkyl glycoside fatty acid esters in nonaqueous media by *Candida sp.* lipase. *J. Am. Oil Chem. Soc.* 70: 43–46.

Mutua, L. N. and Akoh, C. C. 1993b. Lipase-catalyzed modification of phospholipids: Incorporation of n-3 fatty acids into biosurfactants. *J. Am. Oil Chem. Soc.* 70: 125–128.

Na, A., Eriksson, C., Eriksson, S., Osterberg, E., and Holmberg, K. 1990. Synthesis of phosphatidylcholine with (n-3) fatty acids by phospholipase A_2 in microemulsion. *J. Am. Oil Chem. Soc.* 67: 766–770.

Nishio, T., Chikano, T., and Kamimura, M. 1988. Ester synthesis by the lipase from *Pseudomonas fragi. Agric. Biol. Chem.* 52: 1203–1208.

Novo Industri. 1992. Product Information. B 347c-GB, December.

Okumura, S., Iwai, M., and Tjujisaka, Y. 1979. Synthesis of various kinds of esters by four microbial lipases. *Biochim. Biophys. Acta.* 575: 156–165.

Park, Y. H., Pastore, G. M., and Mutsui de Almelda, M. 1988. Hydrolysis of soybean oil by combined lipase system. *J. Am. Oil Chem. Soc.* 65: 252–254.

Patel, R. N., McNamee, C. M., and Szarka, L. J. 1992. Enantioselective enzymatic acetylation of racemic [4-[4α, 6β (E)]]-6-[4,4-bis(4-fluoro-phenyl)-3-(1-methyl-1H-tetrazol-5-yl)-1,3-butadienyl]-tetrahydro-4-hydroxy-2H-pyran-2-one. *Appl. Microb. Biotechnol.* 38: 56–60.

Pecnik, S. and Knez, Z. 1992. Enzymatic fatty ester synthesis. *J. Am. Oil Chem. Soc.* 69: 261–265.

Quinlan, P. and Moore, S. 1993. Modification of triglycerides by lipases:

Process technology and its application to the production of nutritionally improved fats. *Inform* 4: 580–585.

Santaniello, E., Ferraboschi, P., and Grisenti, P. 1993. Lipase-catalyzed transesterification in organic solvents: application to the preparation of enantiomerically pure compounds. *Enzyme Microb. Technol.* 15: 367–382.

Sarney, D. B., Kapeller, H., Fregapane, G., and Vulfson, E. N. 1994. Chemoenzymatic synthesis of disaccharide fatty acid esters. *J. Am. Oil Chem. Soc.* 71: 711–714.

Seino, H., Uchibori, T., Nichitani, T., and Inamasu, S. 1984. Enzymatic synthesis of carbohydrate esters of fatty acids (1) Esterification of sucrose, glucose, fructose and sorbitol. *J. Am. Oil Chem. Soc.* 61: 1761–1765.

Shaw, J-F. and Lo, S. 1994. Production of propylene glycol fatty acid monoesters by lipase-catalyzed reactions in organic solvents. *J. Am. Oil Chem. Soc.* 71: 715–719.

Shieh, C-J., Akoh, C. C., and Koehler, P. E. 1995. Four-factor response surface optimization of the enzymatic modification of triolein to structured lipids. *J. Am. Oil Chem. Soc.* 72: 619–623.

Shishikura, A., Fujimoto, K., Suzuki, T., and Arai, K. 1994. Improved lipase-catalyzed incorporation of long-chain fatty acids into medium-chain triglycerides assisted by supercritical carbon dioxide extraction. *J. Am. Oil Chem. Soc.* 71: 961–967.

Singh, C. P., Shah, D. O., and Holmberg, K. 1994. Synthesis of mono- and diglycerides in water-in-oil microemulsions. *J. Am. Oil Chem. Soc.* 71: 583–587.

Sonnet, P. E., Foglia, T. A., and Feairheller, S. H. 1993. Fatty acid selectivity of lipases: erucic acid from rapeseed oil. *J. Am. Oil Chem. Soc.* 70: 387–391.

Sridhar, R., Lakshminarayana, G., and Kaimal, T. N. B. 1991. Modification of selected edible vegetable oils to high oleic oils by lipase-catalyzed ester interchange. *J. Agric. Food Chem.* 39: 2069–2071.

Svensson, I., Adlercreautz, P., and Mattiasson, B. 1990. Interesterification of phosphatidylcholine with lipases in organic media. *Appl. Microb. Biotechnol.* 33: 255–258.

Vulfson, E. N. 1993. Enzymatic synthesis of food ingredients in low-water media. *Trends Food Sci. Technol.* 4: 209–215.

West, S. I. 1988a. Enzymes in the food processing industry. *Chem. Br.* 12: 1220–1222.

West, S. I. 1988b. Lipase—a new chemical catalyst. *Specialty Chem.* 10: 410–414.

Yamane, T. 1987. Enzyme technology for lipid industry: an engineering overview. *J. Am. Oil Chem. Soc.* 64: 1657–1662.

Yamane, T., Suzuki, T., Sahashi, Y., Vikersveen, L., and Hoshino, T. 1992. Production of n-3 polyunsaturated fatty acid-enriched fish oil by lipase-catalyzed acidolysis without solvent. *J. Am. Oil Chem. Soc.* 69: 1104–1107.

Yang, B. and Parkin, K. L. 1994. Monoacylglycerol production from butter-oil by glycerolysis with a gel-entrapped microbial lipase in microaqueous media. *J. Food Sci.* 59: 47–52.

Yee, L. N., Akoh, C. C., and Phillips, R. S. 1995. Terpene ester synthesis by lipase-catalyzed transesterification. *Biotechnol. Lett.* 17: 67–70.

7

Formation of Lipid Oxidation Products During Deep Fat Frying: Effects on Oil Quality and Their Determination

Edward G. Perkins

University of Illinois
Urbana, Illinois

INTRODUCTION

The primary function of deep frying is as a heat-exchange medium to cook food. Food is immersed in the hot oil until it is cooked. Cooking occurs by heating the outside of the food and, eventually, water in the interior of the food is sufficiently heated to cook the food and is converted to steam. This usually results in a food product with a crisp outer layer and a moist interior. The quality of the oil used in deep frying contributes to the quality of the fried food.

Lipid oxidation at higher temperatures in the presence of oxygen and steam, as in deep fat frying, produces a multiplicity of compounds, which exert both desirable and undesirable effects on food flavor and quality (Porter et al., 1995). Oxidative and chemical changes in frying fats during use are characterized by a decrease in the total unsaturation of the fat with increases in free fatty acid content, foaming, color, viscosity, polar materials, and polymeric material (Fig. 7.1). These increase with time and occur at the expense of the original triglyceride via lipid oxidation through free radical

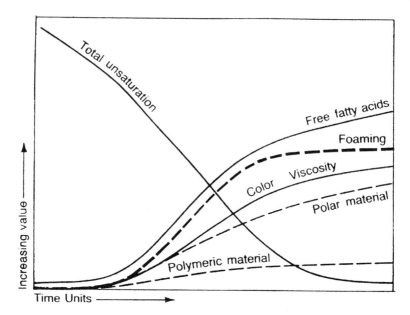

FIG. 7.1   Oxidative and chemical changes in frying fats during use.

mechanisms (Fig. 7.2). Most of the free fatty acids found in frying fats result from hydrolysis of the frying oil by steam generated by interaction of the food product with the hot oil (Fig. 7.3).

Fats at any temperature appear to go through a free radical initiation period (Fig. 7.2). They then move into a free radical–propagation or peroxide-formation phase. The rate of propagation then slows, and a free radical–termination phase is entered wherein reactions with other free radicals can take place. In this phase peroxides are stabilized. After a certain time period, peroxides will begin to decompose into volatile flavor and odor

$$\text{INITIATION} \quad RH \longrightarrow R*$$

$$\text{PROPAGATION} \quad R* + O_2 \longrightarrow ROO*$$

$$ROO* + RH \longrightarrow ROOH + R*$$

$$\text{TERMINATION} \quad R* + R* \longrightarrow \textbf{NONRADICAL}$$
$$\textbf{PRODUCTS}$$

FIG. 7.2   Free radical mechanism of lipid oxidation.

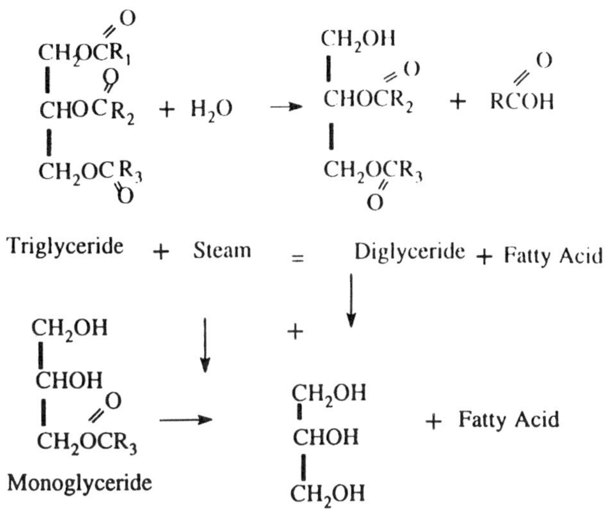

FIG. 7.3 Hydrolysis of frying oil with steam.

components as well as nonvolatile higher molecular weight products (Porter et al., 1995). This process occurs at different rates depending upon the initial unsaturation of the fat and many other associated factors (Pokorny, 1989).

MEASUREMENT OF LIPID OXIDATION

The measurement of lipid oxidation is essential to the determination of its effect on food and food oil quality. Lipid oxidation may be measured with physical methods such as molecular weight, refractive index, viscosity, specific gravity, and dielectric constant. These measurements all increase with heating time. Increases in molecular weight, viscosity, and specific gravity indicate that polymerization is taking place and, in the case of the dielectric constant, that there is oxygen incorporation into the fat.

Spectrophotometry is usually used to detect certain chemical species. Ultraviolet absorption spectrophotometry is useful for determination of unsaturation, particularly in the 232 and 369 nm regions for conjugated dienoic and trienoic fatty acids, respectively (Noor and Augustin, 1984; AOCS, 1989). Infrared absorption spectrophotometry may be used to measure hydroxyl, carboxyl, and ester groups as well as *cis* and *trans* unsaturation. Spectrophotofluorimetry is used to measure the presence of fluorescing materials in heated oils, which are likely due to polymerization and decomposition of the original coloring materials, such as carotenoids and tocopherols, remaining in the oil after processing.

Chemical methods for determination of lipid oxidation (AOCS, 1989) include the iodine value, which decreases as a result of destruction of unsaturation and the saponification value, which will increase as the molecular weight of the sample increases. The peroxide value is less useful in the case of heated fats, since it is an indicator of peroxides present in an oil. The peroxide value primarily indicates the overall quality of a fat during and after storage. At frying temperatures, peroxides do not exist since they would decompose as soon as they are formed. The thiobarbituric acid (TBA) test for the formation of malonaldehyde in fats and oils has also been used to measure lipid oxidation. The success of this test depends upon the simultaneous formation of malonaldehyde from a dihydroperoxide formed from linoleic acid (Noor and Augustin, 1984).

DETERMINATION OF VOLATILE OXIDATION PRODUCTS

The low molecular weight components responsible for flavors and odors in many deep fried food products are formed via decomposition of lipid hydroperoxides by various mechanisms (Porter et al., 1995). For instance, hexanal, a very common aldehyde flavoring component, is formed by the destruction of a 13-hydroperoxide fatty acid derivative. Another very common off flavor component in fats and food products, 2,4-decadienal, is formed by cleavage of the 9-hydroperoxide. Further decomposition of hydroperoxides is responsible for the formation of complete homologous series of saturated and unsaturated hydrocarbons (Fig. 7.4), saturated and unsaturated aldehydes, ketones, alcohols, and carboxylic acids. Frankel (1985) has published extensively in this area. Other components termed pentyl furans (Fig. 7.5) and *trans, cis,* and *trans, trans* dienals and pyrazines may be found in extracts of oils from food products such as French fries (Qian, 1991). Volatiles are generally measured by at least three major methods, coupled with high-resolution gas chromatography (HRGC). In some cases, mass spectrometry also assists in the identification of components (Perkins, 1989; Waltking and Goetz, 1975; Frankel, 1993; Warner and Eskin, 1994). These three methods are static headspace, dynamic headspace, and direct gas chromatographic analysis. Static headspace analysis involves direct injection of the vapor above a liquid (oil) into the HRGC for separation, identification, and quantitation. Headspace analysis is simple and reproducible. Its major disadvantage is that it is dependent upon a complete equilibrium between the liquid phase and the vapor phase above it. Wide ranges in molecular weights of volatile components can cause biased compositions

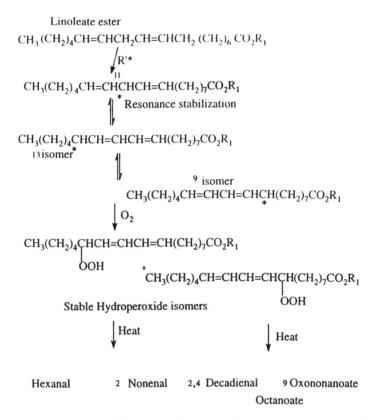

FIG. 7.4   Formation of hexanal, decadienal, and secondary oxidation products.

because of nonequilibrium in the final vapor phase to be sampled (Ioffe and Vitenberg, 1983).

Dynamic headspace analysis in its varied forms is widely used to collect volatiles by purging the sample or flowing a gas over the sample's surface. The gas is then purged onto a specially designed trap, which is then desorbed into the HRGC. Such traps are packed with Tenax GC, Chromasorbs, and Porapac Q (Nunez et al., 1984; Hinshaw, 1990). These packings adsorb organic compounds, which are in turn desorbed by heat and injected into the HRGC for compositional analysis. One advantage of these packings is that water is not adsorbed and does not interfere with the HRGC separations. The use of organic polymer adsorbents can lead to artifacts during desorption, which are possibly caused by thermal degradation of the adsor-

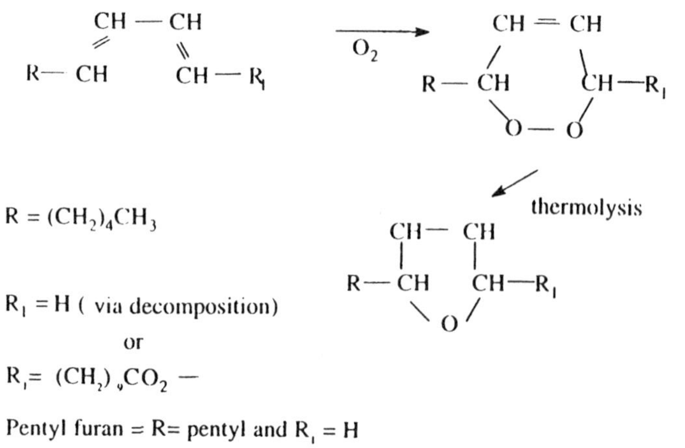

FIG. 7.5   Formation of pentyl furan from free radicals.

bent (Murray, 1977). Although somewhat limited by the design of the desorption apparatus, a typical desorption tube is usually about 0.25 × 3–4 inches. Volatiles may be collected in several ways. Samples of oil containing volatile material may be placed directly onto glass wool at the tube entrance and then purged to remove the volatiles from the oil (Dupuy et al., 1977). Volatiles may be collected by passing a high-purity gas such as argon through an oil (sparging) and into the trap (Warner and Eskin, 1994). This method is routinely used in the analysis of waters for organic material. We have sparged French fries by placing them into a flask fitted with a sparging tube and gas flow meter. Volatiles are collected onto a desorption tube containing Carbopac B, which is then desorbed into the HRGC. The results are as indicated in Figure 7.6 (Qian, 1990). A maximum amount of total volatiles was formed at about 70 hours of deep frying.

Headspace vapor as well as the oil may also be analyzed by direct injection into the HRGC (Warner and Eskin, 1994). However, the band broadening that often results can be prevented by cryofocusing at the head of the column. In all cases volatile analysis may be improved either by cryogenic focusing or cryogenic programming in the gas chromatograph (Scholz and Ptak, 1966; Warner, 1985).

DETERMINATION OF NONVOLATILE MATERIALS

There are many nonvolatile components present in a fat that has been used for deep-frying. Unsaponifiable materials that contain functional groups

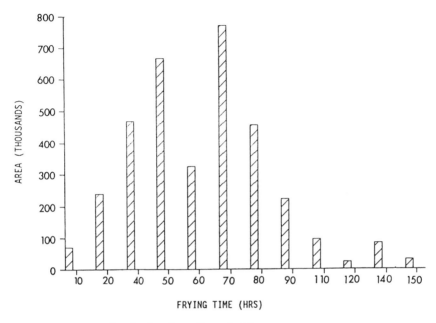

FIG. 7.6   Sparged volatiles from French fries.

such as aldehydes and ketones are found. Material consisting of hydrocarbons is also found. Nonoxidized material consisting of cyclic monomeric products that contain cyclohexyl, cyclopentyl, and cyclohexenyl groups has been detected (Artman, 1969). Dimeric fatty acids containing both cyclic and noncyclic structures have been characterized. Several saturated and unsaturated keto- as well as mono-, dihydroxy-, and ketohydroxy-substituted fatty acids are formed (Artman, 1969). Trimeric triglycerides and a mass of uncharacterized high molecular weight oligomeric triglycerides termed polymers are present. This polymeric material may be polar or nonpolar in nature (Taubold et al., 1973).

Monomers may result from the hydrolysis of triglycerides and may cyclize either in the triglyceride form or as a free fatty acid. They may also form by decomposition of fatty acid hydroperoxides. Nonthermal oxidation products may also be formed and consist of the cyclic monomers formed by an initial cyclization of the fatty acid chain. Both aromatic rings and those containing a cyclohexenyl and cyclopentenyl group may be formed as part of the fatty acid chain (Perkins, 1992).

Nonvolatile thermal oxidation products may be fractionated by solvent partitioning. The polar material will solubilize into a relatively polar solvent.

Nonpolar material must dissolve into a nonpolar solvent, such as hexane. This can be used to separate these compounds on a crude scale. Silicic acid column chromatography using a mixture of 13% diethyl ether in hexane separates "nonpolar" unchanged triglycerides, while elution with diethyl ether removes the polar components (Paquot and Hautfenne, 1987). High vacuum fractional or molecular distillation may be used to separate relatively high molecular weight species. Urea adduction will separate compounds that differ in structure from stearic and linoleic acid. Gas liquid chromatograph (GLC) is used for analysis of the normal nonoxidized fatty acids, but this could also be used for the determination of nonelutable species or polymers (Waltking et al., 1975). Thin-layer chromatography (TLC) in many of its modes such as reverse phase, argentation, or adsorption on silica have been used to separate thermal oxidation products (Sebedio and Perkins, 1995). High-performance liquid chromatography (HPLC) has been successfully used to fractionate thermal oxidation products as well. One can collect component fractions via HPLC and then perform gas chromatography on them (Perkins, 1992). High-performance size exclusion chromatography (HPSEC) will separate lipid oxidation products into their various molecular weight species (Shukla and Perkins, 1991).

Before discussion of the reactions of deep frying and absorption of oxidized components into food, analytical considerations for certain nonvolatile compounds should be addressed. Compounds such as cyclic monomers, dibasic acids, dimers, trimers, and higher molecular weight products, which may contain hydroxy and keto groups, may need to be derivatized for increased volatility. This is usually done by preparing methyl esters, trimethyl silyl esters, or ethers of hydroxyl and carboxyl groups prior to analysis by gas chromatographic methods. The cyclic fatty acids are formed in variable amounts up to 1500–2000 ppm depending upon the unsaturated fatty acids. If linoleic or linolenic acid are the unsaturated fatty acids, the structures shown in Figure 7.7 are formed. A cyclohexyl and/or cyclopentyl ring–containing compound occurs as a series of 17 isomers in heated linseed oil, as shown in Figure 7.7. Isolation of cyclic monomers is accomplished by hydrogenation of the methyl esters of the fat, followed by urea adduction to concentrate cyclic materials. Further purification is carried out by HPLC with ODS silica and the component representing the cyclics collected. Sebedio (1987) has shown that cyclic monomers are eluted after methyl palmitate and before methyl stearate on a reverse phase column with acetonitrile: acetone as mobile phase or as carried out by Rojo and Perkins (1989). If this fraction is collected, hydrogenated, and then the mass spectra of the components separated by capillary gas chromatography–mass spectrometry evaluated, more than 10 different cyclic monomer structures in which the chain lengths range from ethyl to hexyl, as well as *cis, trans* isomers are found (Sebedio et al., 1987a).

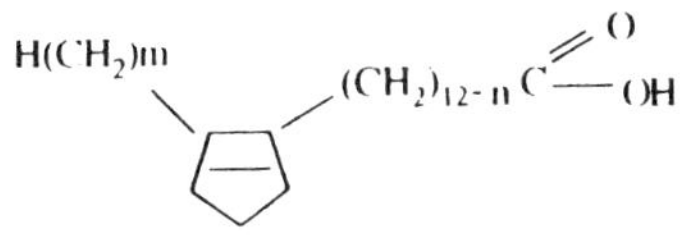

Cyclopentenyl fatty acid (CFA)

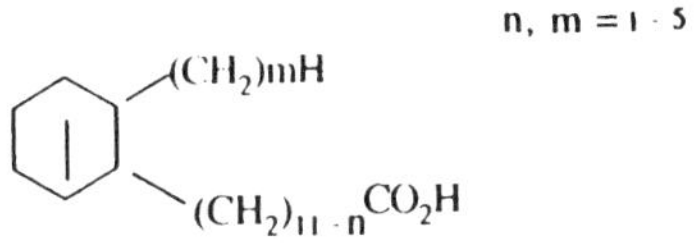

n, m = 1 – 5

Cyclohexenyl fatty acid (CFA)

FIG. 7.7   Structures of cyclic monomers.

Dimeric fatty acids are formed, which may or may not contain two moles of triglyceride. This depends upon whether or not intra- or intermolecular dimerization has taken place. There is evidence for formation of noncyclic and cyclic dimers as well as bicyclic dimers in fats and oils that have been used for frying. Thermal dimers are simply those that are formed by heating and condensation. They are usually cyclic dimers that result from a Diels-Alder reaction. Others often form from condensation reactions of two fatty acid free radicals and do not have a cyclic structure. Seven different dimeric structures ranging from a thermal dimer to a tetrahydroxy dimer have been synthesized (Christopoulou and Perkins, 1989a) (Fig. 7.8a). All synthetic dimers, when made into a model mixture, can be separated by HPLC (Fig. 7.8b) (Christopoulou and Perkins, 1989a). Now that mixtures of isomers of known dimeric structure are available, the dimeric fraction from an oil used for frying may be isolated by preparative size exclusion chromatography and then separated under the same conditions as those developed for model mixtures. All seven types of dimers were present in a soybean oil used for frying. The same types of dimeric components were found in about the same concentrations relative to one another (Christopoulou and Perkins, 1989b) (Fig. 7.8b).

   It appears that the components in the used oils are absorbed by the French fries in concentrations approximating those present in the frying medium. There does not appear to be any preferential uptake by the French fry of any nonvolatile components formed in the frying oils.

DEEP FRYING AND OIL AND FRY QUALITY

In a recent study of the effects of deep frying on the quality of frying oil and French fries, the fatty acid composition of the frying oil showed destruction

Fraction #	MW	# Isomers	Structure	Assignment
I. Peak #1	620	4	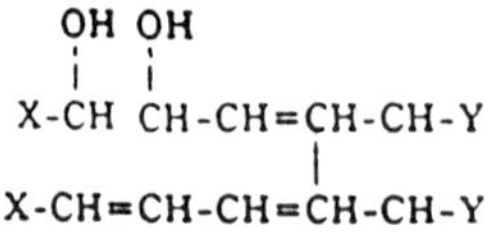 OH OH | | X-CH CH-CH=CH-CH-Y | X-CH=CH-CH=CH-CH-Y	Dehydroxydimer of Me-LN
Peak #2	602	8	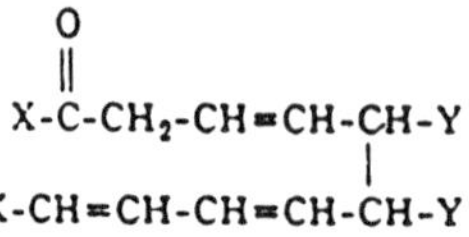 O || X-C-CH$_2$-CH=CH-CH-Y | X-CH=CH-CH=CH-CH-Y	Ketodehydrodimer of Me-LN
II. Peak #1	604	8	OH | X-CH-CH$_2$-CH=CH-CH-Y | X-CH=CH-CH=CH-CH-Y	Monohydrodimer of Me-LN
Peak #2	586	6	X-CH-CH=CH-CH=CH-Y | X-CH-CH=CH-CH=CH-Y	Dehydrodimer of Me-LN
III	588	6	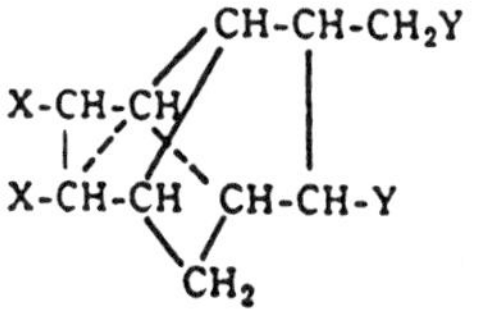	Tricyclic dimers of Me-LN
IV	566	6	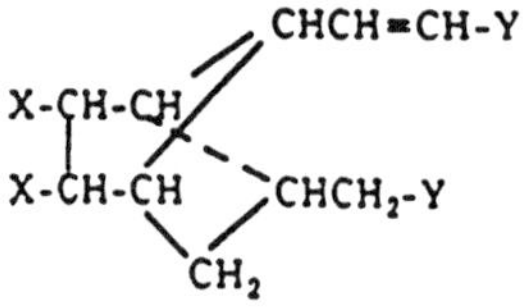	Bicyclic dimer of Me-LN
V. Peak #1	590	10	X-CH$_2$-CH=CH-CH-Y | X-CH$_2$-CH=CH-CH-Y	Dehydrodimer of Me-OL
Peak #2	588	4	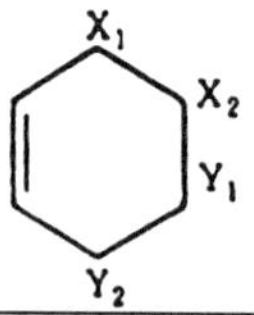	Thermal dimer of Me-LN

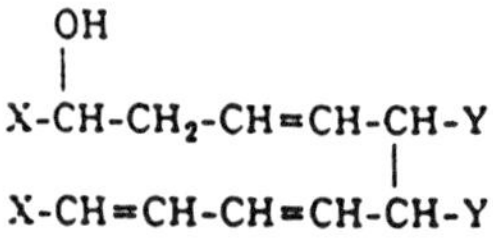

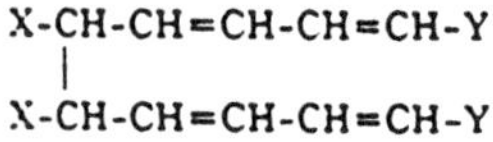

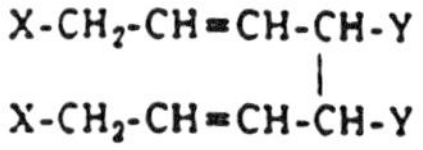

(a)

FIG. 7.8   (a) Structures of dimers. (b) HPLC separation of dimers.

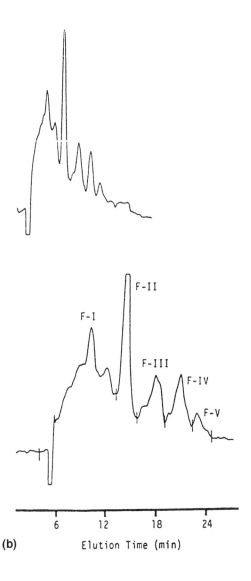

(b)   Elution Time (min)

of linolenic and linoleic acids with frying time (Qian and Perkins, 1991). In addition, the composition of frying oil and French fry components showed that there was a continuous increase in polar materials, polymers, and nonelutable components in both the used oil and in the French fries. There was no significant increase in the amount of oil absorbed by the fries during this study.

The volatile materials present in the frying oil were determined by placing 200 mg of oil from the fryer onto a small column of adsorbent (Chromasorb W) and inserting this into an external closed inlet device (ECID) unit which is connected to a cryogenic HRGC–mass spectrometer (Qian and Perkins, 1991). Volatile components of the frying oil were then eluted from the small column in the ECID and their composition determined. To study the volatile components in the French fries, a 200-g portion of French fries was placed into a chamber such that the volatiles in the headspace within the chamber were carried with purified nitrogen into an ECID cartridge containing Tenax GC to adsorb the volatiles. After a period of time for collection of the volatiles, this cartridge was placed into the ECID unit and then desorbed onto the capillary gas chromatograph column. The components were identified by gas chromatography and mass spectrometry (Qian, 1990). The total volatiles in the frying oil and in the French fries reached the maximum at about 70 hours frying time (Fig. 7.6). The hydrocarbons identified in the frying oil were hexene, hexane, heptane, decane, and nonane, all of which peaked at approximately 70 hours frying time. The major saturated aldehydes in frying oils—pentanal, hexanal, heptanal, octanal, and nonanal—peaked at around 60–70 hours frying time. The same saturated hydrocarbons and aldehydes were present in the French fries and also peaked at about the same time. Alkenals in frying oil and in French fries were 2-heptenal, 2-octenal, 2-nonenal, 2-decenal, and 2-undecenal. These and the alkyl dienals such as *trans,trans* 2,4-heptadienal, *trans,trans* 2,4-decadienal and *trans,cis* decadienals also had a peak formation time at about 70 hours. The content of alpha-pentylfuran in frying oil and French fries peaked at around 58 hours. Pyrazines in French fries cooked in this used oil were identified as methyl pyrazine and 2,5-dimethyl pyrazine. The maximum concentration of these compounds occurred at approximately 70–80 hours in the French fries. They were not present in the original frying oil because they result from interaction between the hot oil and French fries.

In summary, this study showed that the same components in approximately the same concentrations were present in both the frying oils and the corresponding fries at various times of usage of the oils. No evidence was found for the preferential uptake of oils or volatile material in the French fries with time. There also was no evidence for any preferential uptake of free fatty acids or polymeric or polar components with time by these fries. The French fries produced during this study were all of high quality in terms of texture, color, appearance, and flavor.

QUALITY EVALUATION OF FATS

A number of factors influence fat stability and the formation of lipid oxidation products. Increased unsaturation and increased frying time will all result in decreased oxidative stability. The type of food fried influences fat stability. For instance, when chicken is fried, the chicken fat renders into the deep frying medium and changes the fatty acid composition of the oil (Fig. 7.9). Frying fish also replaces some of the shortening fat by highly unsaturated fish oils, thereby influencing fat composition and stability. If both fish and chicken are batter-fried, then components of the batter will further

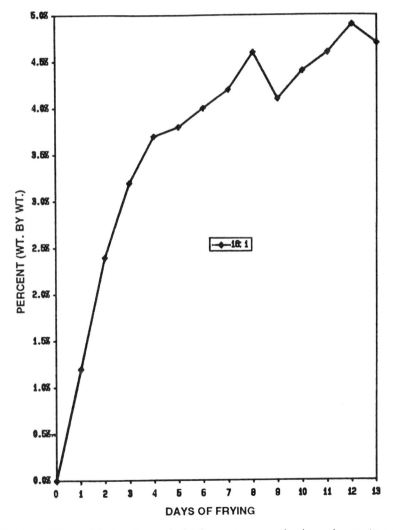

FIG. 7.9 Effect of frying floured chicken wings on the hexadecenoic acid content (% chicken fat) of the frying fat.

degrade the fat more quickly and decrease stability. Nonfat foods such as the potato in French fries will degrade fat stability because of increased aeration of the oil and the accumulation of small food particles that carbonize and, if left in the fat, result in faster deterioration.

The presence of silicones in a frying oil will cause decreased foaming and somewhat increased oil stability by yet unknown mechanisms. A more recent technique used to increase the frying life of an oil is treatment of the frying oil with "active" filtration media (Yates and Caldwell, 1991). Published data indicate that filtration of oils through certain active adsorbents will increase the useful frying life of an oil during actual fryer use by removal of colored materials (Fig. 7.10), free fatty acids, and other oxidation products (Yates and Caldwell, 1991).

QUALITY EVALUATION OF FATS

Quality evaluation of frying fats may be carried out in many ways. The first is sensory evaluation in which the flavor profile of the frying fat, as well as of the food product, is determined using standardized sensory testing. The texture of the product fried in the fat will also indicate the quality of the frying fat. The room odor, or the odor in the room where a deep fryer is used, may give an indication of the quality of the frying fat (Warner, 1985). Peroxide values are an indication of frying fat quality if they are used in a very specific way. Usually peroxides decompose at about 150°C. Therefore at frying temperatures, an accumulation of peroxides does not occur. Peroxide values usually are a measure of lipid oxidation at lower temperatures such as those used for storage of fats or a product. The relationship between storage time and peroxide value can then be used to measure quality.

Volatile profile analysis has been used to evaluate frying fats as well as the food product fried in them. More recently, however, volatiles such as hexanal, pentane, or hexane have been used to characterize the quality of a food product or its frying oil (Warner and Eskin, 1994). The Schall oven test involves simply putting a small amount of the fat into a beaker and placing it into an oven under standardized conditions at 60°C to oxidize the sample. Samples are then taken and peroxide values determined (AOCS, 1989).

Free fatty acids from frying fats can be determined by direct titration (AOCS, 1989). Other components such as soaps may be formed from the reaction of free fatty acids with metal salts present in the oil, but there does not seem to be any published evidence yet on the effect of soap formation upon the quality of the frying fat or the food product fried in it. Industrially, frying oil quality is usually checked quickly by measurement of color (AOCS, 1989) and/or free fatty acid. These tests allow an operator to

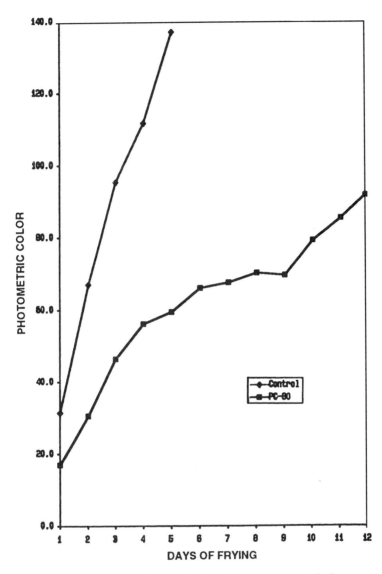

FIG. 7.10   Effects of treating fat used to fry chicken wings with diatomaceous earth (control) and magnesium silicate (Magnesol) on photometric color of the frying fat.

determine when a fat is ending its useful life. The foaming characteristics of the used fat will also lead one to the same conclusion. If one can't fry a food product because of unduly high foaming levels, the oil has ended its useful life.

There are many other tests available to check frying oil quality, all of which purport to tell the operator when to do something with the used fat— either filter it through active filters, discard it, or dilute it with a less degraded fat. Some tests that have been used to check frying oil quality are the saponification color index, 2,6-dichloroindole phenol color test, methylene blue color test, and iodine color scale. These tests allegedly determine when the fat has gone bad and can no longer produce a high-quality food product. For instance, the Rau test from E. Merck is a colorometric test kit containing redox indicators that react with total oxidized compounds in a sample. It has a four-color scale and is used for diagnoses of fat quality. The fourth color scale indicates that an oil is bad and should be discarded (Meyer, 1979). The polar materials quick test kits from Libra laboratories purport to relate the color of a test solution with the percent polar materials present in the fat and the oil quality (Blumental, 1988). Smith et al. (1986) surveyed 56 used shortenings and showed that the relationship of the food oil sensor (FOS) value, polar materials, free fatty acids, and nonelutables by GLC can be used to find ranges for these measurements, which can indicate when frying fats should be discarded. The fat examined was used for frying chicken and French fries. The mean values from the 56 samples that were tested were as follows: 16.4% polar materials vs. 2.5% for fresh fat; 0.76% free fatty acids vs. 0.05% for fresh fat; nonelutable components 6.1% vs. 0.7% in the fresh fat.

A quick colorometric test kit is available with a color scale to be used for measuring oil quality (Blumenthal et al., 1985). The fat is discarded at the highest color scale value. Robern and Gray (1981) developed a spot test to measure free fatty acids in which drops of used fat placed on glass covered with silica gel containing a pH indicator gave a three-color test scale—blue, green, and yellow. This scale can indicate the amount of free fatty acids in a sample prior to its discard. Another test kit for measurement of alkaline contaminant materials in used frying fats has been described by Blumenthal and Stockler (1986). A summary of results for 1800 used fats has been published by Begemann (1986), in which the free acids values, soap color index, smoke point, and any polar compounds present in the fats were estimated in the fresh fats vs. fats with no sensory change and a distinct sensory change vs. a bad fat. The bad fat had an acid value of 9.8 vs. 0.2 for the fresh fat, soap color index 32.5 vs. 0.1 for the fresh fat, smoke point 110 vs. 205°C for the fresh fat, and 64% polar components vs. less than 10% of the fresh fat.

POLAR COMPONENTS

The presence of polar components in a frying fat may be misleading. However, the determination of polar materials in frying fats is an official European method. This text involves separation of used fats into a polar and a nonpolar fraction via silica gel chromatography (Paquot and Hautfenne, 1987). However, the polar fraction contains not only polymeric and monomeric material but also free fatty acids and mono- and diglycerides. These are the major portion of such fractions, and their effects on frying oil and

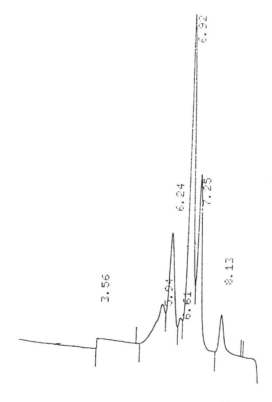

**Col: G2500HXL, THF 1 ml/min
Refractometry Detection**

FIG. 7.11   Separation of the polar fraction of a mixed media frying fat by size exclusion chromatography (monoglyceride at 8.13, diglyceride at 7.25, altered triglyceride at 6.92, dimeric diglyceride at 6.61, dimeric triglyceride at 6.24, and trimeric and oligerimeric glycerides at 5.95).

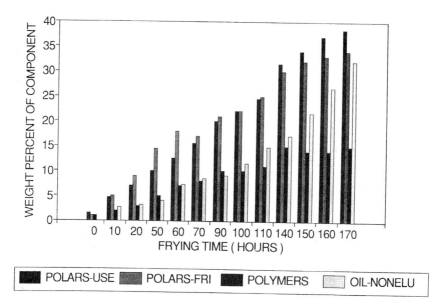

FIG. 7.12   Effect of frying on polar, polymeric, and nonelutable material.

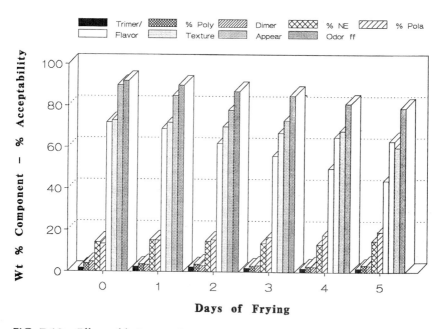

FIG. 7.13   Effect of frying on the sensory and lipid oxidation components of the frying fat.

food product quality are not understood. In Fig. 7.11 the HPSEC curve represents the polar fractions of a used oil at its midlife point. The oil was obtained from a mixed-menu frying operation. Monoglycerides, diglycerides, triglycerides, dimeric diglycerides, dimeric triglycerides, trimeric triglycerides, and oligomeric triglycerides are present. If this fat is analyzed for its nonpolar fraction using the method described above, one peak present is pure triglyceride. This is expected since the silica gel column was eluted with a 13% solution of either in hexane, which should only remove nonpolar or triglyceride material.

Consideration of days of frying vs. weight percent of the component formed during the mixed menu frying study indicates that only total polar material increases uniformly in concentration. The relationship between percent acceptability for flavor, texture, appearance, odor of the product, and weight percent of the component of trimer, percent polymer, percent dimer, percent nonelutables by gas chromatography, and the percent of polar components vs. days of frying in this mixed menu experiment is quite interesting (Fig. 7.12) (Perkins, 1989). Only the polar components increased linearly with days of frying. All of the parameters for flavor, texture, appearance, and odor of product decreased uniformly. Based upon the limited data available, however, the only parameter that correlates well with the sensory evaluation of the product is the percent of total polars formed as shown in Figure 7.13 (Perkins, 1989).

SUMMARY

The effect of lipid oxidation on food and oil quality during deep frying is wide-ranging. The type of food fried in the oil as well as the age of the oil and the conditions under which they are used will influence the quality of the food product. In order to obtain the maximum quality of food product, the oil should be maintained at its maximum quality so that the build-up of polymeric materials, free fatty acids, and color is held at a minimum.

REFERENCES

AOCS. 1989. *Official and Tentative Methods of the American Oil Chemists' Society*, 4th ed. AOCS Press, Champaign, IL.

Artman, N. R. 1969. In *Advances in Lipid Research*, R. Paoletti and D. Kritchevsky (Ed.), p. 245. Academic Press, New York.

Begemann, O. 1986. Erfahrungen in der Beurteilung gebrauchter Fritierfette. *Fette Seifen Anstr.* 88: 124–127.

Blumenthal, M. 1988. Rapid test for the determination of frying oils. *J. Am. Oil Chem. Soc.* 65: 482–483.

Blumenthal, M. Stocker, J., and Summers, P. J. 1985. Alkaline contaminant materials in used frying oils. A new quick test. *J. Am. Oil Chem. Soc.* 63: 687–688.

Christopoulou, C. N. and Perkins, E. G. 1989a. Dimer acids: Synthesis and mass spectrometry of the tetrahydroxy, dihydroxy, and diketo dimers of methyl stearate. *J. Am. Oil Chem. Soc.* 66: 1344–1352.

Christopoulou, C. N. and Perkins, E. G. 1989b. Chromatographic studies on fatty acid chromatography and thin-layer chromatography. *J. Am. Oil Chem. Soc.* 66: 1353–1359.

Christopoulou, C. N. and Perkins, E. G. 1989c. Isolation and characterization of dimers formed in used soybean oil. *J. Am. Oil Chem. Soc.* 66: 1360–1370.

Dupuy, H. P., Rayner, E. T., Wadsworth, J. I., and Legendre, M. C. 1977. Analysis of vegetable oils for flavor quality by direct gas chromatography. *J. Am. Oil Chem. Soc.* 54: 445–446.

Frankel, E. N. 1985. Chemistry of autoxidation: Mechanisms products and flavor significance. In *Flavor Chemistry of Lipid Foods*, D. B. Min and T. H. Smouse (Ed.), pp. 1–37. American Oil Chemists' Society, Champaign, IL.

Frankel, E. N. 1993. In search of better methods to evaluate natural autoxidation and oxidative stability in food lipids. *Trends Food Sci. Technol.* 4: 220–224.

Hinshaw, J. V. 1990. Reader response. Purge-and-trap systems and detectors. *LC-GC* 8: 520–522.

Ioffe, B. V. and Vitenberg, A. G. 1989. In *Headspace Analysis and Related Methods in Gas Chromatography*, p. 9. John Wiley and Son, New York.

Meyer, H. 1979. Eine neue und einfache Schnellmethode zur Erfassung des Oxidationzersetzurgsgrade thermisch belasteter Fett. *Fette Seifen Anstr.* 81: 524–533.

Murray, K. E. 1977. Concentration of headspace, airborne and aqueous volatiles on chromosorb 105 for examination by gas chromatography and gas chromatography-mass spectrometry. *J. Chromatogr.* 135: 49–60.

Noor, N. and Augustin, M. A. 1984. Effectiveness of antioxidants on the stability of banana chips. *J. Sci. Food Agric.* 35: 805–812.

Nunez, A. J., Gonzales, L. F., and Janak, J. 1984. Preconcentration of headspace volatiles for trace organic analysis by gas chromatography. *J. Chromatogr.* 300: 127–162.

Paquot, C. and Hautfenne, A. 1987. *Standard Methods for the Analysis of Oils, Fats and Derivatives*. Blackwell Scientific Publications, Palo Alto, CA.

Perkins, E. G. 1989. In *Flavor Chemistry of Lipid Foods*, D. B. Min and T. H.

Souse (Ed.), pp. 35–57. AOCS Press, American Oil Chemists' Society, Champaign, IL.

Perkins, E. G. 1992. The effects of lipid oxidation on oil and food quality in deep frying. In *Lipid Oxidation in Food*, A. J. St. Angelo (Ed.), ACS Symposium Series 500. American Chemical Society, Washington, DC, pp. 310–322.

Perkins, E. G., Qian, C., Caldwell, J. D., and Yates, R. A. 1989. Applications of high performance size exclusion chromatography (HPSEC) to the analysis of used fats. *J. Am. Oil Chem. Soc.* 66: 483.

Pokorny, J. 1989. Flavor chemistry of deep frying in oil. In *Flavor Chemistry of Lipid Foods*, D. B. Min and T. H. Smouse (Ed.), p. 1, AOCS Press, American Oil Chemists' Society, Champaign, IL.

Porter, N. A., Caldwell, S. E., and Mills, K. A. 1995. Mechanisms of free radical oxidation of unsaturated lipids. *Lipids* 30: 277–290.

Qian, C. 1990. Characterization of deep fried flavor: A preliminary study using French fries. M.S. thesis, University of Illinois, Urbana.

Qian, C. and Perkins, E. G. 1991. Characterization of deep fat frying flavor. *Inform* 2: 323.

Robern, H. and Grey, L. 1981. A colorimetric spot test for heated oils. *Can. Inst. Food Sci. Technol.* 14: 150–152.

Rojo, J. A. and Perkins, E. G. 1989. Cyclic fatty acid monomer: Isolation and purification with solid phase extraction. *J. Am. Oil Chem. Soc.* 66: 1593–1598.

Scholz, R. G. and Ptak, L. R. 1966. Chromatographic method for measuring rancidity in vegetable oils. *J. Am. Oil Chem. Soc.* 43: 596–599.

Sebedio, J. L., LeQuere, J. L., Semon, E., Morin, O., Prevost, J., and Grandgirard, A. 1987b. Heat treatment of vegetable oils. II. GC-MS and GC-FTIR spectra of some isolated cyclic fatty acids monomers. *J. Am. Oil Chem. Soc.* 64: 1324–1333.

Sebedio, J. L. and Perkins, E. G. (Ed.). 1995. *New Trends in Lipid and Lipoprotein Analyses*. AOCS Press, American Oil Chemists' Society, Champaign, IL.

Sebedio, J. L., Prevost, J., and Grandgirard, A. 1987a. Heat treatment of vegetable oils. I. Isolation of the cyclic fatty acids monomers from heated sunflower and linseed oils. *J. Am. Oil Chem. Soc.* 66: 1026–1032.

Shukla, V. K. S. and Perkins, E. G. 1991. The presence of oxidative polymeric materials in encapsulated fish oils. *Lipids* 26: 23–26.

Smith, L. M., Cliford, A. J., Hamblin, C. L., and Creveling, R. K. 1986. Changes in physical and chemical properties of shortenings used for commercial deep fat frying. *J. Am. Oil Chem. Soc.* 63: 1017–1023.

Taubold, R., Hsieh, A., and Perkins, E. G. 1973. Analysis of polymers in fats and oils. *J. Am. Oil Chem. Soc.* 50: 96–100.

Waltking, A. E. and Goetz, A. G. 1983. Instrumental determination of flavor stability of fatty foods and its correlation with sensory flavor responses. *CRC Crit. Rev. Food Sci. Nutr.* 19: 99–100.

Waltking, A. E., Seery, W. E., and Bleffert, G. W. 1975. Chemical analysis of polymerization products in abused fats and oils. *J. Am. Oil Chem. Soc.* 52: 96.

Warner, K. 1985. Sensory evaluation of flavor quality of fats and oils. In *Flavor Chemistry of Fats and Oils*, D. B. Min and T. H. Smouse (Ed.). AOCS Press, American Oil Chemists' Society, Champaign, IL.

Warner, K. and Eskin, M. (Ed.). 1994. *Methods to Assess Quality and Stability of Oils and Fat-Containing Foods*, pp. 118, 121. AOCS Press, American Oil Chemists' Society, Champaign, IL.

Warner, K. and Frankel, E. N. 1985. Flavor stability of soybean oil based on induction periods for the formation of volatile compounds by gas chromatography. *J. Am. Oil Chem. Soc.* 62: 100–110.

Yates, R. A. and Caldwell, J. D. 1991. Evaluation of used oil adsorbent materials by saturation. *Inform* 2:323.

8
Trans Fatty Acids: Labeling, Nutrition, and Analysis

Richard E. McDonald

National Center for Food Safety and Technology
Food and Drug Administration
Summit-Argo, Illinois

Magdi M. Mossoba

Food and Drug Administration
Washington, D.C.

INTRODUCTION

Hydrogenated triglycerides have been a major source of dietary fat throughout the world for over 60 years. Although natural oils contain relatively simple mixtures of *cis* fatty acids, catalytic hydrogenation can form over 50% *trans* geometric isomers. In addition, as hydrogenation proceeds, the double bonds of both *cis* and *trans* isomers move up and down the fatty acid chain. This can produce many isomers in polyunsaturated vegetable oils with the resulting fatty acid isomer mixture so complex that complete quantitation of all fatty acid isomers in partially hydrogenated oils is very difficult.

During commercial hydrogenation, liquid oil is converted into a semisolid or plastic fat that is used to manufacture margarine and shortening. This process is also used to selectively hydrogenate polyunsaturated fatty acids to improve the oxidative stability. Heated oil is exposed to hydrogen at pressures up to 60 psig in the presence of a finely divided nickel catalyst.

This mixture is agitated to disperse the hydrogen into the oil and achieve uniform mixing of the catalyst and oil. The process of hydrogenation has been extensively studied since it was first used to generate edible shortening and margarine. Hydrogenation chemistry including mechanisms and cata-lysts' effects as well as hydrogenation process design has been extensively reviewed (Patterson, 1983; Hastert, 1987). The nutritional implications of hydrogenated oils have also been extensively reviewed (Perkins and Visek, 1983; Emken, 1984; Hunter and Applewhite, 1986; Kanhai, 1988; Enig, 1993; Applewhite, 1994; Kris-Etherton, 1995).

Reports of lipid nutrition studies have received a great deal of media attention, and there have been several requests for the Food and Drug Administration (FDA) to require mandatory labeling of *trans* fatty acids on food products and strict limitations of these isomers in the U.S. diet (Enig, 1993; Willet and Ascherio, 1994). The FDA is now reviewing the labeling of *trans* fatty acids in the light of recent scientific evidence. Nutritional as well as analytical issues should be involved in this review. Some of the food-labeling issues, nutritional considerations, and analytical methods for *trans* fatty acid isomers will be highlighted in this chapter.

LABELING *TRANS* FATTY ACIDS

The Nutritional Labeling and Education Act (NLEA) regulations do not allow labeling of *trans* fatty acid content. The details of the regulations can be found in Title 21, section 101.9, of the Code of Federal Regulations. An overview of some of the unresolved issues concerning *trans* fatty acids was given by Haumann (1995). The FDA has received numerous comments on all sides of the issue concerning the labeling of *trans* fatty acids (Anony-mous, 1995a, b).

The mandatory components of the food label include total fat, saturated fat, and calories from fat. Declaration of total fat may be omitted when the food contains 0.5 g or less per serving size (reference amount customarily consumed). The voluntary parts of the food label include calories from saturated fat, total polyunsaturated fat, and total monounsaturated fat. Only the components specifically listed in the regulations are allowed on the label. This excludes *trans* fatty acids. Although *trans* fatty acids must be included in the calculation for total fat, they *cannot* be included in the calculation for saturated fat, monounsaturated fat, or polyunsaturated fat. This has caused confusion for some consumers, who have contacted the agency to inquire why the sum of the saturated, monounsaturated, and polyunsaturated fatty acids does not equal 100% for many food products.

The NLEA allows several claims on the food label that are related to the total fat and saturated fat content. The claims related to fat content include terms such as *Fat Free, Low in Fat,* and *Reduced Fat,* which have specific fat-content restrictions on their use. For example, a label may contain the *Fat Free* claim if the food product contains less than 0.5 g of fat per labeled serving size. The claims related to saturated fat content include terms such as *Saturated Fat Free, Low in Saturated Fat,* and *Reduced Saturated Fat.* These claims have specific requirements for maximum content of saturated fat as well as other restrictions regarding their use. For example, a label may contain the *Saturated Fat Free* claim if the food product contains less than 0.5 g of saturated fat and less than 0.5 g of *trans* fatty acids per labeled serving size. This is the only situation for which the *trans* fatty acid content is specified by the NLEA. There are no requirements of maximum *trans* fatty acid content for claims of *Low in Saturated Fat* or *Reduced Saturated Fat.* The agency has received some complaints that food companies have reduced the saturated fat content and increased the *trans* fatty acid content of some food products in order to make claims related to saturated fat content.

The FDA is currently considering several options regarding labeling issues for *trans* fatty acids. The desire for harmonization with food-labeling regulations of other countries will be an important factor in the decision-making process. The final decision is made more difficult by a lack of consensus in the scientific community regarding the possible effects of dietary *trans* fatty acids on atherosclerosis. Also, as has been highlighted in previous chapters of this book, the dietary fatty acid profile may also play a role in other aspects of health and nutrition including cancer, immune response, and bone health.

NUTRITIONAL CONSIDERATIONS

The nutritional implications of hydrogenated oils have been debated in the literature for several years. In 1985, the FDA commissioned a study by the Federation of American Societies for Experimental Biology (FASEB) to review the literature on the toxicological, physiological, and nutritional effects of *trans* fatty acids. The FASEB panel issued a report (Senti, 1985) that summarized current information and made several recommendations for more research in this area. The ad hoc panel concluded that the available scientific information suggested little reason for concern with the safety of dietary *trans* fatty acids. However, the report did recommend further research to better define the physiological properties of the isomeric fatty acids in partially hydrogenated vegetable oils. These recommendations included conducting additional studies on the isomeric fatty acid composition of the adipose tissues of humans to provide an improved database for relating adipose tissue composition to dietary intake of fatty acids and their isomers. The panel also recommended conducting additional studies on the accumulation of specific geometric and positional isomers in human tissue as well as conducting additional studies to determine the cholesterolemic and tumor-promoting effects of these isomers. Lastly, the panel recommended that studies be conducted to determine the effect of the major dietary geometric and positional fatty acid isomers in hydrogenated vegetable oils on the modulation of immune function.

Since the FASEB report on *trans* fatty acids was issued, additional reviews have concluded that hydrogenated vegetable oils do not pose a health threat. Kanhai (1988) concluded that the *trans* isomers in processed vegetable oils do not exhibit any unique negative biological qualities in humans and animals when adequate essential fatty acid levels are present in the diet. Applewhite (1994) concluded that there was no reliable evidence of nutritional problems resulting from consumption of partially hydrogenated fat by humans who maintained a balanced diet that contained adequate levels of linoleic acid.

There is some evidence that dietary *trans* fatty acids, like most saturated fatty acids, raise levels of blood cholesterol (Mensink and Katan, 1990; Zock and Katan, 1992; Nestel et al., 1992; Judd et al., 1994) and lipoprotein(a) (Nestel et al., 1992; Mensink et al., 1992). However, a recent study (Clevidence et al., 1995) reported no effect of *trans* fatty acid content on lipoprotein (a) levels. Other researchers have warned of the health risk of consuming *trans* fatty acids, citing epidemiological studies that have reported positive associations between intake of *trans* fatty acids and coronary heart disease (Willet et al., 1993; Ascherio et al., 1994). However, after reviewing epidemiological data, Shapiro (1995) found no association between *trans* fatty acids and coronary heart disease.

A summary report of an expert panel convened by the International Life Sciences Institute concluded that foods containing partially hydrogenated fats are good substitutes for traditional fats rich in saturated fat but are not good substitutes for unhydrogenated vegetable oils (Kris-Etherton, 1995). The report also concluded that the overall effect of hydrogenated fat on serum cholesterol levels depends on the net consumption change of saturated, *trans* and *cis* monounsaturated, and *cis* polyunsaturated fatty acids. More research was recommended to better determine the effects of *trans* fatty acids on serum lipid concentrations and coronary heart disease.

Several studies have shown that dietary fatty acids are incorporated into organ lipids. Astorg and Chevalier (1987) showed that dietary elaidic acid changed the polyunsaturated fatty acid profiles of rat heart phosphatidyl choline and phosphatidylethanolamine, resulting in an inhibition of the biosyntheses of polyunsaturated fatty acids. Other studies (Ren et al., 1988;

Alam et al., 1989) indicate that some membrane-associated cardiac enzymes had reduced activity when rats were fed a diet that included 20% partially hydrogenated soybean oil (PHSBO). Ostlund-Lindquist et al. (1985) also showed that dietary *trans* fatty acids have an effect on membrane enzymes. The study indicated that the mutagenicities of 2-aminofluorene and afla-toxin B_1 were significantly lower in a microsomal liver fraction from rats fed a diet containing 36.6% *trans* fatty acids than in a microsomal liver fraction from rats fed a control diet. Beyers and Emken (1991) showed that different *trans* diene isomers are metabolized differently. The double bond configu-ration of linoleic acid isomers had a major effect on desaturase, elongase, and acyltransferase activities. They suggested that the *cis,trans* 18:2 isomers have biological importance because the *cis,trans* 20:4 metabolites may affect prostaglandin metabolism or be converted to a biologically active prosta-glandin or leukotriene isomer. An evaluation of the nutritional effects of these isomers is difficult since there are many possible geometric and positional fatty acid isomers in processed oils. The nutritional effects of most *trans* diene isomers have not been determined.

Decsi and Koletzko (1995) recently found evidence that *trans* fatty acids are inhibitors of arachidonic acid biosynthesis in healthy children. They rec-ommended limiting dietary *trans* fatty acid intake during childhood since long-chain polyunsaturated fatty acid synthesis is critical during growth.

A two-year Norwegian study (Opstvedt et al., 1988; Pettersen and Opst-vedt, 1988) studied the effect of dietary *trans* fatty acids from PHSBO and partially hydrogenated fish oil (PHFO) on the pre- and postnatal develop-ment of pigs. They reported little effect of PHSBO and PHFO on growth, nervous tissue composition/function, organ weights, and teratogenicity. Fertility was somewhat impaired in pigs on the PHFO diet, although the results were inconclusive. The incorporation of *trans* isomers into organ lipids was highly organ-specific, with none being incorporated into brain phospholipids and only low levels incorporated into heart phosphatidyl-ethanolamine (PE). PHSBO and PHFO increased the levels of 18:2 (n-6) in heart PE and total serum lipids, whereas PHFO also slightly increased the amounts of 20:3 (n-6), 18:3 (n-3), and 20:5 (n-3). A more recent study in Norway by Almendingen et al. (1995) indicated that consumption of PHFO can unfavorably affect lipid risk indicators, such as raising LDL cholesterol and lowering HDL cholesterol. The effects of PHSBO on cholesterol levels were much less significant than the effects of both PHFO and butterfat.

Cyclic fatty acid monomers (CFAMs) that contain *trans* double bonds may be formed when unsaturated oils are heated above 150°C, as occurs during frying. The use of unsaturated oils during food-processing opera-tions such as deep-fat frying has become more prevalent recently as a result of the bad publicity associated with tropical oils and *trans* fatty acids. These unsaturated oils are more susceptible to oxidation during processing and can form several lipid oxidation products including cyclic fatty acid monomers (CFAMs). CFAMs are of interest because they can occur in frying oils at levels up to 0.5%, they are readily absorbed by the digestive system, and their toxicity has not been extensively studied. Sebedio and Grandgirard (1989) reviewed the formation and biological effects of these isomers. CFAMs from heated oil at concentrations as low as 0.15% in rat diets have been shown to cause enlarged livers (Iwaoka and Perkins, 1976). A CFAM from heated linseed oil at a level of 0.1% showed characteristics of inducing hepatic drug-metabolizing enzymes (Siess et al., 1988).

TRANS ISOMERS IN COMMERCIAL PRODUCTS

The main source of fatty acid isomers, including *trans* fatty acids, in the U.S. diet is the partially hydrogenated vegetable oil used to make margarine and shortening. Because the fatty acid isomer composition of commercial sources tends to vary, a disagreement over consumption patterns of *trans* fatty acids has contributed to a debate concerning the level of *trans* fatty acids consumed by the American public. Intake estimates have ranged from a low of 3 g of *trans* fatty acids per capita to over 12 g per day (Hunter and Applewhite, 1986). Enig et al. (1990) proposed a much wider consumption range of 1.6–38.6 g *trans* fatty acids per day. The per capita daily average intake of *trans* fatty acids was estimated to be about 13 g. However, Hunter and Applewhite (1991) and Applewhite (1994) have disagreed with these estimates, claiming that they are too high because they were based on "questionable composition and consumption data" and that the 1989 average consumption of *trans* fatty acids in the U.S. diet was actually about 8 g per person per day. Enig (1993), in a review of *trans* nutrition and consumption, states that the levels of *trans* fatty acids in many diets are too high and that the consumption of these *trans* fatty acids may have "numerous" undesirable effects.

Sahasrabudhe and Kurian (1979) conducted a survey to determine the fatty acid composition of margarines available to consumers in Canada. Of 95 margarine brands analyzed by packed column gas chromatography (GC), 45 had *trans* fatty acid concentrations between 27.2 and 32.8%. The total *trans* content of these margarines ranged from about 8 to 34%. Virtually all products contained less than 5% *trans* dienes, although two margarines were reported to contain 3% *trans*-9,*trans*-12 18:2 diene. This latter observation was refuted by Marchand and Beare-Rogers (1982), who showed that the GC peak previously identified as the *trans*-9,*trans*-12 18:2 isomer also contained the *cis*,*trans* 18:2 and *cis* 18:1 isomers. The concentration of the *trans*-9,*trans*-12 18:2 isomer was less than 0.5%.

The results of fatty acid profile surveys (Enig, 1983; Enig et al., 1990; Ratnayake et al., 1993; Dickey and Caughman, 1995) show that similar food products can contain significantly different *trans* fatty acid concentrations. This finding indicates that foods with dramatically different fatty acid iso-mer profiles can be produced through the choice of ingredients used by food processors. One way to eliminate *trans* fatty acids from hydrogenated products would be to interesterify a mixture of completely hydrogenated vegetable oil with unhydrogenated oil. This procedure may have been used commercially in West Germany, where Heckers and Melcher (1978) con-ducted a study showing that many margarines, shortenings, and cooking fats were essentially free of *trans* fatty acids. List et al. (1995) described a pilot plant process using interesterification of soybean oil-soybean trisaturate blends to produce margarines containing no *trans* fatty acids.

The 1985 FASEB review panel (Senti, 1985) recommended that the fatty acid double bond position, as well as the double bond configuration, be considered during review of the nutritional properties of hydrogenated products. Marchand (1982) determined the positional distribution of the double bonds of *trans*-octadecenoic acids in Canadian margarines. The double bond position ranged from the n-4 to the n-14 position, with most of the isomers at the n-8, n-9, and n-10 positions. It is interesting that different brands of margarines made from the same oil raw materials had significantly different double bond patterns. The different pattern of positional isomers observed in this study was most likely a result of different hydrogenation conditions used by oil processors.

Slover et al. (1985) determined the lipid composition of over 90 commer-cial margarine products in the United States. The total amount of *trans* isomers in these products varied from about 10 to 30%. In general, the tub margarines contained lower levels of *trans* fatty acid isomers than did the stick margarines. The *trans* positional isomers were fairly evenly distributed throughout the fatty acid chain, whereas the *cis* positional isomers were concentrated at the n-9 and n-10 positions. The diene content of the margarines varied greatly, and all dienes were reported to be 9,12-18:2 isomers. Perkins and Smick (1987) determined the *trans* triene isomer content of PHSBO produced for use as salad and cooking oil. Three major *trans* triene isomers accounted for 1.2% of the total fatty acids in PHSBO.

EFFECT OF PROCESSING ON THE FORMATION OF FATTY ACID ISOMERS

There are several explanations for the wide variability of the *trans* isomer content of commercial shortening and margarines. One major factor in-volves the choice of ingredients used by food processors. The practice of blending hydrogenated and unhydrogenated oils to achieve a desirable melting point and functionality has helped to increase the levels of polyunsaturated fatty acids in margarine while decreasing the level of *trans* fatty acids in these margarines. Another major factor that determines *trans* fatty acid compositions and levels in commercial products is the reaction conditions employed during the hydrogenation process. Selectivity is a term used to describe hydrogenation conditions. When nonselective hydrogenation conditions are used, all fatty acid double bonds are hydrogenated at a similar rate. For example, oleic acid (C18:1) is hydrogenated to stearic acid (C18:0) at about the same rate that linoleic acid (C18:2) is hydrogenated to oleic acid. These nonselective conditions produce low concentrations of *trans* fatty acids but also significant amounts of stearic acid. The high melting point of stearic acid results in margarine with a waxy mouthfeel.

When selective hydrogenation conditions are used, fatty acids containing more than one double bond are hydrogenated first and very little stearic acid is formed. Selective conditions are achieved by limiting the amount of hydrogen present at the oil/catalyst interface. This can be accomplished during hydrogenation by increasing the processing temperature, reducing the agitation rate, reducing the hydrogen pressure, and increasing the catalyst concentration. Because the agitation rate is fixed and the amount of catalyst is limited for economic reasons, the major process variables in commercial hydrogenation are temperature and hydrogen pressure. Selective conditions can dramatically increase the level of *trans* and positional isomers in hydrogenated oils. From the aspect of functionality the formation of *trans* fatty acids is desirable because the melting point of these isomers is close to body temperature. Detailed discussions of hydrogenation processing including mechanisms, kinetics, and catalysts' effects are available from several sources (Dutton, 1979; Allen, 1987; Albright, 1987). Nickel-based catalysts are virtually the only catalysts used commercially to hydrogenate vegetable oils. A review of the research that has been conducted using catalysts such as platinum, palladium, and copper chromate was presented by Mounts (1987).

Catalyst poisons have a dramatic effect on the reaction as well as the level and profile of the fatty acid isomers in hydrogenated oil. Catalyst poisons may be minor components of natural fats and oils or may be introduced during processing. These impurities may include organic compounds not removed during oil refining that contain sulfur (S), nitrogen (N), phosphorus (P), or chlorine (Cl). Klimmek (1984) determined the effect of various impurities on the activity of nickel catalysts during fatty acid hydrogenation. The "impurities" investigated included 5-sulfosalicylic acid, hexachlorocyclohexane, lecithin, and *l*-leucine. All these compounds increased catalyst consumption and decreased hydrogenation efficiency. The sulfur and chlorine impurities were the most potent inhibitors of hydrogenation.

The most common catalyst poison is sulfur, which is present in compounds such as hydrogen sulfide, carbon disulfide, and sulfur dioxide. Released sulfur irreversibly reacts with nickel catalyst and occupies sites in the catalyst that would normally be available for hydrogen dissociation. For some applications vegetable oil processors desire a high level of geometric isomerization. These applications include the manufacture of coating fats and vegetable creamers from low-priced oils and the partial hydrogenation of polyunsaturated oils into "hard" margarine-based blending stock. Sulfided nickel catalysts that promote the formation of significantly higher ratios of *trans* to *cis* isomers during hydrogenation of polyunsaturated fatty acids are commercially available for these applications. In one study, up to 10.6% *cis,trans* dienes and 5% *trans,trans* dienes were formed in the presence of a sulfur-containing nickel catalyst (McDonald and Armstrong, 1986).

HYDROGENATED FISH OIL

In Western European and other countries, partially hydrogenated fish oil is used in margarine and other products. Menhaden oil is a fish oil that contains high concentrations of long-chain omega-3 polyunsaturated fatty acids. Although highly hydrogenated menhaden oil has been approved for use in the United States, it has not yet had widespread use in this country.

Menhaden oil can be hydrogenated to produce a fat that has a melting point and mouthfeel similar to those of butter. The chain length of menhaden oil fatty acids varies widely, from 14 to 22 carbons. These fatty acids are very susceptible to oxidation since a large percentage of them are polyunsaturated with five or six double bonds. Therefore, hydrogenation under selective conditions to eliminate the polyunsaturated fatty acids is essential to stabilize the oil. When menhaden oil is selectively hydrogenated, more isomers by at least one order of magnitude are formed than when vegetable oil is hydrogenated because refined menhaden oil contains 20–30% 5,8,11,14,17-eicosapentaenoic acid (EPA) and 4,7,10,13,16,19-docosahexaenoic acid (DHA). So many isomers are produced that some scientists question whether all the isomers in hydrogenated fish oil will ever be identified (Ackman, 1982).

Compositional analysis of hydrogenated fish oil has emphasized the determination of general trends and major structural elements that can be used to evaluate processing, stability, and nutrition factors. Sebedio and Ackman (1983a, b) conducted an extensive analytical study of hydrogenated menhaden oil. The most unsaturated isomers were eliminated at an iodine value of 84.5, although 13.1% diene, 8.3% triene, and 0.4% tetraene isomers still remained in this oil. The 20-carbon monoene, diene, and triene isomers were analyzed further to determine the *cis* and *trans* bond positions. A wide range of monoene, diene, and triene positional isomers were formed. Both *cis* and *trans* double bonds were identified at virtually every position of the fatty acid chain. These results indicate that there are potentially many individual fatty acid isomers present in hydrogenated fish oil. In the past there was concern that high levels of 22:1 isomers would be formed from the hydrogenation of DHA in fish oil. Rapeseed oil containing high levels of erucic acid [C22:1 (n-9)] was reported to be cardiopathogenic in male rats (Kramer et al., 1979). Although the relevance of these results to humans has been disputed, the level of erucic acid in edible oils has been limited to less than 5% in European markets. In the case of fish oil there seems to be little reason for concern, since erucic acid is only a minor component of raw fish oil (Ackman, 1982) and hydrogenated fish oil contains low concentrations of 22:1 isomers.

ANALYSIS OF HYDROGENATED OILS FOR FATTY ACID ISOMERS

The identification and quantitation of the many isomers in hydrogenated oils have provided analytical chemists with a real challenge. There have been several reviews of techniques used to identify and quantitate fatty acids (Scholfield, 1979; Perkins, 1991; Christie, 1992, 1993).

Infrared Spectroscopy

The oldest and still the most common technique for determining *trans* unsaturation is infrared spectroscopy (IR). The strong absorption band at about 965 cm^{-1} arising from the C-H deformation about a *trans* double bond is still used, according to the American Oil Chemists' Society (AOCS) Method Cd 14-95, to determine the total *trans* isomer content of hydrogenated oils. However, there are several disadvantages to using the current AOCS official IR method, including (1) the need to make methyl ester derivatives, (2) the use of the toxic and volatile carbon disulfide, (3) a high bias when triacylglycerols are determined, and (4) low sensitivity and accuracy of determinations when *trans* levels are low. There has, therefore, been a great deal of interest in improving this method. Mossoba and McDonald (1995) described an improved IR method that uses a Fourier transform infrared spectrometer equipped with an attenuated total reflectance (ATR) cell. A horizontal background was obtained by ratioing the single beam spectrum of the test material against that of the unhydrogenated refined oil.

This method eliminated the use of solvents and increased *trans* sensitivity while allowing the analysis to be carried out on neat analytes with little or no sample preparation. The minimum identifiable *trans* level was 0.2%.

Gas Chromatography

Gas chromatography (GC) using packed or capillary columns is very effective in the analysis of complex fatty acid mixtures. The separation efficiency of capillary GC columns is far superior to that of packed columns. A comparison of Figures 8.1 and 8.2 shows that many more individual *trans* isomers can be separately by capillary GC than by packed columns. However, packed columns can still be used for some applications. Gildenberg and Firestone (1985) reported the results of a collaborative study, which showed that GC analysis using an OV-275–packed column was as effective as IR in quantitating total *trans* unsaturation. McDonald et al. (1989) obtained similar results (Table 8.1) for total *trans* monoenes and dienes when both packed and capillary GC methods were used. These results indicate that, although capillary GC is far superior in separating individual isomers, packed columns can still be used to monitor the total *trans* monoene and diene content of hydrogenated oils. However, because of the better resolution provided by capillary columns, most laboratories now use them to separate the complex fatty acid mixtures found in hydrogenated oils. Slover et al. (1985) used a 100-m capillary column to quantitate most of the *cis* and *trans* monoene positional isomers in margarine. Some of the monoene isomers were not separated, and the *trans* diene positional isomers were not identified.

Even with the incredible separation power of long capillary columns, some *cis* and *trans* positional isomers overlap, making the direct quantitation of these isomers impossible by GC alone (Ratnayake and Beare-Rogers, 1990; Wolff, 1994; Adlof et al., 1995). It is therefore necessary to combine GC with other techniques to determine an accurate fatty acid profile of hydrogenated oils. Ackman (1991) describes some of the problems of using GC for qualitative and quantitative analysis of hydrogenated oils. Wolff (1994) used equivalent chain length (ECL) data to show that the *cis*-11 20:1 fatty acid coelutes with *trans* triene isomers when rapeseed oil is analyzed by GC at oven temperatures above 160°C. Christie (1988a) reviewed the use of ECL to identify fatty acid isomers on GC columns.

Ratnayake et al. (1990) described a combined GC and IR method to determine *cis* and *trans* fatty acid monoenes that coelute on GC columns. A collaborative study of this method was completed (Ratnayake, 1995), and the method was adopted as an AOAC Official Method (994.14). First the total *trans* content of the oil is determined by IR. The weight percentages of

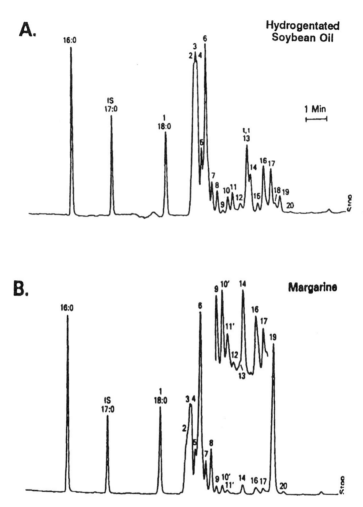

FIG. 8.1 Partial capillary gas chromatogram of the fatty acid methyl esters for (A) hydrogenated soybean oil (Ni-S catalyst) and (B) margarine. Column: CP-Sil 88, 50 m × 0.22 mm. Insert shows a 10× blowup of the flame ionization detector response for several diene peaks. Peak identification: 1 = 18:0; 2–5 = *trans* monoenes; 6–9 = *cis* monoenes; 10–17 = *trans* dienes (see Table 3); 18–20 = *cis* dienes; 21 = *cis* triene. (*From Mossoba et al., 1990.*)

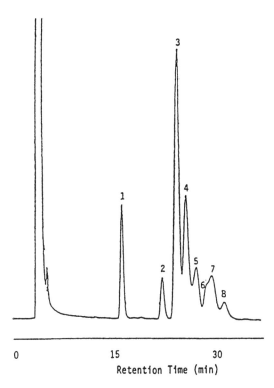

FIG. 8.2   Packed column gas chromatogram of the fatty acid methyl esters of hydrogenated soybean oil (Ni-S catalyst). Column: OV-275, 6.1 m × 2 mm i.d. stainless steel. Peak identification: 1 = 16:0; 2 = 18:0; 3 = *trans* monoene; 4 = *cis* monoene; 5–7 = *trans* dienes; 8 = *cis* diene. (*From McDonald et al., 1989.*)

all the *trans* diene (18:2t and 18:2tt) and triene (18:3t) isomers are then determined by GC using a highly polar 50 or 100 m capillary column. The weight percentage of *trans* monoenes (18:1t) is then determined by the following formula with the appropriate correction factors (0.84, 1.74):

IR *trans* = %18:1t + (0.84 × %18:2t) + (1.74 × %18:2tt) + (0.84 × %18:3t)

After calculation of the *trans* monoenes using this formula, the *cis* monoenes are determined by calculating the difference between the total monoenes determined by GC and the *trans* monoenes.

Although it provides useful information concerning the isomer composition of hydrogenated oils, GC is not very useful for identifying positional

TABLE 8.1   *Trans* Isomer Content of
Hydrogenated Soybean Oil Obtained Using
Capillary and Packed GC Columns

	Composition (%)	
Isomer	Capillary	Packed column
trans Monoenes	38.8	38.9
cis-9,*trans*-12 18:2	4.6	—
trans-9,*cis*-12 18:2	4.7	—
Other *cis*,*trans* 18:2	7.0	13.6[a]
trans-9,*trans*-12 18:2	6.2	9.5[b]
Total *trans*	61.3	62.0
Total *trans* dienes	22.5	23.1

[a]Includes *cis*-9,*trans*-12 and *trans*-9,*cis*-12 18:2 and other
trans dienes.
[b]Includes other *trans* dienes.
Source: McDonald et al., 1989.

fatty acid isomers. The most common method of determining the position
of the double bond in fatty acid isomers has involved splitting the fatty acid
chain at the position of unsaturation by using ozonolysis and oxidative
cleavage to form esters, diesters and other fragments. The fragmentation
pattern is dependent on the conditions used and the position of the double
bond in the fatty acid isomers. The fragments are identified by using GC.
Ozonolysis has been used most often to determine the double bond position in monoenes (Marchand and Beare-Rogers, 1982; Smallbone and
Sahasrabudhe, 1985) but has also been applied to the identification of
diene isomers (Johnston et al., 1978; Dutton et al., 1988). The calculation of
the results of ozonolysis can involve computer solutions of several simultaneous equations as proposed by Dutton et al. (1988).

Carbon-13 Nuclear Magnetic Resonance Spectrometry

The use of high-resolution nuclear magnetic resonance (NMR) spectroscopy is expected to gain much wider use for the identification and quantitation of lipid isomers because the 300 MHz and larger units are becoming
more common. Gunstone (1993) provided a review that describes the use
of ^{13}C-NMR to analyze several classes of lipids including *cis* and *trans* fatty
acid isomers. The ^{13}C-NMR spectrum gives information that can be used to
identify and quantify *cis* and *trans* isomers. The number, position, and

geometric configuration of double bonds in the fatty acid chain determine the chemical shift of the peaks in the spectrum. Table 8.2 shows the published (Bus et al., 1976) ^{13}C-NMR chemical shifts for allylic carbons of linoleic acid geometric isomers. These chemical shifts are unique and separate from shifts for other carbons in the fatty acid chain and, therefore, can be used for identification. Pfeffer et al. (1977) used ^{13}C-NMR to determine the total *trans* monoene, diene, and triene isomer content of shortening. McDonald et al. (1989) used ^{13}C-NMR to confirm the presence of specific *trans* diene isomers in hydrogenated soybean oil.

Matrix Isolation GC/FT-IR

The identification of peaks in a gas chromatogram is based on comparison of the retention time of each peak with the retention times of known standards. Accurate identification or quantitation cannot be made if standards are unavailable or if the GC peaks overlap. The quantitation of fatty acid isomers by GC is difficult because of peak overlap. Sebedio et al. (1987) used light-pipe gas chromatography/Fourier transform infrared spectroscopy (GC/FT-IR) to analyze cyclic fatty acid mixtures. An IR spectrum was obtained for some GC peaks that was useful for peak identification. However, minor peaks could not be identified because of the limited sensitivity of the interface used. Bourne et al. (1984) described an improved technique using a matrix isolation (MI) interface that increased the sensitivity of the GC/FT-IR determination by an order of magnitude. GC/MI/FT-IR is extremely useful for quantitating peak area, determining peak homogeneity, and obtaining structural information on a compound even if positive identification cannot be made. Although conventional light-pipe GC/FT-IR

TABLE 8.2 ^{13}C-NMR Shifts for Allylic Carbons of Linoleic Acid Geometric Isomers

Isomer	Chemical shift (ppm)		
	C_{11}	C_8	C_{14}
trans-9,*trans*-12 18:2	35.7	32.60	32.60
cis-9,*trans*-12 18:2	30.5	27.15	32.60
trans-9,*cis*-12 18:2	30.55	32.60	27.60
cis-9,*cis*-12 18:2	25.75	27.35	27.35

Source: Bus et al., 1976.

techniques provide specific identification of intact molecules, their detection limits are orders of magnitude less than those of techniques that use other GC detectors. Matrix isolation is a technique in which analytes and an inert gas (argon) are rapidly frozen at cryogenic temperatures (12 K) during a GC run. The IR spectra of these molecules are free from indications of intermolecular hydrogen bonding and other band-broadening effects. These combined benefits yield greater sensitivity, which for many applications is on a parity with the sensitivity of gas chromatography/mass spectrometry (GC/MS) (Reedy et al., 1985).

GC/MI/FT-IR was used to quantitate low levels of *trans* diene isomers (Mossoba et al., 1990, 1991), *trans* triene and conjugated isomers (Mossoba et al., 1991), and saturated and monoene isomers (Mossoba et al., 1993) in hydrogenated vegetable and/or fish oils. Figure 8.3 shows the IR spectra (out-of-plane deformation absorption bands) for two *trans* conjugated diene isomer GC peaks. The characteristic absorption bands shown were used to identify the isomers. The conjugated *trans,trans* diene isomer had an out-of-plane deformation absorption band at 990 cm^{-1}, whereas the *cis,trans* isomer had absorption bands at 950 and 986 cm^{-1}. The absorption band for the corresponding methylene-interrupted *trans* diene and the *trans* monoene isomer would have been 971 cm^{-1}. Figure 8.4 shows the unique absorption bands found for a *trans* diene (t9,t12 18:2) and a *cis* diene (c9,c12 18:2) for the carbon-hydrogen stretch (3035 and 3005 cm^{-1} and 3018 cm^{-1}, respectively) and the carbon hydrogen out-of-plane deformation (972 and 730 cm^{-1}, respectively). Table 8.3 indicates that seven *trans* diene isomers in hydrogenated soybean oil were separated and quantitated. There were two *trans,trans* 18:2 positional isomers (peaks 10 and 11) not found in commercial margarine that were present at 3.4 and 4.1% in the hydrogenated soybean oil catalyzed by Ni-S (Fig. 8.1). The retention times of peaks 10' and 11' shown in the chromatogram for margarine and the retention times of these isomers were similar, but the IR spectra indicated that they were *cis* monoene, not *trans* diene, isomers. These data, therefore, provide a good example of the problems of using GC retention times alone to identify *trans* dienes and how the processing conditions during hydrogenation have a significant effect on both the level of *trans* unsaturation and the composition of the isomers formed.

High-Performance Liquid Chromatography

The use of high-performance liquid chromatography (HPLC) to separate complex lipid mixtures can be an effective analytical procedure. HPLC analyses of lipids were reviewed by Shulka (1988). Svensson et al. (1982) analyzed partially hydrogenated vegetable and marine oil for positional and

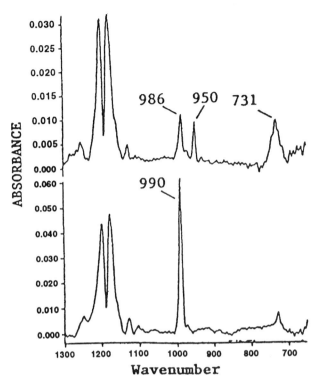

FIG. 8.3 Expanded IR spectral range showing out-of-plane deformation bands for conjugated *cis-trans* (top spectrum) and *trans-trans* (bottom spectrum) 18:2 dienes. (*From Mossoba et al., 1991.*)

geometric isomers of monounsaturated long-chain fatty acids by the combination of reversed-phase HPLC and capillary GC. The fatty acid methyl esters of the *cis* and *trans* isomers were first separated according to chain length by using preparative HPLC. The fractions were analyzed for positional isomer content by using glass capillary GC with a Silar-5 CP stationary phase. Mossoba et al. (1993) used preparative reversed-phase HPLC to separate hydrogenated menhaden oil into five fractions according to chain length. This fractionation helped to minimize peak overlap of *trans* isomers during subsequent GC analysis. GC/MI/FT-IR was then used to identify and quantify five saturated fatty acids and four *trans* monoenes of different chain lengths in the hydrogenated menhaden oil. The *trans* monoenes and saturated fatty acids were quantitated by linear regression analysis from the

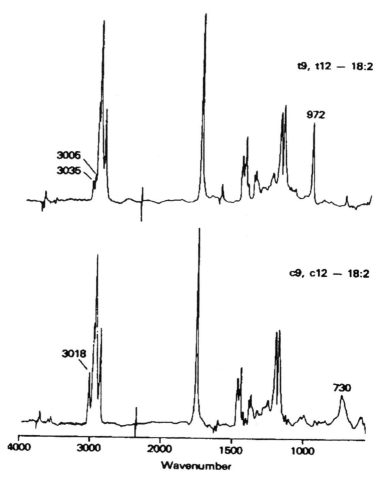

FIG. 8.4 Matrix isolation FT-IR spectra at 4 cm⁻¹ resolution acquired by coadding 300 scans for t9,t12 18:2 (top spectrum) and c9,c12 18:2 (bottom spectrum). (*From Mossoba et al., 1990.*)

intensities of the IR bands at 971 and 1121 cm⁻¹, respectively. Since the band at 971 cm⁻¹ is present only for *trans* geometric isomers, the problem of GC peak overlap from *cis* isomers was eliminated.

Silver Ion Thin-Layer Chromatography

Several chromatography methods have been described that use the long-known principle that the silver ion forms complexes with *cis* double bonds

TABLE 8.3   Quantitation of *Trans* Isomers from Margarines and Hydrogenated Soybean Oil

		Weight (%)			
		Soybean oil		Margarine	
Trans isomer	GC peak	Ni-S[a]	Ni[b]	A	B
t9 18:1	3	29.5	11.1	18.2	17.8
t,t 18:2	10	3.4	—	—	—
t,t 18:2	11	4.1	—	—	—
t,t 18:2	12	2.2	—	0.3	0.3
t9,t12 18:2	13	9.1	<0.1	0.3	0.3
c,t 18:2	14	5.0	2.1	1.5	1.7
c9,t12 18:2	16	6.1	1.9	1.3	1.5
t9,c12 18:2	17	6.0	1.9	1.3	1.4

t = *trans*; c = *cis*.
[a]Hydrogenation catalyzed by sulfided nickel catalyst.
[b]Hydrogenation catalyzed by sulfur-free nickel catalyst.
Source: Mossoba et al., 1990.

more strongly than with *trans* double bonds. Argentation is the general term used to describe this phenomenon. Scholfield (1979) reviewed several argentation methods including thin-layer chromatography (TLC), countercurrent distribution (CCD), and liquid column chromatography.

Argentation TLC has been used for several years to identify *cis* and *trans* isomers in hydrogenated oils (Wood and Snyder, 1966; Carpenter et al., 1976). Preparative argentation TLC is an effective procedure to isolate classes of fatty acid isomers that are then analyzed further by using ozonolysis (Carpenter et al., 1976; Marchand and Beare-Rogers, 1982; Sebedio and Ackman, 1983a, b; Caughman et al., 1987). Two-dimensional TLC analysis employing both argentation and reversed-phase chromatography on a single plate has been used to obtain good resolution of mixtures containing a variety of fatty acid methyl esters (Bergelson et al., 1964; Kennerly, 1988). McDonald et al. (1989) separated hydrogenated soybean oil into six bands by using preparative silver ion TLC and then identified the isomers in each band by using ^{13}C-NMR. Figure 8.5 shows the gas chromatograms obtained for Bands A–D. It was concluded that Band C contained the *cis*-9,*trans*-12 18:2 fatty acid isomer from the characteristic ^{13}C-NMR absorption bands at 32.60, 30.50, and 27.15 ppm (see Table 8.2 and Fig. 8.6).

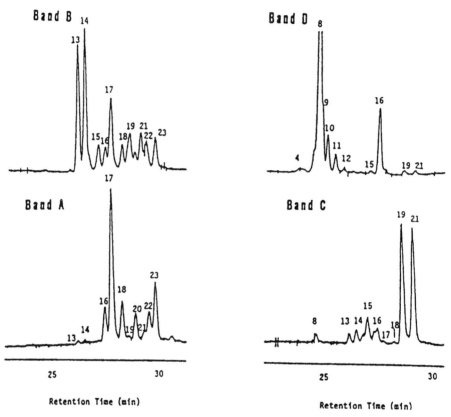

FIG. 8.5   Capillary gas chromatograms showing presence of several components in silver nitrate TLC bands. (*From McDonald et al., 1989.*)

Silver Ion HPLC

According to Christie (1988b), there are a number of disadvantages of incorporating silver ions with the silica gel on TLC plates: (1) large amounts of expensive silver nitrate are required, (2) the method is labor intensive, (3) the separated components can be difficult to visualize, (4) autoxidation can occur on the plate, and (5) some silver ions can be eluted with the fractions. Christie (1987) first described the use of a stable ion-exchange column loaded with silver ions for the separation of triacylglycerols that gave rapid and reproducible results and clean fractions without silver ion contamination. Juaneda et al. (1994) used this method for the separation, collection, and quantification of eight *trans* triene isomers. The recent

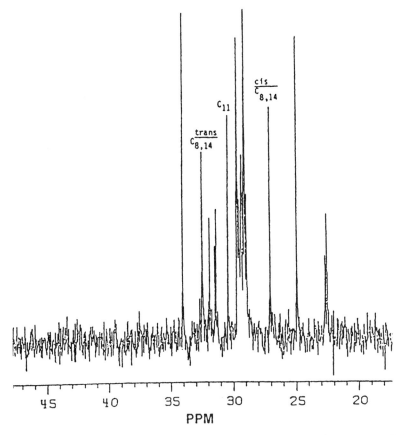

FIG. 8.6 ^{13}C NMR spectrum of Band C from preparative silver nitrate TLC. (*From McDonald et al., 1989.*)

availability of commercial silver ion HPLC columns should dramatically increase the use of this technique. Adlof (1994) used a commercially available HPLC column containing silver ions and an isocratic solvent system of acetonitrile in hexane to separate *cis* and *trans* fatty acid isomers. Adlof et al. (1995) used this procedure to separate hydrogenated soybean oil into four fractions (Fig. 8.7) and subsequently successfully separated individual *cis* and *trans* positional isomers in these fractions, using capillary GC (Fig. 8.8). This method therefore has the potential not only of quantifying the total *cis* and *trans* isomers in hydrogenated oils but also of quantifying the positional monoene isomers.

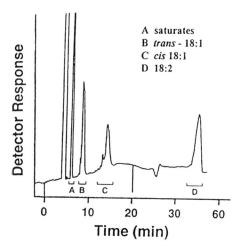

FIG. 8.7   Analysis of partially hydrogenated vegetable oil fatty acid methyl esters by silver ion HPLC. Column: Chrompack ChromSpher lipids, 4.6 mm i.d. × 250 mm. (*From Adlof et al., 1995.*)

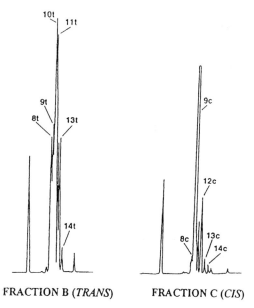

FIG. 8.8   Segment of gas chromatogram (Column: SP2560, 100 m × 0.25 mm) of silver ion HPLC fractions B and C (see Fig. 8.7). (*From Adlof et al., 1995.*)

Gas Chromatography/Mass Spectrometry

Mass spectrometry used in combination with gas chromatography (GC/MS) can be a powerful tool for the location of double bonds in fatty acid isomers. The main obstacle in using GC/MS for this purpose is that double bonds tend to migrate under electron ionization to give inconsistent fragmentation patterns. Schmitz and Klein (1986) reviewed the methods that have been used to overcome this problem such as soft ionization techniques and derivatization. Budzikiewicz (1985) reviewed several chemical ionization methods for the determination of double and triple bond positions. Chemical ionization mass spectrometry (CIMS) is a technique based on the reaction of an unsaturated compound with a reagent gas that yields a characteristic mass spectrum. Brauner et al. (1982) reported that NO^+ reacts with fatty acids that contain three or more methylene-interrupted double bonds by first forming polymethoxy derivatives via reaction with osmium tetroxide and methanol. This procedure can be used to give characteristic fragmentation patterns to determine the double bond positions in fatty acids from marine organisms.

The use of ammonia as a chemical ionization reagent gas was preferable to methane and vinylmethyl ether for analysis of polyunsaturated fatty acids. The formation of pyrrolidide ester derivatives has been a common technique to stabilize double bond migration during electron ionization mass spectrometry (EIMS). Christie's group has reported that picolinyl ester derivatives are even more useful since their more distinctive fragmentation patterns allow unequivocal identification of polyunsaturated fatty acids (Christie et al., 1986, 1987). However, resolution of the picolinyl fatty acid esters by GC was incomplete. Christie and Stefanov (1987) described a reversed-phase HPLC method to obtain simpler picolinyl ester fractions for subsequent identification by GC/MS. By using this method, 39 fatty acid components in cod liver oil were identified. More recently Christie et al. (1993) described a procedure using GC/MS analysis of picolinyl ester derivatives to identify monounsaturated CFAMs in heated oils. They were able to overcome many of the chromatography problems of the picolinyl esters by using silver ion HPLC to fractionate the cyclic monomers before converting them to the picolinyl ester derivatives.

Mossoba et al. (1994) reported that 2-alkenyl-4,4-dimethyloxazoline derivatives of diunsaturated CFAMs gave distinctive mass spectral fragmentation patterns. Unlike the chromatographic resolution of the picolinyl ester derivatives (Christie et al., 1993), the chromatographic resolution of the oxazolines is as good or better than that of the fatty acid methyl esters (Dobson et al., 1995; Mossoba et al., 1995) (Fig. 8.9). Several cyclic fatty acid isomers were identified in heated flaxseed oil (Fig. 8.10). The double bond

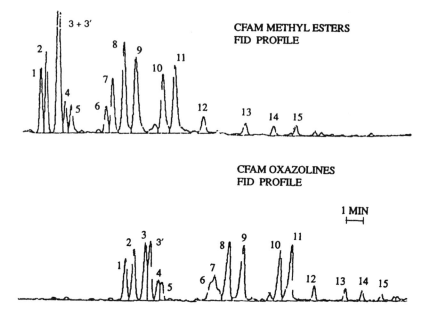

FIG. 8.9   Partial gas chromatogram (Column: CP-Sil 88, 50 m × 0.22 mm) for unsaturated mixtures of CFAM methyl esters (top) and oxazolines (bottom). (*From Mossoba et al., 1995.*)

configuration (*cis* or *trans*) was established by using GC/MI/FT-IR (Table 8.4). The results of this research have shown the feasibility of using the oxazoline derivatives to identify cyclic fatty acid isomers reported to be toxic. The positions of double bonds and 1,2-disubstituted unsaturated five- and six-membered rings along the hydrocarbon chain were established by this method as shown in Fig. 8.11.

Multidimensional Capillary Gas Chromatography

Multidimensional capillary gas chromatography (MDCGC) is a technique used to gain increased resolution for complex mixtures. Two or more columns are connected by a series of column-switching systems. This makes it possible to transfer a single component or a timed cut (called a heartcut) from a precolumn to a second GC column. Various combinations of packed, megabore, and capillary columns with different polarities can be used to achieve good peak separation of complex mixtures. Several reviews describing this technique have been published (Deans, 1981; Gordon et al., 1985;

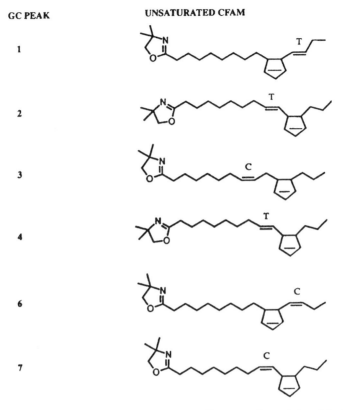

GC PEAK   UNSATURATED CFAM

FIG. 8.10 Structures of CFAMs (containing five-membered rings) in heated flaxseed (linseed) oil. C = *cis*; T = *trans*. (*From Mossoba et al., 1995.*)

Van Hese and Grant, 1988). The separation of the *cis* and *trans* isomers in a complex fatty acid methyl ester mixture by using MDCGC was described by Van Hese and Grant (1988). The components were first separated on the basis of carbon number on a megabore column, and then the components in a heartcut section containing *cis* and *trans* isomers having 18 carbons were separated on a highly polar capillary column. Elder et al. (1986) discussed the potential advantages of using MDCGC in conjunction with mass spectrometry. These advantages include increased resolution of selected components, minimal analyte losses, and reduced analyte isolation/methods development time.

TABLE 8.4 Infrared Bands (cm^{-1}) Attributed to Unsaturation Sites in CFAMS

GC peak[a]	Ring, 5-membered	Chain, trans	Ring, 6-membered	Chain, cis	Chain, trans	Chain, trans	Ring, 6-membered	Ring, 5-membered	Ring, 6-membered
1	3061	3035			3003	970		719	
2	3061	3035			3003	970		719	
3 + 3'	3061			3005				716	
4	3063	3032			3005	979		716	
6	3063			3006				711	
7	3063			3006				711	
8			3032		3000	976			663
9			3032		3005	972			664
10			3032		3005	972			664
11			3032		3004	975			663
12			3031				723		664
13			3031				725		662
14			3025						
15			3025						

[a]See Figure 8.9.

Source: Mossoba et al., 1990.

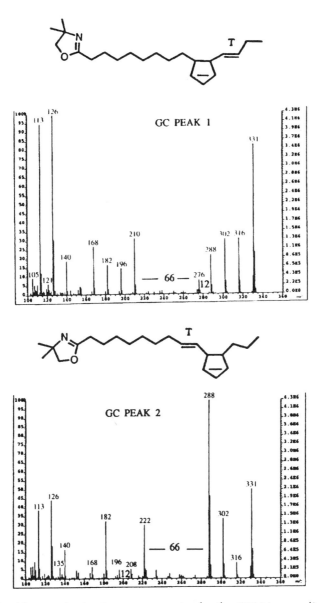

FIG. 8.11   Electron ionization mass spectra for the CFAM oxazoline eluates of gas chromatographic peaks 1, 2, and 10. (*From Mossoba et al., 1995.*)

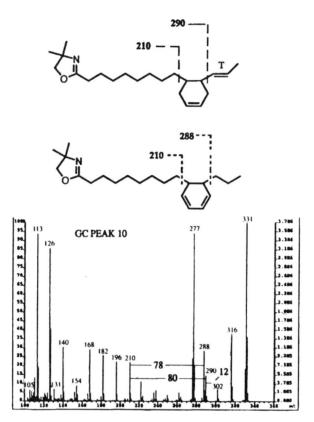

FIG. 8.11   Continued

CONCLUSION

The process of catalytic hydrogenation of vegetable and marine oils dramatically changes their composition by producing many geometric and positional isomers. Although no specific adverse effects on human health have been proven for these isomers, it has been shown that they are incorporated into most organs and tissues. Fatty acid isomers can influence enzyme activity and other biochemical reactions. However, it is not known if these influences cause any short- or long-term beneficial or harmful physiological effects. Unfortunately, careful selection of published data can still be used to provide evidence of either the absolute safety or the adverse physiological effects of hydrogenated oils. It is, therefore, important to continue to conduct more comprehensive studies to better define the physiological properties of the isomeric fatty acids in hydrogenated oils. It is also important to continue to develop improved methods to accurately and conveniently determine total *trans* as well as specific fatty acid isomers in hydrogenated oils.

REFERENCES

Ackman, R. G. 1991. Application of gas-liquid chromatography to lipid separation and analysis: Qualitative and quantitative analysis. In *Analysis of Fats, Oils and Lipoproteins*, E. G. Perkins (Ed.), pp. 270–300. American Oil Chemists' Society, Champaign, IL.

Ackman, R. G. 1982. Fatty acid composition of fish oils. In *Nutritional Evaluation of Long-Chain Fatty Acids in Fish Oil*, S. M. Barlow and M. E. Stansby (Ed.), pp. 25–88. Academic Press, New York.

Adlof, R. O. 1994. Separation of *cis* and *trans* unsaturated fatty acid methyl esters by silver ion high-performance liquid chromatography. *J. Chromatogr.* 659: 95–99.

Adlof, R. O., Copes, L. C., and Emken, E. A. 1995. Analysis of the monoenoic fatty acid distribution in hydrogenated vegetable oils by silver-ion high-performance liquid chromatography. *J. Am. Oil Chem. Soc.* 72: 571–574.

Alam, S. Q., Ren, Y. F., and Alam, B. S. 1989. Effect of dietary *trans* fatty acids on some membrane-associated enzymes and receptors in rat heart. *Lipids* 24: 39–44.

Albright, L. 1987. Partial hydrogenation of triglyceride oils: Relationship between chemical reactions, physical transfer steps, and adsorption steps. In *Hydrogenation: Proceedings of an AOCS Colloquium*, R. Hastert (Ed.), pp. 11–29. American Oil Chemists' Society, Champaign, IL.

Allen, R. R. 1987. Theory of hydrogenation and isomerization. In *Hydrogenation: Proceedings of an AOCS Colloquium*, R. Hastert (Ed.), pp. 1–10. American Oil Chemists' Society, Champaign, IL.

Almendingen, K., Jordal, O., Kierulf, P., Sandstad, B., and Pedersen, J. I. 1995. Effects of partially hydrogenated fish oil, partially hydrogenated soybean oil, and butter on serum lipoproteins and Lp(a) in men. *J. Lipid Res.* 36: 1370–1384.

Anonymous, 1995a. Researchers, CSPI urge FDA action on *trans* fatty acids. Food Chem. News 37(20): 7–8.

Anonymous, 1995. *Trans* fat label changes not warranted, IFT, AIN, ASCN tell FDA. *Food Chem. News* 37(21): 12–13.

Applewhite, T. H. 1994. Margarine products in health and nutrition. *INFORM* 5: 914–921.

Asherio, A., Hennekens, C. H., Buring, J. E., Master, C., Stampfer, M. J., and Willet, W. C. 1994. *Trans* fatty acids intake and risk of myocardial infarction. *Circulation* 89: 94–101.

Astorg, P. O. and Chevalier, J. 1987. Polyunsaturated fatty acids in tissues of rats fed trielaidin and high or low levels of linolenic acid. *Lipids* 22: 1025–1030.

Brauner, A., Budzikienwicz, H., and Boland, W. 1982. Studies in chemical ionization mass spectrometry. *Org. Mass Spectrom.* 17: 161–164.

Bergelson, L. D., Dyatlovitskaya, E. V., and Voronkova, V. V. 1964. Complete structural analysis of fatty acid mixtures by thin-layer chromatography. *J. Chromatogr.* 15: 191–199.

Beyers, E. C. and Emken, E. A. 1991. Metabolites of *cis,trans* and *trans,cis* isomers of linoleic acid in mice and incorporation in tissue lipids. *Biochim. Biophys. Acta* 1082: 275–284.

Bourne, S., Reedy, G., Coffey, P., and Mattson, D. 1984. Matrix isolation GC/FT-IR. *Am. Lab.* 16: 90–101.

Budzikiewicz, H. 1985. Structure elucidation by ion-molecule reactions in the gas phase: The location of C, C-double and triple bonds (1). *Fresenius Z. Anal. Chem.* 321: 150–158.

Bus, J., Sies, I., and Lie Ken Jie, M. S. F. 1976. ^{13}C-NMR of methyl, methylene and carbonyl carbon atoms of methyl alkenoates and alkynoates. *Chem. Phys. Lipids* 17: 501–518.

Carpenter, D. L., Lehmann, B. S., Mason, B. S., and Slover, H. T. 1976. Lipid composition of selected vegetable oils. *J. Am. Oil Chem. Soc.* 53: 713–718.

Caughman, C. R., Boyd, L. C., Keeney, M., and Sampugna, J. 1987. Analysis of positional isomers of monosaturated fatty acids by high performance liquid chromatography of 2,4-dinitrophenylhydrazones of reduced ozonides. *J. Lipid Res.* 28: 338–342.

Christie, W. W. (Ed.). 1993. *Advances in Lipid Methodology—Two.* The Oily Press, Ayr, Scotland.

Christie, W. (Ed.). 1992. *Advances in Lipid Methodology—One.* The Oily Press, Ayr, Scotland.

Christie, W. W. 1988a. Equivalent chain-lengths of methyl ester derivatives of fatty acids on gas chromatography—a reappraisal. *J. Chromatogr.* 447: 305–314.

Christie, W. W. 1988b. Separation of molecular species of triacylglycerols by high-performance liquid chromatography with a silver ion column. *J. Chromatogr.* 454: 273–284.

Christie, W. W. 1987. A stable silver-loaded column for the separation of lipids by high performance liquid chromatography. *J. High Resolut. Chromatogr. Chromatogr. Commun.* 10: 148–150.

Christie, W. W. and Stefanov, K. 1987. Separation of picolinyl ester derivatives of fatty acids by high-performance liquid chromatography for identification by mass spectrometry. *J. Chromatogr.* 392: 259–265.

Christie, W. W., Brechany, E. Y., and Holman, R. T. 1987. Mass spectra of the picolinyl esters of isomeric mono- and dienoic acids. *Lipids* 22: 224–228.

Christie, W. W., Brechany, E. Y., Sebedio, J. L., and LeQuere, J. L. 1993. Silver ion chromatography and gas chromatography-mass spectrometry in the structural analysis of cyclic monoenoic acids formed in frying oils. *Chem. Phys. Lipids* 66: 143–153.

Christie, W. W., Brechany, E. Y., Johnson, S. B., and Holman, R. T. 1986. A comparison of pyrrolidide and picolinyl ester derivatives for the identification of fatty acids in natural samples by gas-chromatography-mass spectrometry. *Lipids* 21: 657–661.

Clevidence, B. A., Judd, J. T., Schaefer, E. J., McNamara, J. R., Muesing, R. A., Wittes, J., and Sunkin, M. E. 1995. Plasma lipoprotein (a) levels in subjects consuming *trans* fatty acids. *FASEB J.* 9: A579.

Deans, D. R. 1981. Use of heart cutting in gas chromatography: A review. *J. Chromatogr.* 203: 19–28.

Decsi, T. and Koletzko, B. 1995. Do *trans* fatty acids impair linoleic acid metabolism in children. *Ann. Nutr. Metab.* 39: 36–41.

Dickey, L. E. and Caughman, C. R. 1995. *Trans* fatty acid content of selected foods. Paper no. 26A, presented at the 86th Annual Meeting of the American Oil Chemists' Society, San Antonio, TX, May 7–11.

Dobson, G., Christie, W. W., Brechany, E. Y., Sebedio, J. L., and LeQuere, J. L. 1995. Silver ion chromatography and gas chromatography-mass spectrometry in the structural analysis of cyclic dienoic acids formed in frying oils. *Chem. Phys. Lipids* 75: 171–182.

Dutton, H. J. 1979. Hydrogenation of fats and its significance. In *Geometrical and Positional Fatty Acid Isomers*, E. A. Emken and H. J. Dutton (Ed.), pp. 1–16. American Oil Chemists' Society, Champaign, IL.

Dutton, H. J., Johnson, S. B., Purch, F. J., Lieken Jie, M. S. F., Gunstone, F. D., and Homan, R. T. 1988. Composition of mixed octadecadienoates via ozonolysis, chromatography and computer solution of linear equations. *Lipids* 68: 481–489.

Elder, Jr., J. F., Gordon, B. M., and Uhrig, M. S. 1986. Complex mixture analysis by capillary-to-capillary column heartcutting GC/MS. *J. Chromatogr. Sci.* 24: 26–32.

Emken, E. A. 1984. Nutrition and biochemistry of *trans* and positional fatty acid isomers in hydrogenated oils. *Annu. Rev. Nutr.* 4: 339–377.

Enig, M. G. 1993. *Trans* fatty acids—an update. *Nutr. Q.* 17(4): 79–94.

Enig, M. G., Atal, S., Keeney, M., and Sampagna, J. 1990. Isomeric *trans* fatty acids in the U.S. diet. *J. Am. Coll. Nutr.* 9: 471–486.

Gildenberg, L. and Firestone, D. 1985. Gas chromatographic determination of *trans* unsaturation in margarine: Collaborative study. *J. Assoc. Off. Anal. Chem.* 68: 46–51.

Gordon, B. M., Rix, C. E., and Borgerding, M. F. 1985. Comparison of state-of-the-art column switching techniques in high resolution gas chromatography. *J. Chromatogr. Sci.* 23: 1–10.

Gunstone, F. D. 1993. High resolution ^{13}C NMR spectroscopy of lipids. In *Advances in Lipid Methodology—Two*, W. W. Christie (Ed.), pp. 1–68. The Oily Press, Ayr, Scotland.

Hastert, R. (Ed.). 1987. *Hydrogenation: Proceeding of an AOCS Colloquium.* American Oil Chemists' Society, Champaign, IL.

Haumann, B. F. 1995. Some food-labeling questions still unresolved. *INFORM* 6: 335–340.

Heckers, H. and Melcher, F. W. 1978. *Trans*-isomeric fatty acids present in West German margarines, shortenings, frying and cooking fats. *Am. J. Clin. Nutr.* 31: 1041–1049.

Hunter, J. E. and Applewhite, T. H. 1986. Isomeric fatty acids in the U.S. diet: Levels and health perspectives. *Am. J. Clin. Nutr.* 44: 707–717.

Hunter, J. E. and Applewhite, T. H. 1991. Reassessment of *trans* fatty acids availability in the U.S. diet: Levels and health perspectives. *Am. J. Clin. Nutr.* 54: 363–369.

Iwaoka, W. T. and Perkins, E. G. 1976. Nutritional effects of the cyclic monomers of methyl linolenate in the rat. *Lipids* 11: 349–353.

Johnston, A. E., Dutton, H. J., Scholfield, C. R., and Butterfield, R. O. 1978. Double bond analysis of dienoic fatty acids in mixtures. *J. Am. Oil Chem. Soc.* 55: 486–490.

Juaneda, P., Sebedio, J. L., and Christie, W. W. 1994. Complete separation of the geometric isomers of linolenic acid by high performance liquid chromatography with a silver ion column. *J. High Resolut. Chromatogr. Chromatogr. Commun.* 17: 321–324.

Judd, J. T., Clevidence, B. A., Muesing, R. A., Wittes, J., Sunkin, M. E., and Podczasy, J. J. 1994. Dietary *trans* fatty acids: Effects on plasma lipids and lipoproteins of healthy men and women. *Am. J. Clin. Nutr.* 59: 861–865.

Kanhai, J. 1988. Hydrogenation of edible oils—toxicological and nutritional implications: A review. *Food Chem.* 27: 191–201.

Kennerly, D. A. 1988. Two dimensional thin-layer chromatographic separation of phospholipid molecular species using plates with both reversed-phase and argentation zones. *J. Chromatogr.* 454: 425–431.

Klimmek, H. K. 1984. Influence of various catalyst poisons and other impurities of fatty acid hydrogenation. *J. Am. Oil Chem. Soc.* 61: 200–204.

Kramer, J. K. G., Hulan, H. W., Conner, A. H., Thompson, B. K., Holfeld, N., and Mills, J. H. L. 1979. Cardiopathogenicity of soybean oil and rapeseed oil triglycerides when fed to male rats. *Lipids* 14: 773–780.

Kris-Etherton, P. M. (Ed.). 1995. Expert panel on *trans* fatty acids and coronary heart disease. *Am. J. Clin. Nutr.* 62: 655S–708S.

List, G. R., Pelloso, T., Orthoefer, F., Chrysam, M., and Mounts, T. L. 1995. Preparation and properties of zero *trans* soybean oil margarines. *J. Am. Oil Chem. Soc.* 72: 383–384.

Marchand, C. M. 1982. Positional isomers of *trans*-octadecenoic acids in margarines. *Can. Inst. Food Sci. Technol. J.* 15: 196–199.

Marchand, C. M. and Beare-Rogers, J. L. 1982. Complementary techniques for the identification of *trans,trans*-18:2 isomers in margarines. *Can. Inst. Food Sci. Technol. J.* 15: 54–57.

McDonald, R. E. and Armstrong, D. J. 1986. *Trans* diene formation during catalytic hydrogenation and isomerization of soybean oil. *J. Am. Oil Chem. Soc.* 63: 467.

McDonald, R. E., Armstrong, D. J., and Kreishman, G. P. 1989. Identification of *trans* diene isomers in hydrogenated soybean oil by gas chromatography, silver nitrate-thin layer chromatography, and ^{13}C-NMR spectroscopy. *J. Agric. Food Chem.* 37: 637–642.

Mensink, R. P. and Katan, M. B. 1990. Effect of dietary *trans* fatty acids on high-density and low-density lipoprotein cholesterol levels in healthy subjects. *N. Engl. J. Med.* 323: 439–445.

Mensink, R. P., Zock, P. L., Katan, M. G., and Hornstra, G. 1992. Effect of dietary and *trans* fatty acids on serum lipoprotein(a) levels in humans. *J. Lipid Res.* 33: 1493–1501.

Mossoba, M. M. and McDonald, R. E. 1995. Quantitation of the *trans* content of hydrogenated oils by infrared spectroscopy. Paper no. 4E, presented at the 86th Annual Meeting of the American Oil Chemists' Society, San Antonio, TX, May 7–11.

Mossoba, M. M., McDonald, R. E., Armstrong, D. J., and Page, S. W. 1991. Identification of minor C18 triene and conjugated diene isomers in hydrogenated soybean oil and margarine by gas chromatography/matrix isolation/Fourier transform infrared spectroscopy. *J. Chromatogr. Sci.* 29: 324–330.

Mossoba, M. M., McDonald, R. E., Chen, J. Y. T., Armstrong, D. J., and Page, S. W. 1990. Identification and quantitation of *trans*-9,*trans*-12 octadecadienoic acid methyl ester and other geometric isomers in hydrogenated soybean oil and margarines by capillary gas chromatography/matrix isolation/Fourier transform infrared spectroscopy. *J. Agric. Food Chem.* 38: 86–92.

Mossoba, M. M., McDonald, R. E., and Prosser, A. R. 1993. Gas chromatography/matrix isolation/Fourier transform infrared spectroscopic determination of *trans*-monounsaturated and saturated fatty acid methyl esters in partially hydrogenated menhaden oil. *J. Agric. Food Chem.* 41: 1988–2002.

Mossoba, M. M., Yurawecz, M. P., Roach, J. A. G., Lin, H. P., McDonald, R. E., Flickinger, B. D., and Perkins, E. G. 1995. Elucidation of cyclic fatty acid monomer structures. Cyclic and bicyclic ring sizes and double bond position and configuration. *J. Am. Oil Chem. Soc.* 72: 721–727.

Mossoba, M. M., Yurawecz, M. P., Roach, J. A. G., McDonald, R. E., Flickinger, B. D., and Perkins, E. G. 1994. Rapid determination of double bond configuration and position along the hydrocarbon chain in cyclic fatty acid monomers. *Lipids* 29: 893–896.

Mounts, T. L. 1987. Alternative catalyst for hydrogenation of edible oils. In *Hydrogenation: Proceedings of an AOCS Colloquium,* R. Hastert (Ed.), pp. 47–64. American Oils Chemists' Society, Champaign, IL.

Nestel, P., Noakes, M., and Belling, B. 1992. Plasma lipoprotein and Lp(a) changes with substitution of elaidic acid for oleic acid in the diet. *J. Lipid Res.* 33: 1029–1036.

Opstvedt, J., Pettersen, J., and Mork, J. 1988. *Trans* fatty acids. I. Growth, fertility, organ weights and nerve histology and conduction velocity in sows and offspring. *Lipids* 23: 713–719.

Ostlund-Lindquist, A. M., Albanus, L., and Croon, L. B. 1985. Effect of dietary *trans* fatty acids on microsomal enzymes and membranes. *Lipids* 20: 620–624.

Patterson, H. B. W. 1983. *Hydrogenation of Fats and Oils.* Elsevier Science Publishing Co., New York.

Perkins, E. G. (Ed.). 1991. *Analysis of Fats, Oil and Lipoproteins.* American Oil Chemists' Society, Champaign, IL.

Perkins, E. G. and Smick, C. 1987. Octadecatrienoic fatty acid isomers of partially hydrogenated soybean oil. *J. Am. Oil Chem. Soc.* 64: 1150–1155.

Perkins, E. G. and Visek, W. J. (Ed.). 1983. *Dietary Fats and Health.* American Oil Chemists' Society, Champaign, IL.

Pettersen, J. and Opstvedt, J. 1988. *Trans* fatty acids. 2. Fatty acid composi tion of the brain and other organs in the mature female pig. *Lipids* 23: 720–726.

Pfeffer, R. E., Luddy, R. E., and Unruh, J. 1977. Analytical ^{13}C-NMR: A rapid, nondestructive method for determining the *cis,trans* composition of catalytically treated unsaturated lipid mixtures. *J. Am. Oil Chem. Soc.* 54: 380–386.

Ratnayake, W. M. N. 1995. Determination of *trans* unsaturation by IR spectrometry and determination of fatty acid composition of partially hydrogenated vegetable oils and animal fats by gas chromatography/infrared spectrophotometry: Collaborative study. *J. Assoc. Off. Anal. Chem.* 78: 783–802.

Ratnayake, N. W. M. and Beare-Rogers, J. L. 1990. Problems of analyzing C18 *cis* and *trans* fatty acids of margarine on the SP-2340 capillary column. *J. Chromatogr. Sci.* 28: 633–639.

Ratnayake, W. M. N., Hollywood, R., O'Grady, E., and Beare-Rogers, J. L. 1990. Determination of *cis* and *trans*-octadecenoic acids in margarines by gas liquid chromatography-infrared spectroscopy. *J. Am. Oil Chem. Soc.* 67: 804–810.

Ratnayake, W. M. N., Hollywood, R., O'Grady, E., and Pelletier, G. 1993. Fatty acids in some common foods in Canada. *J. Am. Coll. Nutr.* 12: 651–660.

Reedy, G. T., Ettinger, D. C., Schneider, J. F., and Bourne, S. 1985. High-resolution gas chromatography/matrix isolation infrared spectrometry. *Anal. Chem.* 57: 1602–1609.

Ren, Y. F., Alam, S. Q., Alam, B. S., and Keefer, L. M. 1988. Adenylate cyclase and beta-receptors in salivary glands of rats red diets containing *trans* fatty *acids. Lipids* 23: 304–308.

Sahasrabudhe, M. R. and Kurian, C. J. 1979. Fatty acid composition of margarines in Canada. *Can. Inst. Food Sci. Technol. J.* 12: 140–144.

Schmitz, B. and Klein, R. A. 1986. Mass spectrometric localization of carbon-carbon double bonds: A critical review of recent methods. *Chem. Phys. Lipids* 39: 285–311.

Scholfield, C. R. 1979. Analysis and physical properties of the isomeric fatty acids. In *Geometrical and Positional Fatty Acids Isomers*, E. A. Emken and H. J. Dutton (Ed.), pp.17–52. American Oil Chemists' Society, Champaign, IL.

Sebedio, J. L. and Ackman, R. G. 1983a. Hydrogenation of a menhaden oil: 1. Fatty acid and C20 monoethylenic isomer compositions as a function of the degree of hydrogenation. *J. Am. Oil Chem. Soc.* 60: 1986–1991.

Sebedio, J. L. and Ackman, R. G. 1983b. Hydrogenation of a menhaden oil:

II. Formation and evolution of the C20 dienoic and fatty acids as a function of the degree of hydrogenation. *J. Am. Oil Chem. Soc.* 60: 1992–1996.

Sebedio, J. L. and Grandgirard, A. 1989. Cyclic fatty acids: Natural sources, formation during heat treatment, synthesis and biological properties. *Prog. Lipid Res.* 28: 303–336.

Sebedio, J. L., LeQuere, J. L., Semon, E., Morin, O., Prevost, J., and Grandgirand, A. 1987. A heat treatment of vegetable oils. II. GC-MS and GC-FTIR spectra of some isolated cyclic fatty acid monomers. *J. Am. Oil Chem. Soc.* 64: 1324–1333.

Senti, F. R. (Ed.). 1985. Health aspects of dietary *trans* fatty acids. Federation of American Societies for Experimental Biology, Bethesda, MD (Contract no. FDA 223-83-2020).

Shapiro, S. 1995. *Trans* fatty acids and coronary heart disease: The debate continues. 2. Confounding and selection bias in the data. *Am. J. Public Health* 85: 410–413.

Shulka, V. K. S. 1988. Recent advances in the high performance liquid chromatography of lipids. *Prog. Lipid Res.* 27: 5–38.

Siess, M. H., Vernevaut, M. F., Grandgirard, A., and Sebedio, J. L. 1988. Induction of hepatic drug-metabolizing enzymes by cyclic fatty acid monomers in the rat. *Food Chem. Toxicol.* 26: 9–13.

Slover, H. T., Thompson, R. H., Jr., David, C. S., and Merola, G. V. 1985. Lipids in margarines and margarine-like foods. *J. Am. Oil Chem. Soc.* 62: 775–786.

Smallbone, B. W. and Sahasrabudhe, M. R. 1985. Positional isomers of *cis*- and *trans*-octadecenoic acids in hydrogenated vegetable oils. *Can. Inst. Food Sci. Technol. J.* 18: 174–177.

Svensson, L., Sisfontes, L., Nyborg, G., and Blomstrand, R. 1982. High performance liquid chromatography of geometric and positional isomers of long chain monounsaturated fatty acids. *Lipids* 17: 50–59.

Van Hese, V. G. and Grant, D. 1988. Automatic multidimensional capillary G.C. *Am. Lab.* 20: 26–33.

Willet, W. C. and Ascherio, A. 1994. *Trans* fatty acids: Are the effects only marginal? *Am. J. Public Health* 84: 722–724.

Willet, W. C., Stampfer, M. J., Manson, J. E., Golgitz, G. A., Speizer, F. E., Rosner, B. A., Sampson, L. A., and Hennekens, C. H. 1993. Intake of *trans* fatty acids and risk of coronary heart disease among women. *Lancet* 341: 581–585.

Wolff, R. L. 1994. Analysis of alpha-linolenic acid geometrical isomers in deodorized oils by capillary gas-liquid chromatography on cyanoalkyl polysiloxane stationary phases: A note of caution. *J. Am. Oil Chem. Soc.* 71: 907–909.

Wood, R. and Snyder, F. 1966. Modified silver ion thin-layer chromatography. *J. Am. Oil Chem. Soc.* 43: 53–54.

Zock, P. L. and Katan, M. B. 1992. Hydrogenation alternatives: Effects of *trans* fatty acids and stearic acid versus linoleic acid on serum lipids and lipoproteins in humans. *J. Lipid Res.* 33: 399–410.

9
Analysis and Health Effects of Cholesterol Oxides

Paul B. Addis

University of Minnesota
St. Paul, Minnesota

Peter W. Park

Crown Laboratories, Inc.
Las Vegas, Nevada

Francesco Guardiola and Rafael Codony

University of Barcelona
Barcelona, Spain

INTRODUCTION

Cholesterol, as an unsaturated lipid (Fig. 9.1), undergoes free radical–mediated oxidation via hydroperoxide formation similar to unsaturated fatty acids. This results in the production of numerous oxygenated derivatives (Table 9.1), which are commonly called oxygenated or oxidized cholesterol, oxysterols, cholesterol oxidation products, or simply cholesterol oxide[s] (CO). Some CO have received much attention due to their undesirable biological properties such as cytotoxicity, atherogenicity, sterol metabolism interference, mutagenicity, and carcinogenicity. The availability of capillary columns for gas chromatography (GC) and rapid progress in high-performance liquid chromatography (HPLC) have provided many methods for determining CO in foods and biological tissues, enhancing our current

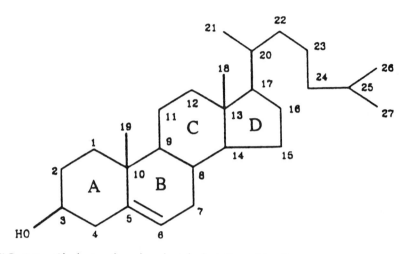

FIG. 9.1   Cholesterol molecule (cholest-5-en-3β-ol).

TABLE 9.1   Abbreviations and Nomenclature

Abbreviation	Trivial name	Systematic name
C	Cholesterol	Cholest-5-en-3β-ol
α-CE	Cholesterol-5α,6α-epoxide	5,6α-Epoxy-5α-cholestan-3β-ol
β-CE	Cholesterol-5β,6β-epoxide	5,6β-Epoxy-5β-cholestan-3β-ol
CEs	Cholesterol-5,6-epoxides (α and β)	
CT	Cholestanetriol	5α-Cholestane-3β,5,6β-triol
4β-HC	4β-Hydroxycholesterol	Cholest-5-en-3β,4β-diol
7-HCs	7-Hydroxycholesterols (α and β)	
7α-HC	7α-Hydroxycholesterol	Cholest-5-en-3β,7α-diol
7β-HC	7β-Hydroxycholesterol	Cholest-5-en-3β,7β-diol
19-HC	19-Hydroxycholesterol	Cholest-5-en-3β,19-diol
20-HC	20-Hydroxycholesterol	Cholest-5-en-3β,20-diol
22R-HC	(22R)-22-Hydroxycholesterol	(22R)-Cholest-5-en-3β,22-diol
24-HC	24-Hydroxycholesterol	Cholest-5-en-3β,24-diol
24S-HC	(24S)-24-Hydroxycholesterol	(24S)-Cholest-5-en-3β,24-diol
25-HC	25-Hydroxycholesterol	Cholest-5-en-3β,25-diol
(25R)-26-HC	(25R)-26-Hydroxycholesterol	(25R)-Cholest-5-en-3β,26-diol
(25S)-26-HC	(25S)-26-Hydroxycholesterol	(25S)-Cholest-5-en-3β,26-diol
26-HC	26-Hydroxycholesterol	Cholest-5-en-3β,26-diol
27-HC	27-Hydroxycholesterol	Cholest-5-en-3β,27-diol
7-KC	7-Ketocholesterol	3β-Hydroxycholest-5-en-7-one
6-KCL	6-Ketocholestanol	3β-Hydroxy-5α-cholestan-6-one
7-KCL	7-Ketocholestanol	3β-Hydroxy-5α-cholestan-7-one

understanding of cholesterol oxidation and its significance in foods. Although still expensive, easier access to mass spectrometry (MS) helped ensure the identity of CO occurring in foods. Interested readers are referred to reviews on cholesterol oxidation chemistry, biological effects of CO, and analysis of CO (Smith, 1981, 1987; Addis, 1986; Smith and Johnson, 1989; Addis and Warner, 1991; Peng and Morin, 1992; Guardiola et al., 1994b, 1995e; Park, 1995).

Research on CO is complex and controversial. We intend to show in this review that enough effort has been expended developing methodology in CO analysis and that it is time to "harmonize" the methodology and conduct some incisive experiments dealing with critical issues such as absorption, assimilation, metabolism, and the health impact of CO. Although consumption of CO is quantitatively not great, it would be a mistake to dismiss health consequences as minimal. CO are not consumed in isolation, and the literature is clear concerning cytotoxicity of CO, other lipid oxidation products, and some native lipids, usually found with CO. Also, lipid oxidation products are produced in vivo by either normal metabolism or pathological processes and aging. Smokers and persons exposed to industrial toxins or who use drugs add additional risks as they will experience amplified lipid oxidation. No studies have inquired about intriguing interactions that could occur among various forms of lipid oxidation and products resulting therefrom.

As in any field of scientific research, methodology is critical and, unfortunately, numerous types of methods are used by researchers on CO. Lack of confirmation of structures by MS, variations in chromatography, and deficiencies in purification procedures have limited the usefulness of some published studies. Detailed accounts of these problems are summarized in this review. There is an urgent need for harmonization of methodology among laboratories studying CO, and fortunately this activity is now underway (Appelqvist, 1995).

CHEMISTRY OF CHOLESTEROL OXIDATION

An understanding of the manifold mechanisms by which CO might be able to adversely affect the well-being of living organisms can be obtained only after developing an appreciation for the various mechanisms of CO formation. It should be emphasized that total body exposure to CO is not derived from food alone. As will be seen, ample evidence exists for CO formation in vivo.

Nonenzymatic Oxidation of Cholesterol

Bergström and Wintersteiner (1941, 1942a, b) reported that cholesterol underwent nonenzymatic oxidative degradation in colloidal aqueous solution. Smith et al. (1967), using thin layer chromatography (TLC), demonstrated occurrence of some 30 CO in aged cholesterol.

Due to the B ring olefinic bond cholesterol being subject to oxygen attack, i.e., autoxidation. Cholesterol autoxidation is initiated by hydrogen abstraction at C-7 forming a C-7 allylic carbon-centered radical (Fig. 9.2). This radical reacts with triplet oxygen ($^3O_2$) producing a peroxyl radical, stabilized by hydrogen abstraction, yielding isomeric 7α- and 7β-hydroperoxides; at equilibrium the β form predominates, being more thermodynamically stable. However, both forms are thermally unstable, leading to 7α-HC, 7β-HC, and 7-KC as secondary products (Teng et al., 1973b).

In addition to 7-hydroperoxides, other hydroperoxides can also be formed by similar free radical mediated processes leading to 20-HC, 24-HC, 25-HC, 26-HC and 27-HC; hydroxycholesterols with a hydroxyl group on tertiary carbons (25-HC and 20-HC) are most common (Fig. 9.2). Probability of a radical on C-4, the other allylic carbon, is low due to steric hindrance by trialkylic C-5 and C-3 hydroxyl (Maerker, 1987).

Oxidative action of H_2O_2 and cholesterol hydroperoxides on cholesterol lead to α- and β-CE (Smith et al., 1978); the β form predominates. By hydrolysis, these epoxides form CT, and in acid medium, β-CE is hydrolyzed more rapidly (Maerker, 1987; Maerker and Bunick, 1986).

Like photooxidation of fatty acids, cholesterol autoxidation can be mediated by singlet oxygen ($^1O_2$), which is generated from triplet oxygen ($^3O_2$) by photochemical action (Bhagavan and Nair, 1992). In this way, the main hydroperoxide formed is 3β-hydroxy-5α-cholest-6-en-5-hydroperoxide, which can be thermally decomposed to cholest-4,6-dien-3-one and 5α-cholest-6-en-3β,5-diol. By stereospecific transposition, 5α-hydroperoxide can isomerize to yield 3β-hydroxy-7α-cholest-5-en-7-hydroperoxide, an intermediate of cholesterol oxidation by $^3O_2$, which finally yields 7-HCs and 7-KC. In this process, small proportions of 3β-hydroxycholest-4-en-6-hydroperoxide can also be obtained, together with their thermal decomposition derivatives (cholest-4-en-3β,6-diols and 3β-hydroxycholest-4-en-6-one).

Cholesterol can be oxidized through action of different tri-(O_3) and diatomic (O_2^+) oxygen species, nitrogen oxides, CCl_4, etc. (Smith, 1981). Gamma radiation can produce oxidation of cholesterol in the A ring (Maerker and Jones, 1992; Hwang and Maerker, 1993a).

Enzymatic Oxidation of Cholesterol

Processes of this type mainly occur in liver and steroidogenic tissues. Some cholesterol oxidation derivatives [7α-HC, 25-HC, (25R)-26-HC and (25S)-26-HC] are intermediates to liver bile acid synthesis, while others [22R-HC, (20R,22R)-cholest-5-en-3β,20,22-triol] are related to steroid hormone synthesis (Crastes de Paulet et al., 1988; Smith, 1990). Cerebrosterol (24S-HC)

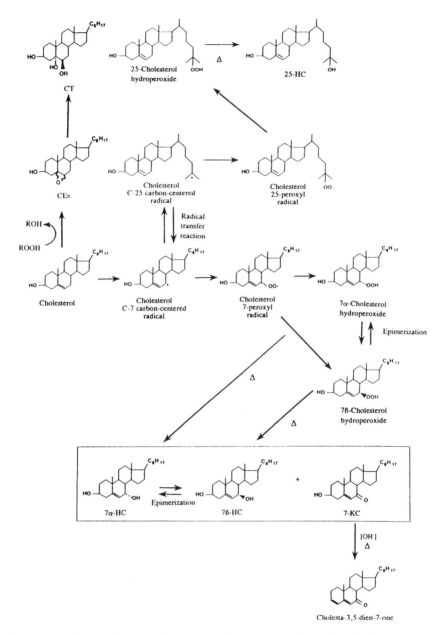

FIG. 9.2 Autoxidation of cholesterol. Formation of oxidized derivatives on the B ring and on the side chain. (*From Smith, 1990.*)

has been isolated from brain, although its function is not well established. Watabe et al. (1980) reported that, in presence of nucleotide adenine dinucleotide phosphate, $FeSO_4$ and adenosine diphosphate, cholesterol was transformed into α-CE, β-CE, and CT in beef liver microsomes, in a ratio of 1.0:4.3:0.7; cytochrome P-450, which is involved in CO formation in the human body, was not involved in formation of CEs. Use of a specific inhibitor of cholesterol-5,6-epoxide hydrolase (5,6α-imino-5α-cholestan-3β-ol) showed that this enzyme was responsible for transformation of CEs to CT. Formation of CT in human erythrocytes in vitro was reported earlier (Danielson and Horning, 1962).

CO can also be formed by microbiological fermentation. *Bacillus coagulans* B1 oxidized 35% of egg cholesterol; α-CE, β-CE, 7α-HC, 7β-HC, 25-HC, CT, 7-KC, and 20-HC were identified (Przybylski et al., 1993). Since enzymatic modification of cholesterol can be exploited as a way to reduce cholesterol in foods, such an approach should evaluate carefully residual CO formed.

Nonenzymatic Oxidation of Cholesterol In Vivo

Until recently, only enzymatic cholesterol oxidation was known in tissue. However, recent studies suggest that nonenzymatic oxidation can also occur; cholesterol could act as an antioxidant, and CO are products of reactions with some endogenous oxidants (see Smith, 1991 review). Cholesterol has an antioxidant effect against some biological oxidant agents in vitro (Teng and Smith, 1973, 1976; Smith and Teng, 1974; Smith and Stroud, 1978; Smith et al., 1978; Gumulka et al., 1982; Smith and Jaworski, 1988; Smith, 1990) and an antioxidant effect on liposomes (Gutteridge, 1978; Szebeni and Toth, 1986; Sevanian and McLeod, 1987) and erythrocytes (Jain and Shohet, 1981; Clemens et al., 1987). Antioxidant action of cholesterol is related to the finding that mortality due to cardiovascular diseases is inversely correlated with the cumulative antioxidant index (Duthie, 1991; Fitch, 1994), defined by Gey (1986) according to plasma concentration of several biological antioxidants:

$$\frac{\text{[Vitamin E] [Vitamin C] [β-Carotene] [Selenium]}}{\text{[cholesterol]}}$$

According to this hypothesis, diets low in natural antioxidants lead to higher participation of cholesterol as an antioxidant, a higher formation of CO, and a higher risk of cardiovascular diseases (Hubbard et al., 1989; Smith and Johnson, 1989; Peng et al., 1991). Furthermore, some epidemiological studies have shown that vitamin E can prevent coronary heart disease, cataracts, and some kinds of cancer (Gey et al., 1987, 1991; Comstock et al., 1991; Knekt, et al., 1991; Robertson et al., 1991), and decrease Parkinson symptoms (Fitch, 1994). Moreover, Kok et al. (1991) observed that diets high in polyunsaturated fatty acids (PUFA) but poor in natural antioxidants were a risk factor for atherosclerosis. High intake of PUFA and low intake of antioxidants is correlated to higher low-density lipoprotein (LDL) oxidation, an atherogenic process (Duthie, 1991; Esterbauer et al., 1991; Luc and Fruchart, 1991). Recent studies suggest that CO in these lipoproteins can have a significant role in atherosclerosis by affecting endothelial permeability and foam cell formation (Peng et al., 1982; Bernheimer et al., 1987; Boissoneault et al., 1991). Activity of vitamin E as a biological antioxidant is well known, and other antioxidants with similar activity include vitamin C, carotenoids, selenium, and polyphenols (Renaud and de Lorgeril, 1992; Frankel et al., 1993). Vitamin C may prevent cataracts, cancer, and atherosclerosis, while β-carotene may be anticarcinogenic (Robertson et al., 1991; Fitch, 1994).

That significant levels of cholesterol oxidation occur in vivo was clearly demonstrated by Addis et al. (1989), who determined highly variable but in some cases very high levels of CO in plasma lipoproteins of fasted human subjects. In addition to the exposure to CO from biological cholesterol oxidation (Addis et al., 1989) are recent findings indicating that high intakes of CO from foods can increase plasma CO levels (Emanuel et al., 1991). Also, intestinal absorption of CO in animals has been demonstrated (Fornas et al., 1984; Bascoul et al., 1985). Recently, Osada et al. (1994) quantified percentages of CO absorption in rats. That CO are associated with LDL, high-density lipoprotein (HDL) and very low-density lipoprotein (VLDL) in plasma (Peng et al., 1982; Addis et al., 1989) suggests that much more research is needed, especially a comparison of the quantification of dietary versus in vivo exposure.

FORMATION OF CHOLESTEROL OXIDES IN FOODS

CO absorption and toxicity findings emphasize the need to inhibit cholesterol oxidation. Factors affecting cholesterol oxidation in foods are cholesterol content, water activity, pH, oxygen, temperature, radiation, photosensitizing agents, metal ions, and storage time (Sander et al., 1989b). Some studies have investigated implications of food processing variables in CO formation, such as addition of salt (Sander et al., 1989b), prooxidant agents (Morgan and Armstrong, 1987; 1992; Chan et al., 1993), and antioxidants (Pearson et al., 1983; Park and Addis, 1986b; Morgan and Armstrong, 1987; Guardiola, 1994; Rankin and Pike, 1993). Drying systems employed to produce spray-dried products are also a key factor in CO formation (Missler et al., 1985; Tsai and Hudson, 1985; Morgan and Armstrong, 1987, 1992; Nourooz-Zadeh and Appelqvist, 1987, 1988b; Guardiola, 1994; Guardiola et al., 1995b). Heating can result in CO in tallow (Ryan et al., 1981; Ryan, 1982;

Pearson et al., 1983; Bascoul et al., 1986b; Park and Addis, 1986a, b; Zhang and Addis, 1990), butter (Csiky, 1982; Nourooz-Zadeh and Appelqvist, 1988a; Sander et al., 1989b; Pie et al., 1990), lard (Chen et al., 1994), and meat products (Higley et al., 1986; Park and Addis, 1987; de Vore, 1988; Nourooz-Zadeh and Appelqvist, 1989; Pie et al., 1991).

CO are detected in various food products, mostly in dairy, egg, meat, and fish products and fried foods. Some bakery products present CO, since butter and egg are ingredients (Table 9.2). The most common CO are α-CE, β-CE, 7α-HC, 7β-HC, 25-HC, CT, and 7-KC (see Fig. 9.2 for oxidative pathways). Generally, the predominant CO is 7-KC; 25-HC and CT are minor. Table 9.3 gives a summary of ranges of values reported for several food products. One should bear in mind that the variety of analytical methods used and, in some studies, uncontrolled variability of food products, in terms of processing and freshness, lead to variable results.

Effect of Radiation on Cholesterol Oxidation in Foods

Bergström and Wintersteiner (1941) described oxidation of cholesterol after exposure to radiation. Later, Fioriti and Sims (1967) identified 7α-HC, 7β-HC, 7-KC, and cholesta-1,4-dien-3-one as oxidation products formed at room temperature by action of ultraviolet (UV) light. Chicoye et al. (1968a) first identified CO (α-CE, 7α-HC, 7β-HC, CT, and 7-KC) in dried egg yolk irradiated with sunlight or fluorescent light. More recent studies have confirmed these findings in different foods. Formation of 7α-HC and 7β-HC was reported in fluorescent irradiation of egg powder (Herian and Lee, 1985) and butter (Luby et al., 1986). Fluorescent irradiation of cheese powder produced α-CE, β-CE, 7β-HC, and 7-KC (Sander et al., 1989b). Csallany et al. (1989) observed 7β-HC, 7α-HC, 25-HC, and 7-KC when ground pork was UV irradiated.

Gamma irradiation is used in some countries for meat preservation in spite of its high oxidative activity. Maerker and Jones (1992) found that cholesterol in aqueous media was oxidized by gamma irradiation to α-CE, β-CE, 7α-HC, 7β-HC, 7-KC, 6-KCL, and 7-KCL. In addition, irradiation of CO showed that β-CE and, in lower proportion, α-CE were transformed to 6-KCL; 7α-HC, 7β-HC, and 7-KC to 7-KCL. This may permit use of 6-KCL and 7-KCL as markers of irradiation. Hwang and Maerker (1993a) reported more detailed studies in this field, finding that gamma irradiation increases CO content in beef, veal, and pork and that storage further increases CO. The same authors (1993b) also showed that presence of 6-KCL is a good marker of irradiation only in chicken, since in beef, veal, and lamb this CO is detected in both irradiated and unirradiated meats (being higher in irradiated). Lebovics et al. (1992) showed that gamma irradiation of spray-dried egg with doses to eliminate *Salmonella* contamination induced CO formation (α-CE, 7α-HC, 7β-HC, and 7-KC).

TABLE 9.2 Foods and Food Products in Which Cholesterol Oxides Have Been Detected

Milk and dairy products	Egg and egg products	Meat and meat products
Chan et al., 1993	Emanuel et al., 1991	Csallany et al. 1989
Cleveland and Harris, 1987	Fontana et al., 1992, 1993	de Vore, 1988
Csiky, 1982	Guardiola, 1994	Higley et al., 1986
Finocchiaro et al., 1984	Guardiola et al., 1995b	Hwang and Maerker, 1993a, b
Jacobson, 1987	Herian and Lee, 1985	Monahan et al., 1992
Kumar and Singhal, 1992	Lebovics et al., 1992	Nourooz-Zadeh and Appelqvist, 1989
Luby et al., 1986	Missler et al., 1985	Park and Addis, 1985b, 1987
Nourooz-Zadeh and Appelqvist, 1988a, b	Morgan and Armstrong, 1987, 1989, 1992	Pie et al., 1991
Pie et al., 1990	Naber and Biggert, 1985	Sander et al., 1989a
Prasad and Subramanian, 1992	Nourooz-Zadeh, 1990	Zubillaga and Maerker, 1991
Sander et al., 1988, 1989a, b	Nourooz-Zadeh and Appelqvist, 1987	
van de Bovenkamp et al., 1988	Pie et al., 1990	
	Sander et al., 1989a	
	Tsai and Hudson, 1984, 1985	
	Tsai et al., 1980	
	van de Bovenkamp et al., 1988	
	Wahle et al., 1993	

Frying media	Fried foods	Bakery products
Bascoul et al., 1986b	Lee et al., 1985	Fontana et al., 1993
Chen et al., 1994	Nourooz-Zadeh and Appelqvist, 1989	Pie et al., 1990
Csiky, 1982	Park and Addis, 1985b	
Kumar and Singhal, 1992	Pie et al., 1991	
Nourooz-Zadeh and Appelqvist, 1988a	Ryan, 1982	
Park and Addis, 1986a, b	Zhang et al., 1991	

Frying media (cont.)	Fish and fish products	Primary reviews on cholesterol oxides in foods and food products
Pie et al., 1990		
Ryan, 1982		
Ryan et al., 1981		
Yan and White, 1990	Chen and Yen, 1994	Addis and Park, 1992
Zhang and Addis, 1990	Osada et al., 1993b	Finocchiaro and Richardson, 1983
	Ohshima et al., 1993	Guardiola et al., 1995e

TABLE 9.3 Range of Cholesterol Oxide Contents Detected in Various Foods and Food Products (same references as in Table 9.2)

Foods and food products	Cholesterol oxides (ppm)						
	α-CE	β-CE	7α-HC	7β-HC	25-HC	CT	7-KC
Whole milk	ND[a]–9.0	ND–1.0	ND	ND	ND	ND	ND
Spray-dried whole milk	ND–0.015	ND–0.07	ND–0.034	ND–0.015	ND	ND	ND–0.010
Spray-dried skimmed milk	ND–0.26	ND–0.09	ND–0.020	ND–0.023	ND	ND	ND–0.025
Butter	ND–7.0	ND–TR[b]	ND	ND–4.0	ND–2.6	ND	ND–TR
Parmesan cheese powders	ND–5.0	ND–6.0	ND	ND–9.0	ND–4.0	ND–9.0	ND–16.0
Cheddar cheese powders	ND–9.0	ND–4.0	ND–6.0	ND–10.0	ND–3.0	ND–17.0	ND–14.0
Egg	ND–0.7	ND–2.0	ND–0.3	ND–0.3	ND	ND	ND–0.8
Frozen egg	0.8	—[c]	—	0.9	0.7	4.1	4.0
Freeze-dried whole egg	ND–0.2	ND	ND–TR	ND–1.2	ND	ND	ND–1.0
Spray-dried whole egg	ND–111.0	ND–62.7	ND–34.4	ND–65.0	ND–10.0	ND–8.8	ND–37.0
Spray-dried egg yolk	1.8–79.0	5.0–68.5	2.6–43.2	1.7–51.0	ND–13.9	ND–0.5	1.8–46.2
Beef	0.05–0.42	0.13–1.06	ND–0.33	ND–0.34	0.14	ND	ND–1.12
Veal	0.03–0.17	0.09–0.47	0.18	0.21	0.05	ND	0.22–0.71

Pork	0.02–0.22	0.03–0.35	ND–0.19	ND–0.28	ND–0.13	0.04	ND–0.92
Chicken	0.07	0.06	ND	ND	—	ND	0.13
Lard	ND–0.3	ND	ND–TR	ND	ND–0.2	—	ND–0.3
Heated butter (10 min, 170°C; 20 min, 180°C)	0.1–2.9	0.1–7.3	0.1–52.2	0.1–19.7	ND–34.0	ND–TR	0.4–11.2
Tallow/Cotton oil (9:1) heated 170°C, 8–32 hr	ND–17.0	ND–4.0	2.0–14.0	ND–1.0	ND–4.0	ND–2.0	1.0–5.0
Tallow/Cotton oil (9:1) heated 170°C, 40–112 hr	1.0–14.0	5.0–12.0	3.0–7.0	1.0–42.0	ND–5.0	1.0–4.0	14.0–53.0
French-fried potatoes	ND–3.0	ND–2.0	ND	1.0–58.8	2.0–7.0	3.0–16.0	4.1–18.0
Salted-dried fish	TR–14.0	TR–49.0	ND–27.0	1.3–98.0	TR–10.7	ND–5.3	0.05–53.0
Boiled-dried fish	TR–18.0	TR–43.3	—	3.7–55.8	0.6–8.5	TR–39.1	4.0–60.6
Canned boiled fish	2.0	7.0	ND	28.0	ND	ND	ND
Smoked fish	2.4	3.3	—	7.3	4.8	2.7	6.3
Butter cakes	0.22–0.45	0.90–1.45	0.29–0.37	0.08–0.44	TR–0.12	TR–0.08	1.55–1.69

[a]Not detected.
[b]Traces.
[c]Not determined.

Effect of Storage Time and Conditions

Storage and conditions of storage may be considered as key factors affecting cholesterol oxidation. Temperature has been reported to be a critical factor (Nourooz-Zadeh and Appelqvist, 1987; Chan et al., 1993), together with light or other radiation (Finocchiaro et al., 1984; Sander et al., 1989b; Chan et al., 1993; Guardiola, 1994), moisture (Nourooz-Zadeh and Appelqvist, 1987; Guardiola, 1994), concentration of prooxidant and antioxidant agents (Morgan and Armstrong, 1987; Chan et al., 1993; Guardiola, 1994), vacuum (Nourooz-Zadeh and Appelqvist, 1987; Guardiola, 1994), or modified atmosphere packaging (Finocchiaro et al., 1984; Missler et al., 1985; Chan et al., 1993), and package size (Nourooz-Zadeh and Appelqvist, 1987).

Fresh and cooked meats stored for a short time at 4°C exhibited increased CO content (Park and Addis, 1987; de Vore, 1988; Zubillaga and Maerker, 1991; Monahan et al., 1992; Hwang and Maerker, 1993a). Meats stored for 3 months at −20°C exhibited only slightly increased CO content (Pie et al., 1991). Nourooz-Zadeh and Appelqvist (1989) found that CO levels did not increase in lard refrigerated for 18 months.

Sander et al. (1988) observed that CO levels in stored butter remained low up to 16 weeks of storage at temperatures from −26 to 16°C. Pie et al. (1990) found that storage of butter at −20°C for 6 months gives slight but significant increases of CO content. Finocchiaro et al. (1984) showed that modified atmosphere packaging of bleached butteroil prevented CO formation during storage. Sander et al. (1989b) found that CO formation was virtually nonexistent during storage of cheese powders for 6 months at 21 or 38°C. Nourooz-Zadeh and Appelqvist (1988a,b) reported a correlation between CO levels and storage time for skimmed milk powder stored for 37 months at room temperature and for butter stored for 4 months at 4°C. Chan et al. (1993) showed that temperature, light, and oxygen concentration influence CO formation during storage of whole milk powder. Nourooz-Zadeh and Appelqvist (1987) observed that refrigerated storage prevented CO formation in powdered egg for 2 months. Guardiola (1994) showed that vacuum packaging and storage under darkness prevented CO formation in egg powder stored for 10 months. CO formation correlated well with UV absorption at 232, 270, and 303 nm, oxidation of carotenoids, PUFA losses, and moisture and water activity.

Processing

Some processes applied to foods, especially heat treatments, can induce cholesterol autoxidation. This effect has been demonstrated for drying processes, except freeze drying. CO in freeze dried egg are not detected (Tsai and Hudson, 1984; Fontana et al., 1992) or are minimal (Nourooz-

Zadeh and Appelqvist, 1987; Morgan and Armstrong, 1989; Guardiola, 1994). CO formation during spray-drying of eggs is much higher in direct-fired dryers than indirect ones (Missler et al., 1985; Tsai and Hudson, 1985; Morgan and Armstrong, 1987; 1992; Nourooz-Zadeh and Appelqvist, 1987). This was attributed to formation of nitrogen oxides (NO, NO_2) in air directly heated by passage through a natural gas flame (Missler et al., 1985; Tsai and Hudson, 1985; Morgan and Armstrong, 1987). Morgan and Armstrong (1987) showed that addition of H_2O_2 to an indirect heating atomizer gave an increase in CO content in dried egg yolk, since N_2O decomposes to NO and NO_2 at high temperatures. Chan et al. (1993) observed that, after 6 months of storage at 20°C, whole milk powders prepared by direct gas-fired heating had greater CO content than those produced by indirect heating systems. CO were absent from both freshly processed whole milk powders. Previous studies had reported that nitrogen oxides (NO_x) can induce oxidation of cholesterol (Sevanian et al., 1979; Smith, 1981) and of unsaturated fatty acids (Pryor and Lightsey, 1981). CO formation in production of powdered egg products is correlated with spray-drying temperature (Morgan and Armstrong, 1987; 1992; Guardiola, 1994; Guardiola et al., 1995b). Guardiola et al. (1995b) showed that CO formation was much lower at 120 and 128°C than at 142°C (outlet temperatures), suggesting a critical temperature between 128 and 142°C at which CO increase significantly. Nourooz-Zadeh and Appelqvist (1988b) studied production of dried milk by roller drying and noted that CO levels between this process and indirect heating spray-drying did not differ.

Smith (1981) reported that H_2O_2 induces formation of CEs and emphasized the role of removal of glucose by glucose-oxidase/catalase and H_2O_2 (used in egg to avoid Maillard browning during spray-drying). Morgan and Armstrong (1987) studied the effect of H_2O_2 at different concentrations during spray-drying of egg yolk and noted induction of CEs in egg yolk powder and their increase during storage due to residual H_2O_2.

Sander et al. (1988) reported no significant CO formation during routine operations to obtain butter and Cheddar cheese. Cleveland and Harris (1987) did not detect CO presence in pasteurized whole, UHT, evaporated, and skim milk, but CO were detected in skim milk powder. Sander et al. (1988, 1989a) detected CEs in whole milk. Nourooz-Zadeh and Appelqvist (1988a) and Sander et al. (1989b) observed that powdered and grated cheese showed considerable CO contents. A significant CO content has been reported in home-made ghee, a clarified butter used by Indian populations, obtained by heating at 150°C for 20–25 minutes (Jacobson, 1987; Kumar and Singhal, 1992; Prasad and Subramanian, 1992). However, when butter was clarified industrially, involving lower heat treatment and use of antioxidants, lower values of CO were found (Prasad and Subramanian, 1992).

Supercritical CO_2 has been demonstrated to greatly reduce both cholesterol and CO in dried egg yolk (Bringe and Cheng, 1995).

Frying and Cooking

In frying, fats undergo extensive oxidative changes. Cholesterol oxidation occurs in lard and tallow used as frying media (Ryan et al., 1981; Ryan, 1982; Pearson et al., 1983; Bascoul et al., 1986b; Park and Addis, 1986a,b; Yan and White, 1990; Chen et al., 1994). In tallow, it has been shown that CO formation increases with time for temperatures between 135 and 165°C, but above 180°C lower levels of CO were found (Park and Addis, 1986a, b); cholesterol thermally decomposes rather than oxidizes at higher temperatures. Zhang and Addis (1990) observed a correlation between CO levels and dielectric properties of frying media (90% tallow/10% cottonseed oil). Ryan et al. (1982) reported that French fried potatoes had an approximately fourfold greater CO content than frying medium. Zhang et al. (1991) studied CO content in French fried potatoes in a fast food restaurant over a period of 30 days; CO levels fluctuated greatly, presumably according to filtration and replacement of frying media, but periodically reached high levels. Significant levels of CT, rarely seen in food products and considered to be highly atherogenic, were noted by Zhang et al. (1991). Lee et al. (1985) reported somewhat similar findings in a study performed in five restaurants. These results underscore the need for effective oil maintenance programs.

Butter is used less as a frying medium, but CO formation occurs when this fat is heated. Sander et al. (1989b) followed CO accumulation in a butteroil heated at 110°C for 24 days. Increases in α-CE, β-CE, 7α-HC, 7β-HC, and 7-KC content occurred for 8 days, after which only 7-KC followed an increasing pattern, while the content of the other four CO remained the same or decreased. Csiky (1982) heated butter at 180°C for 5 to 10 minutes and observed that CO change from traces of 25-HC in fresh butter to quantifiable 7α-HC, 7β-HC, 25-HC, 7-KC, and 4β-HC in heated butter. Nourooz-Zadeh and Appelqvist (1988a) and Pie et al. (1990) found similar results, and it could be concluded that heating at >170°C for 10 minutes induces CO formation in butter. Kumar and Singhal (1992) studied CO formation when ghee is used as a deep frying medium and found extremely high CO levels after intermittent heating at 225°C. The formation of CO was detected in fried bacon by Nourooz-Zadeh and Appelqvist (1989).

de Vore (1988) showed that storage induced higher levels of 7-KC in cooked than in uncooked beef. Park and Addis (1987) observed that cooked, refrigerated beef experienced slight CO formation. Pie et al. (1991) noted that several cooking methods induced CO in meats.

Prevention of Cholesterol Oxidation

Cholesterol is not as labile as PUFA, and protection afforded to PUFA will have a dual benefit with regard to prevention of CO accumulation. Other than direct protection of cholesterol, prevention of PUFA oxidation secondarily protects cholesterol because of the well-established mechanisms of PUFA radicals attacking cholesterol.

Water activity (a_w) is a well-known factor in autoxidation (Karel, 1980). Sander et al. (1989b) observed that addition of increasing amounts of salt in a butter derivative decreased cholesterol autoxidation, possibly due to immobilizing catalytic transition metals at lower a_w values.

Several authors reported that presence of antioxidants (reduced glutathione, propyl gallate, BHA, and BHT) or synergistic combinations (ascorbyl palmitate + d,l-α-tocopherol) prevented CO formation (Pearson et al., 1983; Park and Addis, 1986b; Morgan and Armstrong, 1987; Guardiola, 1994). Propyl gallate is more effective in powdered egg products than BHT, BHA, or a combination of ascorbyl palmitate + d,l-α-tocopherol (Morgan and Armstrong, 1987; Guardiola, 1994).

Wahle et al. (1993) suggested that supplementation of laying hen diets with vitamin E could prevent CO formation during storage of egg powder. Monahan et al. (1992) showed that oxidized corn oil and α-tocopherol acetate in pig diets induce and prevent, respectively, CO formation in cooked pork during storage at 4°C for 2 to 4 days.

HEALTH ASPECTS

CO are a good example of toxicity vs. hazard. The outstanding feature of CO, especially relative to cholesterol itself, is their cytotoxicity; no serious scientist questions this fact. However, given levels of CO intake (van de Bovenkamp et al., 1988) CO may not be a hazard by themselves. However, CO are not consumed in isolation, and therefore if the concern is the health of consumer, we should consider overall exposure of humans to dietary CO and other lipid degradation products, in vivo sources, and other factors such as drugs, smoking, and antioxidant status.

Numerous reviews have been written concerning cytotoxicity and related matters (Addis, 1986; Addis and Warner, 1991; Peng et al., 1992; Addis et al., 1995), and, therefore, this one will be brief and serve the purpose of providing an update. The biological properties of CO are numerous, uniformly detrimental, and appear to in principle increase the risk of coronary heart disease. The property of cytotoxicity is based on numerous other characteristics of CO, such as inhibition of enzymes including hydroxymethylglutaryl coenzyme A reductase, cholesterol-7α-hydroxylase, and cholesterol-5,6-epoxide hydrolase; reduction in membrane fluidity; inhibition of hexose transport; modification of membrane calcium flux; and increase of osmotic fragility of cells. These properties logically explain observed angiotoxicity, and subsequent atherogenicity, if experimental animals are placed on a diet containing CO; they are lethal to endothelial cells and cause atherosclerotic changes in arterial walls (Peng et al., 1992). Plaque accumulated over a period of time minimizes cross-sectional area of lumen; this condition permits thrombi to totally occlude lumen, causing myocardial infarction. Interestingly, CO have been shown to inhibit endothelial cell prostacyclin synthesis, presumably increasing the probability of thrombus formation (Peng et al., 1993).

Other aspects of CO biology tend to increase coronary heart disease. Stimulation of cholesterol esterification and hypercholesterolemia, including increased plasma LDL, have been reported (Addis et al., 1995). Production of LDL particles enriched in cholesterol esters (Warner, 1994) may increase atherogenicity of LDL (Carr et al., 1992, 1995).

The occurrence of variable and, in some cases, high levels of CO in plasma lipoproteins in fasted humans (Addis et al., 1989) and clear evidence of absorption of CO in humans (Emanuel et al., 1991) and rats (Osada et al., 1994) suggest that biologically active CO will exert effects in vivo that have been noted in vitro. The successful incorporation of ^{14}C α-CE into LDL, chylomicrons, and bovine serum albumin suggests manifold mechanisms for transporting CO in the circulation (Addis et al., 1993). However, loading LDL with CO did not increase its susceptibility to oxidative modification (Addis et al., 1993). Peng and Morin (1992) have reviewed the possibility of the cytotoxic effects of CO that have been noted in vitro having significant impact in vivo.

ANALYSIS OF CHOLESTEROL OXIDES

Since the early to mid-1980s, many different methods have been used and sometimes controversial results reported. To achieve an appropriate level of confidence in CO analysis and to facilitate data comparison, a worldwide interlaboratory study is in progress; more than 40 laboratories are engaged in analysis of the same food samples (Appelqvist, 1995). Therefore, we wish to facilitate these activities by presenting an extensive review of CO methodology. Previously, we reviewed analysis of CO (Park and Addis, 1992; Guardiola et al., 1994b; Park, 1995), and, therefore, in this paper we will review and update sample preparation and quantification of CO in foods. Given the complexity of food matrices and structural similarity of CO, it is highly desirable to confirm the identity of CO by nonchromatographic criteria such as MS or proton-nuclear magnetic resonance spectroscopy (^{1}H-NMR).

Lipid Extraction

The most frequently used total lipid extraction solvent is chloroform/methanol [2:1,v/v] (Folch et al., 1957). Most researchers used the same solvent system or modified its strength to extract total fat containing CO (Tsai et al., 1980; Finocchiaro et al., 1984; Herian and Lee, 1985; Lee et al., 1985; Park and Addis, 1985b, 1987; Tsai and Hudson, 1995; Morgan and Armstrong, 1987, 1989, 1992; de Vore, 1988; Sander et al., 1988, 1989a, b; van de Bovenkamp, 1988; Csallany et al., 1989; Ibrahim et al., 1990; Emanuel et al., 1991; Hodis et al., 1991; Pie et al., 1991; Zhang et al., 1991; Lebovics et al., 1992; Pie and Seillan, 1992; Chan et al., 1993; Hwang and Maerker, 1993a, b; Osada et al., 1993b; Ohshima et al., 1993; Wahle et al., 1993; Chen and Yen, 1994; Guardiola, 1994; Sevanian et al., 1994; Guardiola et al., 1995b, d). Other solvents used are acetonitrile (Kou and Holmes, 1985), acetone (Tsai and Hudson, 1984), chloroform (Missler et al., 1985; Lai et al., 1995), methylene chloride/ethanol [1:1,v/v] (Pie et al., 1990), methylene chloride/methanol [9:1,v/v] (Monahan et al., 1992), hexane/isopropanol [3:2 or 2:1,v/v] (Cleveland and Harris, 1987; Nourooz-Zadeh and Appelqvist, 1987, 1988a, b, 1989), or methyl-*tert*-butyl ether (Naber and Biggert, 1985).

Another procedure for fat extraction consists of adsorption of samples on a chromatographic column and a further treatment with selective solvents. Adsorbents are silica gel, Celite 545, or monocalcium phosphate and their blends. Selective elution of CO was achieved by using methylene chloride (Maerker and Jones, 1991, 1992), methylene chloride/methanol [9:1,v/v] (Higley et al., 1986), or sequences of increasingly polar solvents (Zubillaga and Maerker, 1991; Fontana et al., 1992, 1993). This system, called flash chromatography, allowed for lipid extracts of higher purity, since a great proportion of triglycerides, phospholipids, and cholesterol are removed.

Purification of Cholesterol Oxides

Because CO are minor components in the complex lipid fraction obtained, purification is necessary and is usually accomplished by saponification or chromatographic fractionation. In some cases both operations are combined in different ways to provide purified CO extracts. Choice of a suitable system must consider sample composition and affects sensitivity and selectivity of method.

Saponification. Most authors apply saponification to lipid fractions previously extracted, but application of direct saponification, which saves time and solvent, is also used (Naber and Biggert, 1985; Gruenke et al., 1987; Koopman et al., 1987; van Doormaal et al., 1989). Recently, Rose-Sallin et al. (1995) used cold direct saponification on milk powders. However, in contrast to saponification of lipid extract, direct saponification was always followed by further chromatographic purification prior to chromatographic determination. When egg products after direct saponification were subjected to HPLC determination (Naber and Biggert, 1985), the resulting chromatograms displayed severe interferences.

Hot saponification is often practiced to hasten isolation of nonsaponifiables (Finocchiaro et al., 1984; Herian and Lee, 1985; Naber et al., 1985; Bascoul et al., 1986b; Higley et al., 1986; Jacobson, 1987; Lebovics et al., 1992; Prasad and Subramanian, 1992; Osada et al., 1993b). However, it has long been known that 7-KC degrades to cholesta-3,5-dien-7-one (Fig. 9.2) during hot saponification (Bergström and Wintersteiner, 1941; Pennock et al., 1962; Ryan et al., 1981; Bascoul et al., 1986b; Chicoye et al., 1968b, c; Higley et al., 1986; Maerker and Unruh, 1986). Although this dienone artifact has been detected after a mild saponification of plasma (Hodis et al., 1991; Sevanian et al. 1994), as a degradation product of heated pure cholesterol (Korahani et al., 1981), and of cholesterol heated with phosphatidylethanolamine or triacylglycerols (Nawar et al., 1991), one should evaluate analytical procedures with care; even brief warming, e.g., dipping alkaline reaction mixtures in a waterbath at 65°C for 5 minutes to disperse lipid extracts containing 7-KC, was sufficient to destroy 10% of 7-KC, whereas cold saponification (18 hr at room temperature) recovered more than 95% (Guardiola et al., 1995a). This likely explains the low recovery, about 11 to 40% of 7-KC after cold saponification, by van de Bovenkamp et al. (1988).

Tsai et al. (1980) reported that α-CE is hydrolyzed to CT by heating in alkaline medium, conflicting with Chicoye et al. (1968a). Park and Addis (1986a) documented virtually full recovery of α-CE during cold saponification, which was confirmed by others (Pie et al., 1990; Guardiola et al., 1995d). Even when α-CE was subjected to hot KOH (70°C for 30 min), recovery was 93.9 to 97.3% (Kudo et al., 1989).

Bascoul et al. (1986b) reported no formation of CO from cholesterol saponification with hot methanolic KOH for 2 hours, whereas others reported cholesterol oxidation in similar conditions (Naber and Biggert, 1985; Maerker and Unruh, 1986). Park and Addis (1986a) detected no CO from cold saponification of tallow, and others confirmed that artifactual oxidation of cholesterol is not a practical concern (Pie et al., 1990; Pie and Seillan, 1992; Guardiola et al., 1994a, 1995d). Guardiola et al. (1995d) confirmed by GC-MS absence of cholesterol oxidation during application of three purification procedures including cold saponification, silica cartridge clean-up, or cold saponification coupled with silica cartridge clean-up. However, the temperature must be kept below 35°C during solvent removal since traces of some CO (7β-HC and 7-KC) were found when evaporation was carried to dryness at 45°C. Nourooz-Zadeh (1990) prepared fresh egg yolk using two purification methods—cold saponification and column chromatographic clean-up—and observed slightly more C-7 CO by cold saponification. The author suggested a further study to determine if increased level of CO after cold saponification was due to contribution from esterified CO or an artifact.

Recently, Rose-Sallin et al. (1995), using deuterated cholesterol, estimated overall artifactual CO formation to be approximately 0.2% (ca. 0.15% 7-KC) during sample preparation, including cold saponification. Although artifactual oxidation during sample preparation may not be extremely high, it is important enough to warrant attention. Maerker and Unruh (1986) observed slight formation of α-CE, β-CE, and 7-KC without saponification; oxidation was not avoided by addition of phenolic antioxidants during preparative HPLC. From these results, it was concluded that cholesterol oxidation occurred during HPLC enrichment and GC determination. Some authors work with addition of BHT from the first step in order to prevent cholesterol oxidation (Pie et al., 1990, 1991; Hodis et al., 1991; Monahan et al., 1992; Pie and Seillan, 1992; Sevanian et al., 1994).

Chromatographic Fractionation. Column chromatography and preparative TLC and HPLC can purify unsaponifiable extracts or isolate CO from accompanying bulk lipids. Tsai et al. (1980) and Tsai and Hudson (1985) devised small silicic acid column chromatography to purify epoxides from lipid extracts of egg yolk. Park and Addis (1985b) devised a similar process to enrich 7-HCs and 7-KC. Taking advantage of commercial clean-up column availability, de Vore (1988) replaced hand-packed silica columns of Park and Addis (1985b). The use of silica cartridges, which save solvents and time, has increased in recent years (Morgan and Armstrong, 1987, 1989, 1992; Nawar et al., 1991; Monahan et al., 1992; Chan et al., 1993; Osada et al., 1993a; Lai et al., 1995). Guardiola et al. (1995d) compared efficiency of silica cartridges in purification of CO using four different systems of elution with increasing polarities. Hwang and Maerker (1993a) coupled two silica columns with TLC on silica plates for lipid extract purification. C18 (Kou and Holmes, 1985; Chen et al., 1994) and aminopropyl (Przybylski et al., 1993) cartridges have been infrequently used. Size exclusion chromatography (Lipidex-5000) is also used in purification of lipid extracts, usually coupled to an ion exchange column, TEAP-Lipidex (Nourooz-Zadeh and Appelqvist, 1987). The same authors coupled these columns to a previous purification with a silica cartridge (Nourooz-Zadeh and Appelqvist, 1988a, 1989). However, other authors (Nawar et al., 1991) suggest that size exclusion columns are efficient but too time-consuming. CO collected through column chromatography represent oxidation of only free cholesterol.

Zubillaga and Maerker (1991) used TLC (silica plates) alone to purify lipid extract proceeding from flash chromatography extraction. Preparative TLC has been also used in analysis of standard mixtures of CO (Korahani et al., 1981; Teng, 1990, 1991; Maerker and Jones, 1991).

Preparative HPLC, alone (Csiky et al., 1982) or coupled to silica columns (Missler et al., 1985), has been used for lipid purification prior to CO determination. Nourooz-Zadeh (1990) coupled aminopropyl and C18 cartridges to preparative HPLC to purify egg yolk lipid extract. Fontana et al. (1992, 1993) reported a double preparative HPLC purification of lipid extract prior to ^{1}H-NMR 500 MHz determination.

Further purification of nonsaponifiables by chromatographic fractionation has been frequently used for supplemental clean-up of nonsaponifiables using various adsorbents such as silica cartridges (Guardiola et al., 1995b,d), aminopropyl cartridges (Rose-Sallin et al., 1995), alumina columns (Ibrahim et al., 1990), diol columns (Hodis et al., 1991; Sevanian et al., 1994), or silica plates (Finocchiaro et al., 1984; Pie et al., 1990, 1991; Pie and Seillan, 1992; Wahle et al., 1993; Chen and Yen, 1994). Finally, some studies coupled hot saponification to further purification with different combinations of silica and argentated (Florisil-AgNO$_3$) columns (Herian and Lee, 1985; Lee et al., 1985; Higley et al., 1986).

Quantification and Tentative Identification of Cholesterol Oxides

The low content of CO in samples requires high sensitivity and efficient resolution. GC and HPLC are used most frequently. Given the complexity of CO and propensity of foods to contain interferences, GC-MS or LC-MS is highly desirable for structure confirmation. Fontana et al. (1992) reported application of a new method using ^{1}H-NMR 500 MHz spectroscopy in order to ensure identification and quantification in a single operation. However, this was accomplished off-line, unlike GC-MS, because the method relied on HPLC for separation and collection of each CO prior to NMR quantification.

CO Determination by GC. GC is the most widespread method for CO determination in foods and biological materials. CO are usually converted to trimethylsilyl ethers (TMSE) to avoid peak tailing and to improve thermal stability of some hydroxycholesterols (van Lier and Smith, 1968; Teng et al., 1973a; Park and Addis, 1985a). Reproducible derivatization depends on silylating reagent, conditions, and ratio of silylating reagent/hydroxyl groups. Partial silanization produces multiple chromatographic peaks from a single CO. Frequently used reagents include hexamethyldisilazane (HMDS), N,O-bis(trimethylsilyl)acetamide (BSA), N,O-bis(trimethylsilyl)-trifluoroacetamide (BSTFA), and N-trimethylsilylimidazole (TMSI). Trimethylchlorosilane (TMCS) is a common catalyst. The most popular blend is BSA/TMSI TMCS [3:3:2, v/v/v, Sylon BTZ], due to its strong derivatization power. Complete silanization (except CT) can be obtained with this reagent in 20 to 30 minutes at room temperature (Park and Addis, 1989). Guardiola et al. (1995c) have shown variable absorptions of CO in various microtube materials during silanization.

Some studies (Korahani et al., 1981; Park and Addis, 1985a; Pie et al., 1990) reported that elution order and resolution of these TMSE derivatives differ according to polarity of stationary phase. Figure 9.3 shows a comparative CO separation on two common phases (100% methyl silicone and 5% phenyl 95% methyl silicone). Both columns provide good resolution. Split injection is usually employed in CO analysis, although some authors use on-column injection, which avoids potential injection port discrimination (Missler et al., 1985; Maerker and Bunick, 1986; Maerker and Unruh, 1986; van de Bovenkamp et al., 1988; Zubillaga and Maerker, 1989, 1991; Maerker and Jones, 1991, 1992; Wahle et al., 1993; Hwang and Maerker, 1993a,b).

The internal standard technique is frequently employed for quantification by GC. The internal standard is added at the start in order to reflect entire method. 5α-Cholestane is most frequently used (Guardiola et al., 1994b; Park, 1995). However, when columns or plates of silica are used in purification, the lower polarity of 5α-cholestane makes it impossible to elute it together with CO in a single fraction, and it must be added after purification, which only serves to correct GC determination variability. Other compounds used as internal standard that have polarities similar to CO include 19-HC, 6-KCL, 7-ketopregnenolone, and 5α-androstan-3β-ol-17-one acetate (Missler et al., 1985; Morgan and Armstrong, 1987, 1989; Pie et al., 1990, 1991; Nawar et al., 1991; Pie and Seillan, 1992; Guardiola et al., 1995b,d). Guardiola et al. (1995d) assayed use of four standards (11α-hydroxyprogesterone, 11β,17α-dihydroxyprogesterone, 19-HC, 6-KCL), selecting 19-HC as most suitable for internal standard purposes using silica purification.

The quantification of CO from chromatographic peak areas obtained through flame ionization detector (FID) can be achieved through use of relative response factors (RRF):

$$RRF = (W_{XS} \cdot A_{IS}) / (A_{XS} \cdot W_{IS})$$

where W_{XS} = CO standard weight, W_{IS} = internal standard weight, A_{XS} = CO standard area, and A_{IS} = internal standard area. RRF of derivatized and underivatized CO are given in Table 9.4. Some moderate disagreement

1. 5α-Cholestane
2. Cholesta-3,5-dien-7-one
3. Cholesterol
4. 7α-Hydroxycholesterol
5. Cholesterol-5α,6α-epoxide
6. 7ß-Hydroxycholesterol
7. 4ß-Hydroxycholesterol
8. Cholestanetriol
9. 7-Ketocholestrol
10. 25-Hydroxycholesterol

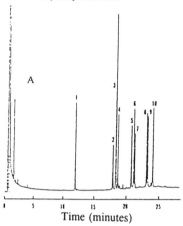

Time (minutes)

1. 7α-Hydroxycholesterol
2. Cholesterol
3. 19-Hydroxycholesterol
4. Cholesta-3,5-dien-7-one
5. 7ß-Hydroxycholesterol
6. Cholesterol-5α,6α-epoxide
7. Cholesterol-5ß,6ß-epoxide
8. 20-Hydroxycholesterol
9. Cholestanetriol
10. 25-Hydroxycholesterol
11. 7-Ketocholesterol
12. 26-Hydroxycholesterol

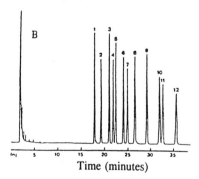

Time (minutes)

FIG. 9-3   Separation of TMSE of cholesterol oxides on different polarity columns. (A) Methyl silicone (15 m × 0.25 μm film thickness, 200 to 260°C at 3°C/min). (*From Park and Addis, 1985a.*) (B) 5% phenyl 95% methyl silicone (30 m × 1.0 μm film thickness, 280°C). (*From Pie et al., 1990.*)

TABLE 9.4 Relative Response Factors of Cholesterol and Key Cholesterol Oxides Reported by Different Authors

| | TMSE derivatives | | | | | | | Underivatized | |
| | Split | | | | | | On-column | On-column | |
Standards	Guardiola et al. (1995d)[a]	Park and Addis (1985a)[a]	Sevanian et al. (1994)[a]	Lai et al. (1995)[b]	Nawar et al. (1991)[c]	Pie et al. (1990)	van de Bovenkamp et al. (1988)[a]	Maerker and Jones (1991)[b]	Maerker and Jones (1992)[f]
Cholesterol	0.88	1.00	—	—	0.74	0.92[d]	—	0.87	0.97
α-CE	1.03	1.13	0.77	1.03	0.85	1.10[e]	1.23	1.10	1.05
7β-HC	0.98	0.98	1.09	1.05	0.86	0.99[e]	0.93	1.11	1.14
CT	0.99	1.03	0.79	1.50	—	1.13[e]	1.07	—	1.36
7-KC	1.24	1.13	0.81	1.08	0.91	1.20[e]	1.10	1.03	1.11
25-HC	0.94	0.98	0.81	1.48	—	1.14[e]	0.93	—	—

[a] Internal standard 5α-cholestane.
[b] Internal standard 3β-hydroxy-5α-cholestan-6-one (6-ketocholestanol).
[c] Internal standard 5α-androstan-3β-ol-17-one.
[d] Internal standard 5α-cholestan-3β-ol (cholestanol).
[e] Internal standard cholest-5-en-3β,19-diol (19-hydroxycholesterol).
[f] Internal standard cholesta-5,24-dien-3β-ol (desmosterol).

exists among researchers, but it is difficult to understand a large difference (as much as 60 to 90%) in RRF within epimeric pairs such as epoxides and hydroxycholesterols as recently reported by Lai et al. (1995).

In a recent work, Sevanian et al. (1994) compared detection limits and RRF for CO obtained by GC-FID and GC-MS. When MS was used as detector, RRF were calculated using most intense characteristic ion for each compound (selected ion monitoring mode). Results showed that the sensitivity of both detectors is very similar.

Cholesterol Oxide Determination by HPLC. The main advantages of HPLC are nondestructive detection and low separation temperatures, avoiding thermal decomposition. However, HPLC detectors are not as universal as FID, which can add complexity to the determination of some CO. Some authors evaluated variability of CO resolution on different silica columns and with several mobile phases (Tsai and Hudson, 1981; Teng, 1990, 1991). Tsai and Hudson (1981) assayed 24 steroid standards on a μ-Porasil column testing different mobile phases, hexane/isopropanol, hexane/ethyl acetate, and hexane/tetrahydrofuran. Among three mobile phases, hexane/isopropanol (100:3, v/v) gave the best resolution. An interesting conclusion was that k' (capacity factor) was influenced by location of a second oxygenated group and its stereospecific orientation.

Teng (1990, 1991) studied μ-Porasil, Ultrasphere SIL, and Zorbax SIL columns, and mobile phases of hexane/isopropanol, from 100:2 to 100:3 (v/v); he concluded that resolution depends on number of silanol groups on stationary phase surface. μ-Porasil and Zorbax SIL showed better resolution than Ultrasphere SIL but did not separate 7-HC epimers. If cholesterol hydroperoxides need to be determined, Ultrasphere SIL provides better resolution and shorter analysis time.

Good separation of all CO is difficult if isocratic conditions are employed. Using isocratic elution, Tsai and Hudson (1984, 1985) determined only α-CE and β-CE in egg products. Other authors determined only C-7 CO (Herian and Lee, 1985; Park and Addis, 1985b; Csallany et al., 1989). de Vore (1988) quantified only 7-KC in beef. Lee et al. (1985) showed that HPLC (LiChrosorb Si 60, hexane/isopropanol, 100:10, v/v) was unable to resolve CO and β-sitosterol oxidation products. Gradient elution achieves better resolution of complex CO mixtures. Maerker et al. (1988b) obtained narrow, symmetrical peaks and good resolution on μ-Porasil among a wide variety of CO species with solvent programming. Csiky (1982) obtained good simultaneous determination of 7α-HC, 7β-HC, 25-HC, 7-KC, and 4β-HC from a butter sample, applying a gradient 0 to 10% of butanol in hexane on a Nucleosil NO$_2$ column.

Sevanian et al. (1994) resolved 11 compounds with polarities between

5α-cholestane and CT in plasma using normal- and reverse-phase HPLC with various elution solvents. Naber et al. (1985) and Fillion et al. (1991) reported poor resolution between 7-HC and CE epimers for reverse-phase HPLC. Reverse-phase HPLC worked very well for Finocchiaro et al. (1984) in dairy products, resolving simultaneously 7α-HC, 7β-HC, α-CE, β-CE, and CT (μ-Bondapak C18, acetonitrile/water, 9:1, v/v).

The UV spectrophotometer is the most widely used detector for HPLC determination of CO. Most CO show absorption maximum below 210 nm. While 7-KC has a strong absorption at 233 nm (Fig. 9.4); CEs and CT do not adsorb in the UV region. Nonabsorbing CO can be derivatized with benzoyl chloride or 3,5-dinitrobenzoyl chloride. Carey and Persinger (1972) and Fitzpatrick and Siggia (1973) introduced these procedures, but they were optimized by Fillion et al. (1991). In addition, *p*-nitrobenzoylation and picration have been used for CE epimers (Lee et al., 1984; Sugino et al., 1986). However, these techniques have not been widely used because stability of derivatives is critical and a high variability of results is introduced by

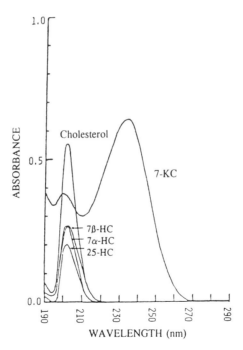

FIG. 9.4   UV absorption spectra of some cholesterol oxides. (*From Csallany et al., 1989.*)

derivatization. Less frequently used are other detectors like MS (Sevanian et al., 1994) or FID (Maerker et al., 1988a, b).

The external standard is most frequently used method of quantification in HPLC. However, when underivatized CO are detected by UV spectrometry, use of more than one external standard is needed due to UV response differences among CO. Park and Addis (1987) used 7-ketopregnenolone as an internal standard for 7-HCs and 7-KC quantification.

Confirmation of Cholesterol Oxide Identity

As CO are a complex family of compounds, identification of individual compounds must be confirmed. The most universal method for confirmation of tentatively identified compounds is MS (electronic impact), comparing mass spectra from tentatively identified CO, or their TMSE derivatives, with standards. ^{1}H-NMR and infrared spectroscopy are also used in CO identification (Tsai and Hudson, 1984; Fontana et al., 1992, 1993).

CO determination is mostly done by GC of TMSE derivatives, and MS is easily coupled to GC systems; therefore, spectra corresponding to these derivatives are common in the literature. Table 9.5 provides a summary of relevant data.

7-HCs TMSE. Mass spectra of both epimers are very similar, and their differentiation must be achieved by comparing retention times. Their spectra are very simple, with a predominant peak at m/z 456 (M-90) and some

TABLE 9.5 Summary of Literature on Cholesterol Oxide Mass Spectra

Cholesterol oxides		
Nonderivatized	Derivatized as TMSE	Other cholesterol oxide derivatives
Cleveland and Harris, 1987	Aringer and Eneroth, 1974	Pannecoucke et al., 1992
deVore, 1988	Brooks et al, 1968, 1973	
Finocchiaro et al., 1984	Guardiola, 1994	
Gray et al., 1971	Nourooz-Zadeh and Appelqvist, 1987, 1989	Primary reviews on cholesterol oxide mass spectra
Kou and Holmes, 1985	Park and Addis, 1985a, 1986a, 1987, 1989	
Park and Addis, 1985b		
Sevanian et al., 1994	Osada et al., 1993a	Guardiola et al., 1994b
Tsai and Hudson, 1984	Rose-Sallin et al., 1995	Park and Addis, 1992
	Zhang et al., 1991	Park, 1995

minor but characteristic peaks at m/z 546 (M), 441 (M-90-15), 366 (M-90-90), and 351 (M-90-90-15). Their differentiation from other dihydroxycholesterols is simple (Table 9.5). 4β-HC gives characteristic peaks with relative intensity > 10% at m/z 546 (M), 531 (M-15), 456 (M-90), 417 (M-129), 366 (M-90-90), and 351 (M-90-90-15) and a peak with high intensity at m/z 129, which is characteristic of sterols with a double bond in position 5 and a 3β-hydroxyl group (Dumazer et al., 1986).

Side-Chain HCs TMSE.   25-HC shows base peak at m/z 131 and other minor but characteristic peaks at m/z 546 (M), 531 (M-15), 456 (M-90), 441 (M-90-15), 366 (M-90-90), 351 (M-90-90-15), 327 (M-90-129), and 271 (Table 9.5). 20-HC is characterized by a base peak at m/z 201, corresponding to complete side chain, including trimethylsilyl group, and peak at m/z 461 (M-85) according to Brooks et al. (1973).

CEs TMSE.   Both epimers show similar spectra, with peaks at m/z 474 (M) and 384 (M-90) as most characteristic and peaks at m/z 459 (M-15) and 456 (M-18). Peaks at m/z 366 (M-90-18) and 369 (M-90-15) are always observed for α-CE, but for β-CE Park and Addis (1986a) only observed a peak at m/z 369. Aringer and Eneroth (1974) and Nourooz-Zadeh and Appelqvist (1987) observed both. This is not a problem, because both CEs are easily differentiated by their chromatographic retention times. In addition, for these two derivatives, little agreement in terms of relative intensities of characteristic ions is found among mass spectra literature (Table 9.5).

7-KC TMSE.   Most studies report molecular ion (m/z 472) as base peak; other characteristic ions are 382 (M-90) and 367 (M-90-15). Other peaks are only cited by some authors, like 457 (M-15), 187, 174, and 161 (Table 9.5). The base peak is m/z 472 with magnetic sector MS (Brooks et al., 1968; Park and Addis, 1985a) but is m/z 129 if a quadrupole MS is used (Park and Addis, 1986a; Guardiola, 1994).

CT TMSE.   As this CO has three hydroxyl groups, different spectra can be obtained if silanization is not complete. A treatment at 60°C for 60 hours with BSA/TMSI/TMCS (3:3:2, v/v/v) was needed to complete it (Brooks et al., 1968). When salinization was carried out at room temperature for 1 hour, only bis-TMSE was obtained, suggesting that 5α-hydroxyl group is sterically hindered. The mass spectra of tris- and bis-TMSE are very similar. However, relative intensity of characteristic ions was quite different. The base peak for bis-TMSE was m/z 129, while for tris-TMSE was 456 (M-90-90) (Brooks et al., 1973). Later, Park and Addis (1989) showed that if the derivatization was done at 70°C for an extended period, tris-TMSE peak emerged at the expense of bis-TMSE peak by GC. When both peaks were subjected to MS, almost identical mass spectra were obtained. However, m/z

636 (M) and 621 (M-15) from tris-TMSE and 564 (M) from bis-TMSE were clearly observed, providing critical information for differentiation between these two TMSE. Common peaks for both spectra are m/z 546, 531, 456, 441, 403, 367, and 321. For bis-TMSE the peak at m/z 351 has been reported by Park and Addis (1987) and Guardiola (1994). As derivatization conditions used in CO determination by GC usually leads to bis-TMSE, its spectra is very common in literature and little agreement in terms of relative intensities of characteristic ions is found among authors (Table 9.5).

Although less frequent, MS may be coupled to HPLC for underivatized CO. In addition, direct insertion of pure analyte obtained by HPLC into ionization chamber can be made. Therefore we present some data on characteristic spectra of underivatized CO.

7-HCs.   Both epimers show very similar spectra, with base peak at m/z 384 (M-18). Other characteristic peaks are 402 (M), 366 (M-18-18), 351 (M-18-18-15), and 247 (M-42-side chain) reported by Park and Addis (1985b), Finocchiaro et al. (1984), and Sevanian et al. (1994). The peak at 369 (M-18-15) has been reported as significant by some authors (Finocchiaro et al., 1984; Sevanian et al., 1994).

25-HC.   Kou and Holmes (1985) observed these characteristic ions: m/z 402 (M), 384 (M-18) and 369 (M-18-15). Sevanian et al. (1994) reported characteristic peaks at m/z 402 and 400.

CEs.   Spectra data on both epimers are very similar (Table 9.5), with characteristic peaks at m/z 402 (M), 384 (M-18), 369 (M-18-15), 271 (M-18-side chain), 247 (M-42-side chain), and 229 (M-18-42-side chain). However, Tsai and Hudson (1984) observed that at m/z 331 (M-C_4H_7O) appears a specific peak for α-CE and also that β-CE shows a minor peak at m/z 356, which is very intense for α-CE.

7-KC.   Base peak appears at m/z 400 (M), and other minor characteristic peaks are m/z 382 (M-18), 367 (M-18-15), 287 (M-side chain), 205, 192, and 174 (Park and Addis, 1985b; de Vore, 1988; Sevanian et al., 1994).

CT.   Finocchiaro et al. (1984) observed these characteristic ions: m/z 420 (M), 402 (M-18), 387 (M-18-15), 366 (M-18-18), 351 (M-18-18-15), 271 (M-18-side chain), 247 (M-42-side chain), and 229 (M-18-18-42-side chain).

SUMMARY

This review covers new developments in research on cholesterol oxides (CO), including food composition, methods of analysis, and biological and health aspects. We find it premature to speculate about deleterious health effects of dietary CO. However, in attempting to summarize the accomplishments of more than two decades of vigorous, difficult research, one must be impressed with what has been learned about cholesterol relative to CO. Cholesterol is clearly free of the many biological effects of CO, consistent with its role as perhaps the most important single chemical entity in animal tissue. As a corollary, CO research has demonstrated that the role of (pure) cholesterol in coronary heart disease must be minor if it exists at all. Virtually all of the untoward effects previously attributed to cholesterol have been found to be due to contaminating CO. These are no small accomplishments. As a conclusion, if cholesterol is cited as being atherogenic, for example, intellectual honesty requires that CO be cited as being far more atherogenic, based on the tremendous amount of research reported. Likewise, intellectual honesty dictates that anyone dismissing the potential health effects of CO must do so for cholesterol as well. Unfortunately, cholesterol and other lipids, as well as CO and other lipid oxidation products, are not consumed in isolation. The many interactions of these dietary components pose a formidable research problem. Fortunately, development of an improved understanding of CO analysis and techniques paves the way to better understanding of the health effects of CO and other lipid oxidation products.

ACKNOWLEDGMENTS

Published as paper no. 22,182 of the Scientific Journal Series of the Minnesota Agricultural Experiment Station, Project 18-23H. The authors thank Dr. Abdulwahab Asamarai for technical advice. This study was supported in part by a research grant from "Comissió Interdepartamental de Recerca i Innovació Tecnològica" (CIRIT).

REFERENCES

Addis, P. B. 1986. Occurrence of lipid oxidation products in foods. *Food Chem. Toxicol.* 24: 1021–1030.

Addis, P. B., Carr, T. P., Hassel, C. A., Huang, Z. Z., and Warner, G. J. 1995. Atherogenic and anti-atherogenic factors in the human diet. In *Free Radicals and Oxidative Stress: Environment, Drugs and Food Additives*, C. Rice-Evans and B. Halliwell (Ed.), pp. 259–271. Portland Press, London.

Addis, P. B., Emanuel, H. A., Bergmann, S. D., and Zavoral, J. H. 1989. Capillary GC quantification of cholesterol oxidation products in plasma lipoproteins of fasted humans. *Free Radical Biol. Med.* 7: 179–182.

Addis, P. B., and Park, S. W. 1992. Cholesterol oxide content of foods. In *Biological Effects of Cholesterol Oxides*, S. K. Peng and R. J. Morin (Ed.), pp. 71–88. CRC Press, Boca Raton, FL.

Addis, P. B. and Warner, G. J. 1991. The potential health aspects of lipid oxidation products in food. In *Free Radicals and Food Additives*, O. I. Aruoma and B. Halliwell (Ed.), pp. 77–119. Taylor and Francis Ltd., London.

Addis, P. B., Warner, G. J., and Hassel, C. A. 1993. Dietary lipid oxidation products: Are they atherogenic? *Can. J. Cardiol.* 9: 6B–10B.

Appelqvist, L-Å. 1995. Harmonization of oxysterol analysis in food and blood. Worldwide interlaboratory study with more than 40 laboratories involved. Department of Food Science, Swedish University of Agricultural Sciences, Uppsala, Sweden.

Aringer, L. and Eneroth, P. 1974. Formation and metabolism in vitro of 5,6-epoxides of cholesterol and β-sitosterol. *J. Lipid Res.* 15: 389–398.

Bascoul, J., Domergue, N., and Crastes de Paulet, A. 1985. Intestinal absorption of cholesterol autoxidation products in dietary fats. *J. Am. Oil Chem. Soc.* 62: 623a.

Bascoul, J., Domergue, N., Mourot, J., Debry, G., and Crastes de Paulet, A. 1986a. Intestinal absorption and fecal excretion of 5,6α-epoxy-5α-cholesta-3β-ol by the male Wistar rat. *Lipids* 21: 744–747.

Bascoul, J., Domergue, N., Olle, M., and Crastes de Paulet, A. 1986b. Autoxidation of cholesterol in tallows heated under deep frying conditions: Evaluation of oxysterols by GLC and TLC-FID. *Lipids* 21: 383–387.

Bergström, S. and Wintersteiner, O. 1941. Autoxydation of sterols in colloidal aqueous solutions. The nature of the products formed from cholesterol. *J. Biol. Chem.* 141: 597.

Bergström, S. and Wintersteiner, O. 1942a. Autoxydation of sterols in colloidal aqueous solution III. Quantitative studies on cholesterol. *J. Biol. Chem.* 145: 309–322.

Bergström, S. and Wintersteiner, O. 1942b. Autoxydation of sterols in colloidal aqueous solution IV. Influence of esterification and of constitutional factors. *J. Biol. Chem.* 145: 327–333.

Bernheimer, A. W., Robinson, W. G., Linder, R., Mullins, D., Yip, Y. K., Cooper, N. S., Seidman, I., and Uwajima, T. 1987. Toxicity of enzymically oxidized low-density lipoprotein. *Biochem. Biophys. Res. Commun.* 148: 260–266.

Bhagavan, H. N. and Nair, P. P. 1992. Antioxidants in dietary fats. In *Fatty Acids in Foods and Their Health Implications*, C. K. Chow (Ed.), pp. 329–336. Marcel Dekker, Inc., New York.

Boissonneault, G. A., Hennig, B., Wang, Y., Ouyang, C-M, Krahulik, K., Cunnup, L., and Oeltgen, P. R. 1991. Effect of oxysterol-enriched low density lipoprotein on endothelial barrier function in culture. *Am. Nutr. Metab.* 35: 226–232.

Bringe, N. A. and Cheng, J. 1995. Low-fat, low-cholesterol egg yolk in food application. *Food Technol.* 49: 94–106.

Brooks, C. J. W., Henderson, W., and Steel, G. 1973. The use of trimethylsilyl ethers in the characterization of natural sterols and steroid diols by gas chromatography-mass spectrometry. *Biochim. Biophys. Acta* 296: 431–445.

Brooks, C. J. W., Horning, E. C., and Young, J. S. 1968. Characterization of sterols by gas chromatography-mass spectrometry of the trimethylsilyl ethers. *Lipids* 3: 391–402.

Carey, M. A. and Persinger, H. E. 1972. Liquid chromatographic determination of traces of aliphatic carbonyl compounds and glycols as derivatives that contain the dinitrophenyl group. *J. Chromatogr. Sci.* 10: 537–543.

Carr, T. P., Hamilton Jr., R. L., and Rudel, L. L. 1995. ACAT inhibitors decrease secretion of cholesterol esters and apolipoprotein B by perfused livers of African green monkeys. *J. Lipid Res.* 34: 25–36.

Carr, T. P., Parks, J. S., and Rudel, L. L. 1992. Hepatic ACAT activity in African green monkeys is highly correlated to plasma LDL cholesteryl ester enrichment and coronary artery atherosclerosis. *Arterioscler. Thromb.* 12: 1274–1283.

Chan, S. H., Gray, J. I., Gomaa, E. A., Harte, B. R., Kelly, P. M., and Buckley, D. J. 1993. Cholesterol oxidation in whole milk powders as influenced by processing and packaging. *Food Chem.* 47: 321–328.

Chen, Y. C., Chiu, C. P., and Chen, B. H. 1994. Determination of cholesterol oxides in heated lard by liquid chromatography. *Food Chem.* 50: 53–58.

Chen, J. S. and Yen, G. C. 1994. Cholesterol oxidation products in small sundried fish. *Food Chem.* 50: 167–170.

Chicoye, E., Powrie, W. D., and Fennema, O. 1968a. Photoxidation of cholesterol in spray-dried egg yolk upon irradiation. *J. Food Sci.* 3: 581–587.

Chicoye, E., Powrie, W. D., and Fennema, O. 1968b. Isolation and characterization of cholesterol-5β,6β-oxide from an aerated aqueous dispersion of cholesterol. *Lipids* 3: 335–339.

Chicoye, E., Powrie, W. D., and Fennema, O. 1968c. Synthesis, purification and characterization of 7-ketocholesterol and epimeric 7-hydroxycholesterols. *Lipids* 3: 551–556.

Clemens, M. R., Ruess, M., Bursa, Z., and Waller, H. D. 1987. The relationship between lipid composition of red blood cells and their susceptibility to lipid peroxidation. *Free Radic. Res. Commun.* 3: 265–271.

Cleveland, M. Z. and Harris, N. D. 1987. Oxidation of cholesterol in commercially processed cow's milk. *J. Food Prot.* 50: 867–871.

Comstock, G. W., Helzlsouer, K. J., and Bush, T. L. 1991. Prediagnostic serum levels of carotenoids and vitamin E as related to subsequent cancer in Washington County, Maryland. *Am. J. Clin. Nutr.* 53 (suppl.): 260–264S.

Crastes de Paulet, A., Astruc, M. E., and Bascoul, J. 1988. Les oxystérols: propriétés biologiques et problèmes nutritionnels. In *Biologie des lipides chez l'homme*, L. Dousty-blazy and F. Mendy (Ed.), pp. 154–174. Editions Médicales Internationales, Paris.

Csallany, A. S., Kindom, S. E., Addis, P. B., and Lee, J. H. 1989. HPLC method for quantitation of cholesterol and four of its major oxidation products in muscle and liver tissues. *Lipids* 24: 645–651.

Csiky, I. 1982. Trace enrichment and separation of cholesterol oxidation products by absorption high performance liquid chromatography. *J. Chromatogr.* 24: 381–389.

Danielson, H. and Horning, M. G. 1962. On the oxidation of cholesterol by blood in vitro. *Acta Chim. Scand.* 16: 774–775.

de Vore, V. R. 1988. TBA values and 7-ketocholesterol in refrigerated raw and cooked ground beef. *J. Food Sci.* 53: 1058–1061.

Dumazer, M., Farines, M., and Soulier, J. 1986. Identification de stérols par spectrométrie de masse. *Rev. Fr. Corps Gras* 33: 151–156.

Duthie, G. G. 1991. Antioxidant hypothesis of cardiovascular disease. *Trends Food Sci. Technol.* (August) 205–207.

Emanuel, H. A., Hassel, C. A., Addis, P. B., Bergmann, S. D., and Zavoral, J. H. 1991. Plasma cholesterol oxidation products (oxysterols) in human subjects fed a meal rich in oxysterols. *J. Food Sci.* 56: 843–847.

Esterbauer, H., Dieber-Rotheneder, M., Striegl, G., and Waeg, G. 1991. Role of vitamin E in preventing the oxidation of low-density lipoprotein. *Am. J. Clin. Nutr.* 53 (suppl.): 314–321S.

Fillion, L., Zee, J. A., and Gosselin, C. 1991. Determination of a cholesterol oxide mixture by a single-run high-performance liquid chromatographic analysis using benzoylation. *J. Chromatogr.* 547: 105–112.

Finocchiaro, E. T., Lee, K., and Richardson, T. 1984. Identification and quantification of cholesterol oxides in grated cheese and bleached butteroil. *J. Am. Oil Chem. Soc.* 61: 877–883.

Finocchiaro, E. T. and Richardson, T. 1983. Sterol oxides in foodstuffs: A review. *J. Food Prot.* 46: 917–925.

Fioriti, J. A. and Sims, R. J. 1967. Autoxidation products from cholesterol. *J. Am. Oil Chem. Soc.* 44: 221–224.

Fitch, B. 1994. Antioxidants: Health implications. *Inform* 5: 242–251.

Fitzpatrick, F. A. and Siggia, S. 1973. High resolution liquid chromatography of derivatized nonultraviolet absorbing hydroxy steroids. *Anal. Chem.* 45: 2310–2314.

Folch, J., Lees, M., and Sloane-Stanley, G. H. 1957. A simple method for the isolation and purification of total lipids from animal tissues. *J. Biol. Chem.* 226: 497–509.

Fontana, A., Antoniazzi, F., Ciavatta, M. L., Trivellone, E., and Cimino, G. 1993. ^{1}H-NMR study of cholesterol autooxidation in egg powder and cookies exposed to adverse storage. *J. Food Sci.* 58: 1286–1290.

Fontana, A., Antoniazzi, F., Cimino, G., Mazza, G., Trivellone, E., and Zanone, B. 1992. High resolution NMR detection of cholesterol oxides in spray-dried egg yolk. *J. Food Sci.* 57: 869–879.

Fornas, E., Martínez-Sales, V., Camañas, A., and Baguena, J. 1984. Intestinal absorption of cholesterol autoxidation products in the rat. *Arch. Farmacol. Toxicol.* 10: 175–182.

Frankel, E. N., Waterhouse, A. L., and Kinsella, J. E. 1993. Inhibition of human LDL oxidation by resveratrol. *Lancet* 341: 1103.

Gey, K. F. 1986. On the antioxidant hypothesis with regard to arteriosclerosis. *Bibl. Nutr. Dieta* 37: 53–91.

Gey, K. F., Brubacher, G. B., and Stahelin, H. B. 1987. Plasma levels of antioxidant vitamins in relation to ischemic heart disease and cancer. *Am. J. Clin. Nutr.* 45: 1368–1377.

Gey, K. F., Puska, P., Jordan, P., and Moser, U. K. 1991. Inverse correlation between plasma vitamin E and mortality from ischemic heart disease in cross-cultural epidemiology. *Am. J. Clin. Nutr.* 53 (suppl,): 326–334S.

Gray, M. F., Lawrie, T. D. V., and Brooks, C. J. W. 1971. Isolation and identification of cholesterol α-oxide and other minor sterols in human serum. *Lipids* 6: 836.

Gruenke, L. D., Graig, J. C., Petrakis, N. L., and Lyon, M. B. 1987. Analysis of cholesterol, cholesterol-5,6-epoxides and cholestane-3β,5α,6β-triol in nipple aspirates of human breast fluid by gas chromatography/mass spectrometry. *Biomed. Environ. Mass Spectrom.* 14: 335–338.

Guardiola, F. 1994. Fomación de oxiesteroles en el huevo en polvo durante el proceso d atomización and el almacenamiento. Ph.D. Thesis, Unidad de Nutrición y Bromatología, Facultad de Farmacia, Barcelona, Spain.

Guardiola, F., Codony, R., Rafecas, M., and Boattella, J. 1994a. Selective gas chromatographic determination of cholesterol in eggs. *J. Am. Oil Chem. Soc.* 71: 867–871.

Guardiola, F., Codony, R., Rafecas, R., and Boatella, J. 1994b. Metodología analítica para la determinación de oxiesteroles. *Grasas y Aceites* 45: 164–192.

Guardiola, F., Addis, P. B., and Park, P. W. 1995a. Unpublished data. Department of Food Science and Nutrition, University of Minnesota, Saint Paul, MN.

Guardiola, F., Codony, R., Miskin, D., Rafecas, R., and Boatella, J. 1995b. Oxysterol formation in egg powder and relationship with other quality parameters. *J. Agric. Food Chem.* In press.

Guardiola, F., Codony, R., Rafecas, M., and Boatella, J. 1995c. Adsorption of oxysterols on different microtube materials during silanization prior to gas chromatographic determination. *J. Chromatogr. A* 705: 696–699.

Guardiola, F., Codony, R., Rafecas, M., and Boatella, J. 1995d. Comparison of three methods for the determination of oxysterols in Spray-dried egg. *J. Chromatogr. A* 705: 289–304.

Guardiola, F., Codony, R., Rafecas, R., and Boatella, J. 1995e. Formación de derivados oxidados del colesterol en alimentos. *Grasas y Aceites.* 46: 202–212.

Gumulka, J., Pyrek, J. S., and Smith, L. L. 1982. Interception of discrete oxygen species in aqueous media by cholesterol: formation of cholesterol epoxides and secosterols. *Lipids* 17: 197–203.

Gutteridge, J. M. C. 1978. The membrane effects of vitamin E, cholesterol and their acetates on peroxidative susceptibility. *Res. Commun. Chem. Pathol. Pharmacol.* 22: 563–572.

Herian, A. M. and Lee, K. 1985. 7α- and 7β-Hydroxycholesterols formed in a dry egg nog mix exposed to fluorescent light. *J. Food Sci.* 50: 276–277.

Higley, N. A., Taylor, S. L., Herian, A. M., and Lee, K. 1986. Cholesterol oxides in processed meats. *Meat Sci.* 16: 175–188.

Hodis, H. N., Crawford, D. W., and Sevanian, A. 1991. Cholesterol feeding increases plasma and aortic tissue cholesterol oxide levels in parallel: Further evidence for the role of cholesterol oxidation in atherosclerosis. *Atherosclerosis* 89: 117–126.

Hubbard, R. W., Ono, Y., and Sánchez, A. 1989. Atherogenic effect of oxidized products of cholesterol. *Prog. Food Nutr. Sci.* 13: 17–44.

Hwang, K. T. and Maerker, G. 1993a. Quantitation of cholesterol oxidation products in unirradiated and irradiated meats. *J. Am. Oil Chem. Soc.* 70: 371–375.

Hwang, K. T. and Maerker, G. 1993b. Determination of 6-ketocholestanol in unirradiated and irradiated chicken meats. *J. Am. Oil Chem. Soc.* 70: 789–792.

Ibrahim, N., Unklesbay, N., Kapila, S., and Puri, R. K. 1990. Cholesterol content of restructured pork/soy hull mixture. *J. Food Sci.* 55: 1488–1490.

Jacobson, M. S. 1987. Cholesterol oxides in Indian ghee: Possible cause of unexplained high risk of atherosclerosis in Indian immigrant populations. *Lancet* September 19: 656–658.

Jain, S. K. and Shohet, S. B. 1981. Apparent role of cholesterol as an erythrocyte membrane antioxidant. *Clin. Res.* 29: 336a.

Karel, M. 1980. Lipid oxidation secondary reactions and water activity of foods. In *Autoxidation in Food and Biological Systems*, M. G. Simic and M. Karel (Ed.), pp. 191–206. Plenum Press, New York.

Knekt, P., Aromaa, A., Maatela, J., Aaran, R-K., Nikkari, T., Hakama, M., Hakulinen, T., Peto, R., and Teppo, L. 1991. Vitamin E and cancer prevention. *Am. J. Clin. Nutr.* 53 (suppl.): 283–286S.

Kok, F. J., van Poppel, G., Melse, J., Verheul, E., Schouten, E. G., Kruyssen, D. H. C. M., and Hofman, A. 1991. Do antioxidants and polyunsaturated fatty acids have a combined association with coronary atherosclerosis? *Atherosclerosis* 31: 85–90.

Koopman, B. J., van Der Molen, J. C., and Wolthers, B. G. 1987. Determination of some hydroxycholesterols in human serum samples. *J. Chromatogr.* 416: 1–13.

Korahani, V., Bascoul, J., and Crastes de Paulet A. 1981. Capillary column gas-liquid chromatographic analysis of cholesterol derivatives. Application to the autoxidation products of cholesterol. *J. Chromatogr.* 211: 392–397.

Kou, I. L. and Holmes, R. P. 1985. The analysis of 25-hydroxycholesterol in plasma and cholesterol containing foods by high performance liquid chromatography. *J. Chromatogr.* 330: 339–346.

Kudo, K., Emmons, G. T., Casserly, E. W., Via, D. P., Smith, L. C., Pyrek, J. S., and Schroepfer, Jr., G. J. 1989. Inhibitors of sterol synthesis. Chromatography of acetate derivatives of oxygenated sterols. *J. Lipid Res.* 30: 1097–1111.

Kumar, N. and Singhal, O. P. 1992. Effect of processing conditions on the oxidation of cholesterol in ghee. *J. Sci. Food Agric.* 58: 267–273.

Lai, S. M., Gray, J. I., and Zabik, M. 1995. Evaluation of solid phase extraction and gas chromatography for determination of cholesterol oxidation products in spray dried whole egg. *J. Agric. Food Chem.* 43: 1122–1126.

Lebovics, V. K., Gaál. Ö., Somogyi, L., and Farkas, J. 1992. Cholesterol oxides in gamma-irradiated spray-dried egg powder. *J. Sci. Food Agric.* 60: 251–254.

Lee, K., Herian, A. M., and Higley, A. 1985. Sterol oxidation products in french fries and in stored potato chips. *J. Food Prot.* 48: 158–161.

Lee, K., Herian, A. M., and Richardson, T. 1984. Detection of sterol epoxides in foods by colorimetric reaction with picric acid. *J. Food Prot.* 47: 340–342.

Luby, J. M., Gray, J. I., Harte, B. R., and Ryan, T. C. 1986. Photooxidation of cholesterol in butter. *J. Food Sci.* 51: 904–923.

Luc, G. and Fruchart, J. C. 1991. Oxidation of lipoproteins and atherosclerosis. *Am. J. Clin. Nutr.* 53 (suppl.): 206–209S.

Maerker, G. 1987. Cholesterol autoxidation—current status. *J. Am. Oil Chem. Soc.* 64: 388–392.

Maerker, G. and Bunick, F. J. 1986. Cholesterol oxides II. Measurement of the 5,6-epoxides during cholesterol oxidation in aqueous dispersions. *J. Am. Oil Chem. Soc.* 63: 771–777.

Maerker, G. and Jones, K. C. 1991. Unusual product ratios resulting from the gamma-irradiation of cholesterol in liposomes. *Lipids* 26: 139–144.

Maerker, G. and Jones, K. C. 1992. Gamma-irradiation of individual cholesterol oxidation products. *J. Am. Oil Chem. Soc.* 69: 451–455.

Maerker, G. and Jones, K. C. 1993. A-ring oxidation products from γ-irradiation of cholesterol in liposomes. *J. Am. Oil Chem. Soc.* 70: 255–259.

Maerker, G., Nungesser, E. H., and Bunick, J. 1988a. Reaction of cholesterol 5,6-epoxides with simulated gastric juice. *Lipids* 23: 761–765.

Maerker, G., Nungesser, E. H., and Zulak, I. M. 1988b. HPLC separation and quantitation of cholesterol oxidation products with flame ionization detection. *J. Agric. Food Chem.* 36: 61–63.

Maerker, G. and Unruh, J. 1986. Cholesterol oxides. I. Isolation and determination of some cholesterol oxidation products. *J. Am. Oil Chem. Soc.* 63: 767–773.

Missler, S. R., Wasilchuk, B. A., and Merritt, C. 1985. Separation and identification of cholesterol oxidation products in dried egg preparations. *J. Food Sci.* 50: 595–598, 646.

Monahan, F. J., Gray, J. I., Booren, A. M., Miller, E. R., Buckley, D. J., Morrissey, P. A., and Gomaa, E. A. 1992. Influence of dietary treatment on lipid and cholesterol oxidation in pork. *J. Agric. Food Chem.* 40: 1310–1315.

Morgan, J. N. and Armstrong, D. J. 1987. Formation of cholesterol-5,6-epoxides during spray-drying of egg yolk. *J. Food Sci.* 52: 1224–1227.

Morgan, J. N. and Armstrong, D. J. 1989. Wide-bore capillary gas chromatographic method for quantification of cholesterol oxidation products in egg yolk powder. *J. Food Sci.* 54: 427–429, 457.

Morgan, J. N. and Armstrong, D. J. 1992. Quantification of cholesterol oxidation products in egg yolk powder spray-dried with direct heating. *J. Food Sci.* 57: 43–45, 107.

Naber, E. C., Allred, J. B., Winget, J., and Stock, A. E. 1985. Effect of cholesterol oxidation products on cholesterol metabolism in laying hen. *Poult. Sci.* 64: 675–680.

Naber, E. C. and Biggert, M. D. 1985. Analysis for and generation of cholesterol oxidation products in egg yolk by heat treatment. *Poult. Sci.* 64: 341–347.

Nawar, W. W., Kim, S. K., Li, Y. J., and Vadji, M. 1991. Measurement of oxidative interactions of cholesterol. *J. Am. Oil Chem. Soc.* 68: 496–498.

Nourooz-Zadeh, J. 1990. Determination of the autoxidation products from free or total cholesterol: A new multistep enrichment methodology including the enzymatic release of esterified cholesterol. *J. Agric. Food Chem.* 38: 1667–1673.

Nourooz-Zadeh, J. and Appelqvist, L-Å. 1987. Cholesterol oxides in Swedish foods and food ingredients: Fresh eggs and dehydrated egg products. *J. Food Sci.* 52: 57–62, 67.

Nourooz-Zadeh, J. and Appelqvist, L-Å. 1988a. Cholesterol oxides in Swedish foods and food ingredients: Butter and cheese. *J. Am. Oil Chem. Soc.* 65: 1635–1641.

Nourooz-Zadeh, J. and Appelqvist, L-Å. 1988b. Cholesterol oxides in Swedish foods and food ingredients: Milk powder products. *J. Food Sci.* 53: 74–79, 87.

Nourooz-Zadeh, J. and Appelqvist, L-Å. 1989. Cholesterol oxides in Swedish foods and food ingredients: lard and bacon. *J. Am. Oil Chem. Soc.* 66: 586–592.

Osada, K., Kodama, T., Yamada, K., and Sugano, M. 1993a. Oxidation of cholesterol by heating. *J. Agric. Food Chem.* 41: 1198–1202.

Osada, K., Kodama, T., Cui, L., Yamada, K., and Sugano, M. 1993b. Levels and formation of oxidized cholesterols in processed marine foods. *J. Agric. Food Chem.* 41: 1893–1898.

Osada, K., Sasaki, E. and Sugano, M. 1994. Lymphatic absorption of oxidized cholesterol in rats. *Lipids* 29: 555–559.

Ohshima, T., Li, N., and Koizumi, C. 1993. Oxidative decomposition of cholesterol in fish products. *J. Am. Oil Chem. Soc.* 70: 595–600.

Pannecoucke, X., van Dorsselaer, A., and Luu B. 1992. Mass spectrometric studies of phosphodiesters linked to oxysterols and nucleosides, a family of biologically potent oxygenated sterols. *Org. Mass Spectrom.* 27: 140–144.

Park, P. W. 1995. Toxic compounds derived from lipids. In *Analyzing Foods for Nutrition Labeling and Hazardous Contaminants*, I. J. Jeon and W. G. Ikins (Ed.). pp. 363–433. Marcel Dekker, Inc., New York.

Park, S. W. and Addis, P. B. 1985a. Capillary column gas-liquid chromatographic resolution of oxidized cholesterol derivatives. *Anal. Biochem.* 149: 275–283.

Park, S. W. and Addis, P. B. 1985b. HPLC determination of C-7 oxidized cholesterol derivatives in foods. *J. Food Sci.* 50: 1437–1441, 1444.

Park, S. W. and Addis, P. B. 1986a. Identification and quantitative estimation of oxidized cholesterol derivatives in heated tallow. *J. Agric. Food Chem.* 34: 653–659.

Park, S. W. and Addis, P. B. 1986b. Further investigation of oxidized cholesterol derivatives in heated fats. *J. Food Sci.* 51: 1380–1381.

Park, S. W. and Addis, P. B. 1987. Cholesterol oxidation products in some muscle foods. *J. Food Sci.* 52: 1500–1503.

Park, S. W. and Addis, P. B. 1989. Derivatization of 5α-cholestane-3β,5,6β-triol into trimethylsilyl ether sterol for GC analysis. *J. Am. Oil Chem. Soc.* 66: 1632–1634.

Park, P. S. W. and Addis, P. B. 1992. Methods of analysis of cholesterol oxides. In *Biological Effects of Cholesterol Oxides*. S. K. Peng and R. J. Morin (Ed.), pp. 33–70. CRC Press, Boca Raton, FL.

Pearson, A. M., Gray, J. I., Wolzak, A. M., and Horenstein, N. A. 1983. Safety implications of oxidized lipids in muscle foods. *Food Technol.* 37: 121–129.

Peng, S. K., Hu, B. and Morin, R. J. 1991. Angiotoxicity and atherogenicity of cholesterol oxides. *J. Clin. Lab. Anal.* 5: 144–152.

Peng, S. K., Hu, B., Peng, A. Y., and Morin, R. J. 1993. Effect of cholesterol oxides on prostacyclin production and platelet adhesion. *Artery* 20: 122–134.

Peng, S. K. and Morin, R. J. (Ed.). 1992. *Biological Effects of Cholesterol Oxides*. CRC Press, Boca Raton, FL.

Peng, S. K., Sevanian, A., and Morin, R. A. 1992. Cytotoxicity of cholesterol oxides. In *Biological Effects of Cholesterol Oxides*, S. K. Peng and R. J. Morin (Ed.), pp. 147–166. CRC Press, Boca Raton, FL.

Peng, S. K., Taylor, C. B., Mosbach, E. H., Huang, W. Y., Hill, J., and Mikkelson, B. 1982. Distribution of 25-hydroxycholesterol in plasma lipoprotein and its role in atherogenesis. A study in squirrel monkeys. *Atherosclerosis* 41: 395–402.

Pennock, H. F., Neiss, G., and Mahler, H. R. 1962. Developing avian embryo. V. Ubiquinone and some other unsaponifiable lipids. *Biochem. J.* 85: 530–537.

Pie, J. E. and Seillan, C. 1992. Oxysterols in cultured bovine aortic smooth muscle cells and in the monocyte-like cell line. *Lipids* 27: 270–274.

Pie, J. E., Spahis, K., and Seillan, C. 1990. Evaluation of oxidative degradation of cholesterol in food and food ingredients: Identification and quantification of cholesterol oxides. *J. Agric. Food Chem.* 38: 973–979.

Pie, J. E., Spahis, K., and Seillan, C. 1991. Cholesterol oxidation in meat products during cooking and frozen storage. *J. Agric. Food Chem.* 39: 250–254.

Prasad, C. R. and Subramanian, R. 1992. Qualitative and comparative studies of cholesterol oxides in commercial and home-made Indian ghees. *Food Chem.* 45: 71–73.

Pryor, W. A. and Lightsey, J. W. 1981. Mechanisms of nitrogen dioxide reactions: Initiation of lipid peroxidation and the production of nitrous acid. *Science* 214: 435–437.

Przybylski, R., Eskin, N. A. M., and Cullimore, D. R. 1993. Transformation of egg cholesterol during bacterial transformation. *Food Chem.* 48: 195–199.

Rankin, S. A. and Pike, O. A. 1993. Cholesterol autoxidation inhibition varies among several natural antioxidants in a aqueous model system. *J. Food Sci.* 58: 653–655, 687.

Renaud, S. and de Lorgeril, M. 1992. Vin, alcool, plaquettes et coronaropathies: le paradoxe français. *Lancet* (édition française) 225: 22–25.

Robertson, J. M., Donner, A. P., and Trevithick, J. R. 1991. A possible role for vitamins C and E in cataract prevention. *Am. J. Clin. Nutr.* 53 (suppl.): 346–351S.

Rose-Sallin, C., Huggett, A. C., Bosset, J. O., Tabacchi, R., and Fay, L. B. 1995. Quantification of cholesterol oxidation products in milk powders using [^{2}H$_7$]cholesterol to monitor cholesterol autoxidation artifacts. *J. Agric. Food Chem.* 43: 935–941.

Ryan, T. C., Gray, J. I., and Morton, I. D. 1981. Oxidation of cholesterol in heated tallow. *J. Sci. Food Agric.* 32: 305–308.

Ryan, T. C. 1983. Oxidation of cholesterol in heated tallow. *Food Technol.* 37: 121–129.

Sander, B. D., Smith, D. E., and Addis, P. B. 1988. Effects of processing stage and storage conditions on cholesterol oxidation products in butter and Cheddar cheese. *J. Dairy Sci.* 71: 3173–3178.

Sander, B. D., Addis, P. B., Park, S. W., and Smith, D. E. 1989a. Quantification of cholesterol oxidation products in a variety of foods. *J. Food Prot.* 52: 109–114.

Sander, B. D., Smith, D. E., Addis, P. B., and Park, S. W. 1989b. Effects of prolonged and adverse storage conditions on levels of cholesterol oxidation products in dairy products. *J. Food Sci.* 54: 874–879.

Sevanian, A. and McLeod, L. L. 1987. Cholesterol autoxidation in phospholipid membrane bilayers. *Lipids* 22: 627–636.

Sevanian, A., Mead, J. F., and Stein, R. A. 1979. Epoxides as products of lipid autoxidation in rat lungs. *Lipids* 14: 634–643.

Sevanian, A., Seraglia, R., Traldi, P., Rossato, P., Ursini, F., and Hodis, H. 1994. Analysis of plasma cholesterol oxidation products using gas- and high-performance liquid chromatography/mass spectrometry. *Free Radic. Biol. Med.* 17: 397–409.

Smith, L. L. 1981. *Cholesterol Autoxidation.* Plenum Press, New York.

Smith, L. L. 1987. Cholesterol autoxidation 1981–1986. *Chem. Phys. Lipids* 44: 87–125.

Smith, L. L. 1990. Mechanisms of formation of oxysterols: a general survey. In *Free Radicals, Lipoproteins, and Membrane Lipids*, A. Crastes de Paulet, L. Douste-Blazy, and R. Paoletti (Ed.), pp. 115–132. Plenum Press, New York.

Smith, L. L. 1991. Another cholesterol hypothesis: Cholesterol as antioxidant. *Free Radical Biol. Med.* 11: 47–61.

Smith, L. L. and Jaworski, K. 1988. Cholesterol epoxidations by defined oxygen species. *Basic Life Sci.* 49: 313–317.

Smith, L. L. and Johnson, B. H. 1989. Biological activities of oxysterols. *Free Radical Biol. Med.* 7: 285–332.

Smith, L. L., Kulig, J. M., Miller, D., and Ansari, G. A. S. 1978. Oxidation of cholesterol by dioxygen species. *J. Am. Chem. Soc.* 100: 6206–6211.

Smith, L. L., Matthews, W. S., Price, J. C., Bachmann, R. C., and Reynolds, B. 1967. Thin-layer chromatographic examination of cholesterol autoxidation. *J. Chromatogr.* 27: 187–205.

Smith, L. L. and Stroud, J. P. 1978. Sterol metabolism XLII. On the interception of singlet molecular oxygen by sterols. *Photochem. Photobiol.* 28: 479–485.

Smith, L. L. and Teng, J. I. 1974. Sterol metabolism XXIX. On the mechanism of microsomal lipid peroxidation in rat liver. *J. Am. Chem. Soc.* 96: 2640–2641.

Sugino, K., Terao, J., Murakami, H., and Matsushita, S. 1986. High-performance liquid chromatographic method for the quantification of cholesterol epoxides in spray-dried egg. *J. Agric. Food Chem.* 34: 36–39.

Szebeni, J. and Toth, K. 1986. Lipid peroxidation in hemoglobin-containing liposomes. Effects of membrane phospholipids composition and cholesterol content. *Biochim. Biophys. Acta* 857: 139–145.

Teng, J. I. 1990. Oxysterol separation by HPLC in combination with thin layer chromatography. *Chromatogram* (November): 8–10.

Teng, J. I. 1991. Column variations in the analysis of oxysterols using normal-phase high performance liquid chromatography. *LC-GC Int.* 4: 34–36.

Teng, J. I., Kulig, M. J., and Smith, L. L. 1973a. Sterol metabolism. XXII. Gas chromatographic differentiation among cholesterol hydroperoxides. *J. Chromatogr.* 75: 108–113.

Teng, J. I., Kulig, M. J., Smith, L. L., Kan, G., and van Lier, J. E. 1973b. Sterol metabolism. XX. Cholesterol 7β-hydroperoxide. *J. Org. Chem.* 38: 119–123.

Teng, J. I. and Smith, L. L. 1973. Sterol metabolism XXIV. On the unlikely participation of singlet molecular oxygen in several enzyme oxygenations. *J. Am. Chem. Soc.* 95: 4060–4061.

Teng, J. I. and Smith, L. L. 1976. Sterol metabolism. XXXVII. On the oxidation of cholesterol by dioxygenases. *Bioorg. Chem.* 5: 99–119.

Tsai, L. S. and Hudson, C. A. 1981. High performance liquid chromatography of oxygenated cholesterols and related compounds. *J. Am. Oil Chem. Soc.* 58: 931–934.

Tsai, L. S. and Hudson, C. A. 1984. Cholesterol oxides in commercial dry egg products: Isolation and identification. *J. Food Sci.* 49: 1245–1248.

Tsai, L. S. and Hudson, C. A. 1985. Cholesterol oxides in commercial dry egg products: Quantitation. *J. Food Sci.* 50: 229–231, 237.

Tsai, L. S., Ijichi, K., Hudson, C. A., and Meehan, J. J. 1980. A method for the quantitative estimation of cholesterol α-oxide in eggs. *Lipids* 15: 124–128.

van de Bovenkamp, P., Kosmeijer-Schuil, T. G., and Katan, M. B. 1988. Quantification of oxysterols in Dutch foods: Egg products and mixed diets. *Lipids* 23: 1079–1085.

van Doormaal, J. J., Smit, N., Koopman, B. J., van der Molen, J. C., Wolthers, B. G., and Doorenbos, H. 1989. Hydroxycholesterols in serum from hypercholesterolaemic patients with and without bile acid sequestrant therapy. *Clin. Chim. Acta* 181: 273–279.

Van Lier, J. E. and Smith, L. L. 1968. Sterol metabolism II. Gas chromatographic recognition of cholesterol metabolites and artifacts. *Anal. Biochem.* 24: 419–430.

Wahle, K. W. J., Hope, P. P., and McIntosh, G. 1993. Effects of storage and various intrinsic vitamin E concentrations on lipid oxidation in dried egg powders. *J. Sci. Food Agric.* 61: 463–469.

Warner, G. J. 1994. Effect of dietary oxysterols on cellular cholesterol metabolism in the human hepatoma cell line, HepG2. Ph.D. Thesis, University of Minnesota, St. Paul, MN.

Watabe, T., Kanai, M., Isobe, M., and Ozawa, N. 1980. Cholesterol α- and β-epoxides as obligatory intermediates in the hepatic microsomal metabolism of cholesterol to cholestane-triol. *Biochim. Biophys. Acta* 619: 414–419.

Yan, P. S. and White, P. J. 1990. Cholesterol oxidation in heated lard enriched with two levels of cholesterol. *J. Am. Oil Chem. Soc.* 67: 927–931.

Zhang, W. B. and Addis, P. B. 1990. Prediction of levels of cholesterol oxides in heated tallow by dielectric measurement. *J. Food Sci.* 55: 1673–1675.

Zhang, W. B., Addis, P. B., and Krick, T. P. 1991. Quantification of 5α-cholestane-3β,5-6β-triol and other cholesterol oxidation products in fast food French fried potatoes. *J. Food Sci.* 56: 716–718.

Zubillaga, M. P. and Maerker, G. 1989. Cholesterol oxides III. Autoxidation of cholesterol in sodium stearate and sodium linoleate dispersions. *J. Am. Oil Chem. Soc.* 66: 1499–1503.

Zubillaga, M. P. and Maerker, G. 1991. Quantification of three cholesterol oxidation products in raw meat and chicken. *J. Food Sci.* 56: 1194–1202.

10
Chemistry of Lipid Oxidation

David B. Min and Hyung-Ok Lee

The Ohio State University
Columbus, Ohio

INTRODUCTION

The lipid oxidation of food has been largely responsible for the flavor stability, nutritional quality, and acceptability of foods (Labuza, 1971; Frankel, 1980; Warner et al., 1986). Lipid oxidation is due to the combination of triplet oxygen and singlet oxygen oxidation. Triplet oxygen lipid oxidation has been extensively studied to improve the oxidative stability of foods during last 50 years (Labuza, 1971; Frankel, 1980). However, it does not fully explain the initiation step of lipid oxidation (Frankel et al., 1985; Lee and Min, 1990). Rawls and Van Santen (1970) suggested that singlet oxygen is involved in the initiation of lipid oxidation because singlet oxygen can directly react with double bonds of fatty acids without the formation of free radicals and its reaction rate with linoleic acid is at least 1450 times higher than that of triplet oxygen. Singlet oxygen can be formed by chemical, enzymatic, photochemical, and physical methods and initiate the oxidation of lipids in foods. Photosensitized reaction, which is initiated by sensitizers and light, is the most common pathway to produce singlet oxygen in foods (Carlsson et al., 1976; Min et al., 1989; Lee and Min, 1990). This has great impact on the oxidation of foods that contain sensitizers. Chlorophylls and their decomposition products in vegetable oils are known to be efficient photochemical sensitizers for singlet oxygen formation (Terao and Matsushita, 1977; Min and Lee, 1988). Terao and Matsushita (1977) indicated that singlet oxygen reacts directly with unsaturated fatty acids of vegetable oils to form a mixture of conjugated and nonconjugated hyroperoxides. The decomposition of hydroperoxides produces off-flavor volatile compounds and potentially toxic oxidation compounds (Neff et al., 1982, 1983). The undesirable singlet oxygen lipid oxidation can be minimized by preventing the formation of singlet oxygen by quenching singlet oxygen physically and chemically (Min and Lee, 1988). Foote (1979) reported that physical quenching can be explained by energy and charge transfer mechanisms. Carotenoids quench the singlet oxygen through energy transfer from singlet oxygen to carotenoids with nine or more conjugated double bonds. It is exothermic, and these carotenoids are efficient singlet oxygen quenchers. The physical quenching of singlet oxygen by tocopherols is due to the charge transfer mechanism.

CHEMISTRY OF TRIPLET AND SINGLET OXYGENS

The molecular orbital theory best describes the electron structures of triplet oxygen and singlet oxygen (Korycka-Dahl and Richardson, 1978; Bradley and Min, 1992). Molecular oxygen, which consists of two oxygen atoms, has 10 molecular orbitals containing 12 valence electrons. Valence electrons are added sequentially to the orbitals in order of increasing energy to obtain molecular orbitals. The molecular orbitals of triplet and singlet oxygens are shown in Figures 10.1 and 10.2, respectively.

Pauli's exclusion principle states that only two electrons can occupy each molecular orbital. Hund's rule states that one electrons is placed into each orbital of equal energy before the addition of second electron as shown in Figure 10.1. Pauli's exclusion principle also states that electrons in a given orbital must have opposite spins. An electron in an atom or molecule produces magnetic momentum and mechanical angular momentum. This behavior is a result of the motion of electron around the nucleus and from the spin of the electron. The ground state of a molecule is singlet if the resultant spin (S) is zero dictating the multiplicity of the state, 2S + 1, to be one. An excited state is formed by removing one of the electrons from the uppermost filled orbital of the ground state to a vacant orbital of higher energy. The ground state of most stable molecules containing an even number of electrons is diamagnetic because of the arrangement of the

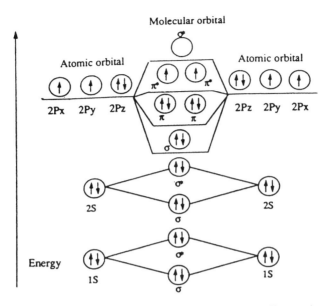

FIG. 10.1   Molecular orbital of triplet oxygen. (*From Bradley and Min, 1992.*)

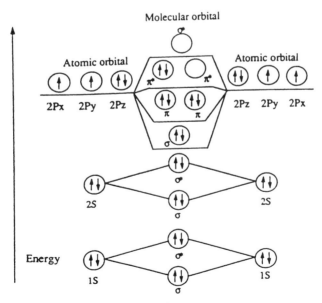

FIG. 10.2   Molecular orbital of singlet oxygen. (*From Bradley and Min, 1992.*)

electrons into pairs with opposed spin magnetic moments. The ground state for most molecules is singlet until a molecule is excited to a triplet state that is paramagnetic due to the total spin magnetic moment of the two unpaired electrons. The stable molecular oxygen, however, is a triplet. The two highest energy electrons of triplet oxygen illustrate the diradical nature of oxygen with an unpaired electron in each of the two highest degenerate orbitals.

Singlet oxygen, whose electrons are paired, is a violation of Hund's rule, creating an electronic repulsion as shown in Figure 10.2. Two of the most common singlet oxygen states are an activated $^1\Sigma$ state which lies 37.5 kcal above the ground state and an activated $^1\Delta$ state with 22.4 kcal above the ground state. The $^1\Sigma$ state of molecular oxygen has two electrons with opposite spins in different orbitals and is so reactive that it is not able to survive relaxation to the ground state. The less energetic $^1\Delta$ state of singlet oxygen is sufficiently stable enough to react with other singlet state molecules. The $^1\Delta$ state is responsible for most singlet oxygen reactions, therefore, the $^1\Delta$ singlet oxygen is subsequently used to designate singlet state oxygen (Foote, 1968).

The $^1\Delta$ state singlet oxygen is suggested to be responsible for initiating lipid oxidation because of its energy of 22.4 kcal above the ground state, its relatively long lifetime of several microseconds, and its highly electrophilic nature seeking electrons from electron-rich compounds to occupy its vacant molecular orbital. Once this active singlet oxygen is formed, it reacts with lipids to form hydroperoxides, which produce free radicals that in turn can initiate a free radical chain reaction (Rawls and Van Santen, 1970). Singlet oxygen can be produced chemically (Khan and Martell, 1967; Rosenthal, 1985), enzymatically (McCord and Fridovich, 1969), by gaseous discharge (Bader and Orgryzlo, 1964; Wayne, 1969), and by decomposition of hydroperoxides (Held et al., 1978). The single oxygen formation by photochemical methods in the presence of natural photosensitizers is most important in food systems (Carlsson et al., 1972; Clements et al., 1973).

MECHANISM OF PHOTOSENSITIZED OXIDATION

The interaction of light, photosensitizers, and oxygen is the major cause of the formation of singlet oxygen in foods. Pigments present in food, such as chlorophyll, hematoporphyrins, and riboflavin, are known to be efficient photosensitizers due to their conjugated double bond system, which easily absorbs visible light energy (Usuki et al. 1984). Once singlet oxygen is formed, it reacts directly with compounds that contain high densities of electrons, forming a mixture of conjugated and nonconjugated hydroperoxides that readily break down to produce undesirable compounds (Terao and Matsushita, 1977; Neff et al., 1983).

The effects of light on the flavor stability of food can be explained by both photolytic autoxidation or photosensitized oxidation. Photolytic autoxidation is the production of free radicals primarily from lipids during exposure to light. Photosensitized oxidation, however, occurs in the presence of photosensitizers and visible light. This potentially undesirable reaction begins with the absorption of light by photosensitizers, which is dependent upon the arrangement of electrons around the atomic nuclei in the molecule. As light energy is absorbed, an electron is boosted to a higher energy level, and the sensitizer is referred to as an excited singlet state, as shown in Figure 10.3. Only picoseconds are required for a chlorophyll molecule to absorb energy and be transformed into an excited singlet state. When light energy is removed, the electrons rapidly lose energy during the return of electron to the lower energy ground state.

The excited singlet sensitizer can lose energy as heat or emit light to decay to the ground state. The nature of the emission of light is dependent on the state multiplicity of the molecule. If the state from which the emission originates and terminates has the same multiplicity, the emission is called *fluorescence.* Excitation of molecules by light and their fluorescent decays are extremely fast processes. Finally, the excited singlet sensitizer may be converted to an excited triplet state sensitizer via intersystem crossing mechanism. The excited triplet state sensitizer undergoes degradation to a lower triplet energy state, which then decays to the ground state of the singlet state by emitting light. Since the emission originates from the triplet state and terminates in a singlet state, the emission is called *phosphorescence.* It is the excited triplet state sensitizer that is the reactive intermediate in

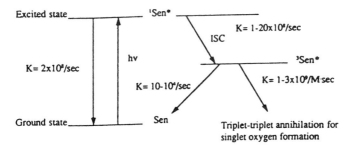

FIG. 10.3   Excitation and deactivation of photosensitizers. (*From Bradley and Min, 1992.*)

photosensitized oxidation. The excited triplet sensitizer may follow Type I and Type II reaction pathways, as shown in Figure 10.4.

The Type I pathway is characterized by hydrogen atom transfer or electron transfer between an excited triplet sensitizer and a substrate, resulting in the production of free radicals or free radical ions. The triplet sensitizer serves as a photochemically activated free radical initiator. These free radicals may then react with triplet oxygen to produce oxidized compounds, which readily break down to form free radicals that can initiate free radical chain reactions. The rate of the Type I reaction is dependent on the type and concentration of the sensitizer and substrate. For example, the sensitizer benzophenone abstracts hydrogen from a simple alcohol 10,000 times faster than eosin, however, both eosin and benzophenone react at similar rates with more powerful reductants like N,N-dimethylaniline (Foote, 1976). It is generally accepted that readily oxidizable compounds such as phenols or amines or readily reducible compounds such as quinones favor this sensitizer-substrate pathway.

The Type II pathway is an example of the energy transfer process in that the excited triplet sensitizer reacts with triplet oxygen via a triplet-triplet annihilation mechanism to form singlet oxygen. This reaction occurs very quickly and accounts for almost all of the transfer of energy from the excited triplet sensitizer to triplet oxygen. Electron transfer from the excited triplet sensitizer to triplet oxygen may also occur leading to superoxide anion formation and an oxidized sensitizer. Less than one percent of the triplet oxygen is converted to superoxide anion by collision with the triplet sensitizer. Electron-rich compounds such as olefins, dienes, and aromatic compounds favor the Type II pathway. The rate of the Type II reaction mainly depends on the solubility and concentration of oxygen present in the food

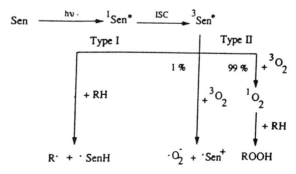

FIG. 10.4   Type 1 and Type II pathways. (*From Foote, 1979; Bradley and Min, 1992.*)

system. Oxygen is more soluble in lipids and nonpolar solvents than in water. Therefore, traces of the sensitizer chlorophyll in vegetable oils would tend to promote photosensitized oxidation by the Type II pathway (Samuel and Steckel, 1974). Water-based solutions, on the other hand, would tend to favor the sensitizer-substrate reaction of Type 1 due to the low concentration of oxygen available to interact with the excited triplet sensitizer.

The competition between substrate and triplet oxygen for the excited triplet sensitizer largely determines whether the reaction pathway is Type I or Type II. Photosensitized oxidation may change the types of pathway during the course of reaction as the concentration of substrate and oxygen changes. In aqueous-lipid biphasic systems, the longer half-life of singlet oxygen in the lipid phase favors oxidation of compounds that partition into the lipids.

REACTION MECHANISMS OF TRIPLET AND SINGLET OXYGEN WITH LINOLEIC ACID

Triplet oxygen, which is a diradical compound, does not react directly with the singlet state linoleic acid. The linoleic acid should be in free radical form by losing hydrogen atom to react with triplet oxygen, as shown in Figure 10.5. Since the radical formation of linoleic acid requires energy, the reaction between linoleic acid and triplet oxygen is relatively slower than the singlet oxygen oxidation of linoleic acid, which is not a free radical reaction. The triplet oxygen reaction with linoleic acid produces only conjugated hydroperoxides.

Singlet oxygen is a very electrophilic and nonradical compound. Singlet oxygen reacts with electron-rich compounds by 1,4-cycloaddition to dienes and heterocyclic compounds, the ene reaction with olefins, the oxidation of sulfides to sulfoxides, and the photosensitized oxidation of phenols to unstable hydroperoxy-dienones (Foote, 1976). Among these reactions, the ene reaction is the most important in singlet oxygen oxidation of foods. The reaction between singlet oxygen and linoleic acid is shown in Figure 10.6. The concerted ene mechanism of the six-center transition state is involved in the reaction between singlet oxygen and linoleic acid. One end of the singlet oxygen molecule reacts with the α-olefinic carbon, while the other end abstracts the γ-allylic hydrogen (Korycka-Dahl and Richardson, 1978).

The concerted six-membered ring formation might yield a hydroperoxide from the *cis* addition of singlet oxygen. The geometry of possible six-membered transition state in the reaction between singlet oxygen and linoleate leads to the formation of conjugated and nonconjugated *cis* and *trans* hydroperoxides (Korycka-Dahl and Richardson, 1978). The ene reac-

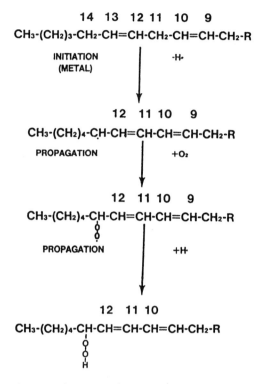

14 13 12 11 10 9
CH3-(CH2)3-CH2-CH=CH-CH2-CH=CH-CH2-R
INITIATION
(METAL)
-H·
12 11 10 9
CH3-(CH2)4-CH-CH=CH-CH=CH-CH2-R
PROPAGATION
+O2
12 11 10 9
CH3-(CH2)4-CH-CH=CH-CH=CH-CH2-R
PROPAGATION
+H·
12 11 10
CH3-(CH2)4-CH-CH=CH-CH=CH-CH2-R

FIG. 10.5 Reaction mechanism of triplet oxygen with linoleic acid.

1O2
OOH
Conjugated
1O2
OOH
Nonconjugated

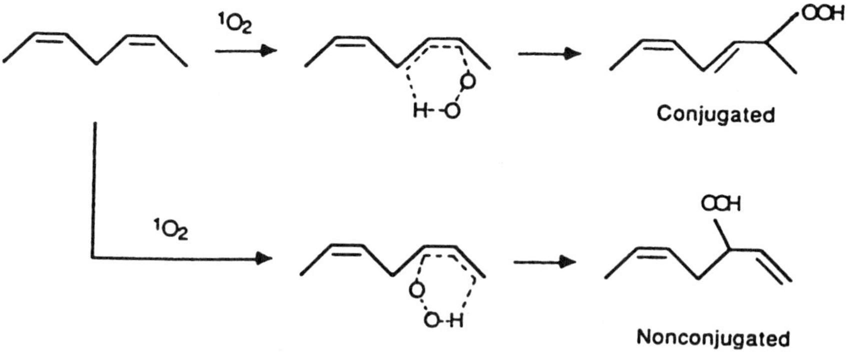

FIG. 10.6 Reaction mechanism of singlet oxygen with linoleic acid.

tion producing conjugated and nonconjugated hydroperoxides can be used to distinguish the singlet oxygen oxidation from the free radical autoxidation of lipid, which does not produce nonconjugated hydroperoxides.

PHOTOSENSITIZED SINGLET OXYGEN OXIDATION IN FOODS

The effect of light has long been known to play an important role in the flavor stability of vegetable oils and other fat-containing products such as margarine, butter, and mayonnaise (Clements et al. 1973). Most food pigments and colorants are potential initiators of singlet oxygen oxidation in food due to their ability to absorb light in the visible light range, exhibit fluorescence and phosphorescence reflecting both a singlet and triplet state, and have a high quantum yield of a long-lived triplet state (Umehara et al., 1979). Photosensitizers include synthetic dyes (acridine orange, crystal violet, eosin, erythrosine, methylene blue, proflavin, rose bengal), naturally occurring pigments (chlorophyll, flavin, porphyrin), coenzymes and biochemical compounds (pyridoxals and psoralens), metallic salts (cadmium sulfide, zinc oxide, zinc sulfide), polycyclic aromatic hydrocarbons (anthracene and rubene), and transition metal complexes such as ruthenium bipyridine (Kearsley and Rodriguez, 1981; Rosenthal, 1985). Yang and Min (1994) reported the effects of colorants on singlet oxygen oxidation determined by measuring the headspace oxygen depletion of soybean oil as shown in Table 10.1. The result showed that eosin B, Red No. 3, rose bengal, and methylene blue did not produce singlet oxygen under dark as was expected. The sensitizers produced different amounts of singlet oxygen under light. Methylene blue produced about 10 times more singlet oxygen than eosin B.

The effects of FD&C colorants on the singlet oxygen oxidation of soybean oil is shown in Table 10.2 (Yang and Min, 1994). Blue No. 1 and 2, Green No. 3 and 5, Yellow No. 6, and Red No. 40 did not produce singlet oxygen as the concentration increased from 0 to 1, 5, 20, 100, and 200 ppm and the storage time increased from 0 to 1, 2, and 4 hours under light. These colorants did not act as photosensitizers to produce singlet oxygen during storage under light. Of the seven FD&C colorants studied, only Red No. 3 acted as a photosensitizer.

Biologically important lipids that are susceptible to photosensitized oxidation include unsaturated fatty acids, phospholipids, triglycerides, cholesterol, vitamin D, steroids, and prostaglandins. Photosensitized oxidation of unsaturated fatty acids is mainly responsible for the photooxidative degradation of foods (Spikes, 1977). Erythrosine showed the photosensitizing effect of oxidation of pork luncheon meat, and it accelerated the deteriora-

TABLE 10.1 Effects of FD&C Colorants on the Headspace Oxygen of Soybean Oil During Storage Under Light

FD&C colorant (ppm)	Headspace oxygen (%)		
	1 hr	2 hr	4 hr
Blue No. 1[a]			
0	21.28	21.01	20.87
5	21.25	20.92	20.10
20	21.27	21.32	21.08
100	21.28	21.19	20.93
200	21.29	21.33	21.10
Red No. 3			
0	21.28	21.01	20.87
5	16.89	12.25	6.30
20	14.39	8.57	5.64
100	12.24	6.87	4.64
200	11.20	6.85	4.58

[a]The headspace oxygen results of Blue No. 3, Green No. 3 and 5, Yellow No. 6, and Red No. 40 were very similar to those of Blue No. 1.
Source: Yang and Min, 1994.

TABLE 10.2 Effects of Colorants on the Headspace Oxygen Content of Oil Sample Bottles Under Light for 2 Hours

	Headspace oxygen content[a]			
	Under Light		Under Dark	
	0 ppm	100 ppm	0 ppm	100 ppm
Control	100	100	100	100
Eosin B	100	92	100	100
Red No. 3	100	27	100	100
Rose bengal	100	31	1000	100
Methylene blue	100	23	100	100

[a]Oxygen content of air is expressed as 100%.
Source: Yang and Min, 1994.

tion of the meat flavor on exposure to fluorescent lamps (Chan, 1977). Soybean phosphatidyl choline and synthetic dilinoleoyl phosphatidyl choline reacted with singlet oxygen in the presence of light and methylene blue as a sensitizer (Terao and Matsushita, 1977). Cholesterol is readily oxidized by singlet oxygen to form 3-β-hydroxy-5α-hydroperoxy-Δ^6-cholestene, the decomposition of which leads to free radical chain oxidation of unsaturated fatty acids (Doleiden et al., 1974). Photosensitized oxidation of vegetable oils that contain natural photosensitizers and are commonly sold under light display is a major concern in the edible oil industry (Labuza, 1971; Stevenson et al., 1984; Warner et al., 1986). Salad dressings contain 30–40% vegetable oil (Swern, 1982). Specifically, soybean oil, which has a 90% share of the prepared dressings market is susceptible to oxidation due to the high concentration of linoleic acid and the presence of 1–1.5 ppm chlorophyll (Brekke, 1984). Chlorophylls and their decomposition products in vegetable oils are potential photosensitizers generating singlet oxygen in the presence of light and triplet oxygen (Endo et al., 1984; Lee and Min, 1988). Singlet oxygen reacts rapidly with unsaturated fatty acids to produce a mixture of conjugated and nonconjugated hydroperoxides, which decompose to produce undesirable volatile compounds (Neff et al., 1982, Gunstone, 1984) as shown in Figure 10.6. Most studies have been done in model systems that consist of one or two free fatty acids exposed to light in the presence of a sensitizer. Lee and Min (1990) reported the effects of chlorophyll on the photosensitized oxidation of soybean oil by measuring volatile flavor compounds in the headspace of soybean oil samples during light exposure as shown in Figure 10.7. As the chlorophyll concentration was increased, the headspace volatile content significantly increased during light exposure. No increase in flavor volatiles was observed for the soybean oil samples stored in the dark under the same experimental conditions.

The prooxidant effect of chlorophyll on the light-induced oxidation in soybean oil is due to the singlet oxygen formation via chlorophyll in the presence of light and atmospheric oxygen. Pheophytin, pheophorbide, clorophyllin, and protoporphyrin are similar in structure to chlorophyll and also have exhibited photosensitizing capabilities (Endo et al., 1984; Usuki et al., 1984; Min et al., 1989). Pheophorbide and pheophytin are formed by the loss of phytol and magnesium and magnesium from chlorophyll, respectively.

The oxidative deterioration of virgin olive oil sold as an unrefined greenish oil is related to the amount of chlorophyll contained in the oil. Olive oil in its natural state contains chlorophyll, carotenes, tocopherols, and other phenolic compounds. The presence of 6 ppm chlorophyll acted as a photosensitizer resulting in rapid oxidation of the oil during exposure to fluorescent light. The presence of β-carotene and nickel chelates substantially

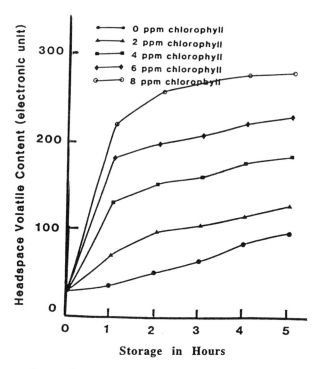

FIG. 10.7   Effects of chlorophyll on the headspace volatile compounds of soybean oil under light at 10°C.

inhibited oxidation in the first hours of illumination, thus supporting the content that chlorophyll is involved in the formation of singlet oxygen, which is quenched by β-carotene and nickel chelates (Lee and Min, 1991).

The relative reactivities of fatty acids of vegetable oils with singlet oxygen are highest with arachidonate followed by linolenate, linoleate, and oleate with ratios of 3.5:2.9:1.9:1.1, respectively (Doleiden et al., 1974). The relative reaction rates of triplet oxygen with methyl esters of linolenate, linoleate, and oleate are 25:12:1, respectively. Singlet oxygen oxidation of oleate produces equal amounts of 9- and 10-isomeric hydroperoxides without the formation of 8- and 11-isomeric hydroperoxides by free radical autoxidation. Singlet oxygen oxidation of linoleate produces a mixture of conjugated and nonconjugated hydroperoxides (Carlsson et al., 1976; Terao and Matsushita, 1977; Neff et al., 1982; Warner et al., 1986). Linolenate produces a mixture of conjugated and nonconjugated hydroperoxides (Carlsson et al.,

1976; Terao and Matsushita, 1977; Korycka-Dahl and Richardson, 1978; Foote, 1979; Neff et al., 1982; Warner et al., 1986).

Hydroperoxides produced during photosensitized oxidation of vegetable oils undergo further reactions to form secondary products (Neff et al., 1983). These secondary products include hydroperoxy epidioxides, dihydroperoxides, hydroperoxy bisepidioxides, hydroperoxy bicyclic endoperoxides, keto-dienes, and epoxy esters. Many changes can occur in the flavor quality of milk and dairy products during exposure to light (Singleton et al., 1963; Gaylord et al., 1985). Light penetrates milk to an appreciable depth, which increases its susceptibility to photosensitized reactions (Finley and Shipe, 1968; Maniere and Dimick, 1976). Riboflavin is a prevalent water-soluble vitamin present in milk that easily absorbs light energy to become an excited triplet sensitizer. Singlet oxygen, therefore, has been implicated in the riboflavin-sensitized photooxidation of milk fat (Foote, 1976; Aurand et al., 1977). Aurand et al. (1977) suggested the formation of singlet oxygen in milk based on the inhibitory effects of a singlet oxygen quenchers such as 1,3-diphenylisobenzofuran or 1,4-diazabicyclo-[2,2,2]-octane on oxidation of milk fat as catalyzed by copper ions, enzymes, and light. Bradley and Min (1995) reported that 1,4-diazabicyclo-[2,2,2]-octane or dimethyl furan minimized the singlet oxygen lipid oxidation of milk containing 40 μM riboflavin during 3 hours of illumination, as shown Tables 10.3 and 10.4, respectively. They also reported that 1,4-diazabicyclo-[2,2,2]-octane and dimethyl furan quenched singlet oxygen only instead of riboflavin in milk to minimize the riboflavin-photosensitized oxidation in milk. The single oxygen quenching rates of 1,4-diazabicylo-[2,2,2]-octane and

TABLE 10.3 Depleted Headspace Oxygen of Milkfat Containing Dimethyl Furan with 40 μM Riboflavin During 3 Hours of Illumination

Dimethyl furan	Depleted headspace oxygen (μmol O_2/ml)			
	0.10 M[e]	0.14 M	0.21 M	0.41 M
0.00	1.79[a]	2.32[a]	2.90[a]	4.10[a]
0.01	0.77[b]	1.02[b]	1.33[b]	2.33[b]
0.03	0.47[c]	0.62[c]	0.91[c]	1.58[c]
0.05	0.34[d]	0.44[d]	0.67[d]	1.18[d]

[a–d]Different superscripts are significantly different at $p < 0.05$.
[e]Milk fat concentration in the sample.
Source: Bradley and Min, 1995.

TABLE 10.4 Depleted Headspace Oxygen of Milkfat
Containing 1,4-Diazabicyclo-[2,2,2]-octane with 40
μM Riboflavin During 3 Hours of Illumination

DABCO (M)	Depleted headspace oxygen (μmol O_2/mL)			
	0.10 M[c]	0.14 M	0.21 M	0.41 M
0.00	1.79[a]	2.32[a]	2.90[a]	4.10[a]
0.01	0.95[b]	1.20[b]	1.71[b]	2.64[b]
0.03	0.70[c]	0.94[c]	1.26[c]	2.18[c]
0.05	0.52[d]	0.64[d]	0.97[d]	1.73[d]

[a-d]Different superscripts are significantly different at $p <$ 0.05.
[c]Milk fat concentration in sample.
Source: Bradley and Min, 1995.

dimethyl furan were 1.5×10^7 $M^{-1}sec^{-1}$ and 2.6×10^7 $M^{-1}sec^{-1}$, respectively (Bradley and Min, 1995).

Riboflavin, an easily oxidizable compound, would tend to flavor the Type I pathway of photosensitized oxidation. However, it has been suggested that riboflavin can undergo both Type I and II reactions. Riboflavin has also been shown to produce superoxide anion in the serum of bovine milk after exposure to fluorescent lights and has been reported to destroy other milk components such as vitamin C (Spikes and Livingstone, 1969; Korycka-Dahl and Richardson, 1979).

Riboflavin photosensitizes the oxidation of the amino acid methionine to yield methional (Tada et al., 1971; Sattar et al., 1977). Jung et al. (1995) reported that the photosensitized oxidation of methionine produced dimethyl disulfide during the exposure of milk to sunlight. Methionine is probably not the only amino acid in milk proteins photosensitized in the presence of light and riboflavin. Directly related to the photodegradation of milk proteins is the deactivation of milk lipase. Eighty percent of initial lipase activity was lost after 30 minutes of exposure to sunlight due to riboflavin-photosensitized oxidation (Dimick, 1976). Light-induced changes in cheese have also been reported in the presence of riboflavin (Deger and Ashoor, 1987).

The exposure of butter to light accelerates the deterioration of fats (Luby et al., 1986). The severity of deterioration depends upon factors such as the light source, wavelength of light, exposure time, temperature of butter, distance of butter from light source, and salt and β-carotene contents of the butter. Cholesterol is the major steroid component in milk fat. Cholesterol in milk produced 5-cholesten-3β, 7α-diol, and 7β-epimer, and 6-cholesten-3β, 5α-diol after the exposure to light. The latter compound is only known to form following singlet oxygen attack on cholesterol. When cholesterol undergoes photosensitized oxidation in pyridine, 6-cholesten-3β-ol-5α-hydroperoxide is the major breakdown product (Kulig and Smith, 1973; Flanagan and Feretti, 1974). Potential sensory problems may be reduced by light-barrier packaging, such as aluminum foil. The main factor contributing to photochemical oxidation of butter is direct exposure to light, whereas temperatures and storage times used in the dairy industry have little effect on the quality of butter (Luby et al., 1986).

Other possible mechanisms for the production of singlet oxygen during processing and storage of dairy products include the reaction of residual hypochlorite with hydrogen peroxide, chemical or enzymatic reactions involving metalloproteins, self-reduction of secondary peroxy radicals, and oxidation of superoxide by oxidizing agents. The incorporation of a safe singlet oxygen quencher in foods and beverages could substantially improve their shelf life.

QUENCHING MECHANISMS AND KINETICS OF SINGLET OXYGEN LIPID OXIDATION

Quenching of singlet oxygen means both chemical and physical quenching (Foote, 1979). Singlet oxygen reacts with quenchers to form oxidized quenchers in chemical quenching, but physical quenching degenerates singlet oxygen to triplet oxygen. Although chemical and physical quenchings can occur together, chemical quenching is a chemical reaction rather than a quenching. Physical quenching is explained by energy transfer and/or charge transfer mechanisms (Foote, 1979). Energy transfer quenching involves the formation of triplet oxygen and triplet quencher as follows:

$$^1O_2 + {}^1Q \rightarrow {}^3O_2 + {}^3Q$$

The energy of the quencher in this process is very near or below that of singlet oxygen. The quenching of singlet oxygen by β-carotene is a good example of energy transfer quenching (Foote, 1979).

The compounds with low oxidation potentials and low triplet energies undergo charge transfer quenching. In charge transfer quenching, a singlet oxygen reacts with electron donors to form a charge transfer complex as follows:

$$Q + {}^1O_2 \rightarrow [Q^+ - O_2^-]^1 \rightarrow [Q^+ - O_2^-]^3 \rightarrow Q + {}^3O_2$$

The complex of the singlet state is relaxed to a triplet state by the intersystem crossing mechanism and then dissociates. The involvement of electron transfer in this mechanism implies that the more easily oxidizable compounds are the better charge transfer quenchers. These types of quenchers are amines, phenols, sulfides, iodide, and azide (Foote, 1979).

Singlet oxygen lipid oxidation can be minimized by singlet oxygen quenching and/or triplet sensitizer quenching, as shown in Figure 10.8. The excited singlet state sensitizer quenching is negligible due to its short lifetime. Therefore, the steady-state kinetic equation for the lipid oxidation products (AO_2) is as follows from Figure 10.8:

$$\frac{d[AO_2]}{dt} = K\left(\frac{K_o[^3O_2]}{K_o[^3O_2] + K_Q[Q]}\right)\left(\frac{K_r[A]}{K_r[A] + (K_q + K_{ox-Q})[Q] + K_d}\right)$$

where AO_2 = oxidized lipid, K = the rate constant of triplet sensitizer formation, K_r = the reaction rate constant of lipid with singlet oxygen. A = lipid, k_q = the reaction rate constant of physical singlet oxygen quenching by quencher Q, k_{ox-Q} = the reaction rate constant of chemical quenching by quencher, Q = quencher, k_d = the decaying rate constant of singlet oxygen.

In the case where there is only singlet oxygen quenching ($k_Q[Q] \ll k_o[^3O_2]$), the equation is as follows:

$$\frac{d[AO_2]}{dt} = K\left(\frac{K_r[A]}{K_r[A] + (K_q + K_{ox-Q})[Q] + K_d}\right)$$

where K = the rate of singlet oxygen formation.

The plot of $(d[AO_2]/dt)^{-1}$ vs. $[A]^{-1}$ at various concentrations of Q gives a constant y-intercept of K^{-1}, which is independent of [Q]. When there is no quencher, the slope (S_o) becomes $K^{-1}(k_d/k_r)$ and the ratio of S_o to y-intercept gives k_d/k_r. Since k_d is known for the solvent, k_r can be calculated from k_d/k_r. If there is a quencher, the slope (S_Q) to y-intercept gives $\{(K_{ox-Q}[Q] + k_Q[Q] + k_d)/k_r\}$ and is thus [Q] dependent. The ratio of slope (S_Q) to y-intercept gives $\{(K_{ox-Q}[Q] + k_q[Q] + k_d)/k_r\}$. The slope of S_Q/y-intercept vs. [Q] has another y-intercept of k_d/k_r and slope of $(K_{ox-Q} + k_q)/k_r$, from which the total singlet oxygen quenching rate constant ($K_{ox-Q} + k_q$) of the quencher can be determined.

If there is only a triplet sensitizer, $(K_{ox-Q} + k_q)[Q] \ll K_r[A] + k_d$, the reaction equation becomes as follows:

$$\frac{d[AO_2]}{dt} = K\left(\frac{K_o[^3O_2]}{K_o[^3O_2] + K_Q[Q]}\right)\left(\frac{K_r[A]}{K_r[A] + K_d}\right)$$

where K = the rate constant of triplet sensitizer formation.

The plot of $(d[AO_2]/dt)^{-1}$ vs. $[A]^{-1}$ at various concentrations of Q gives

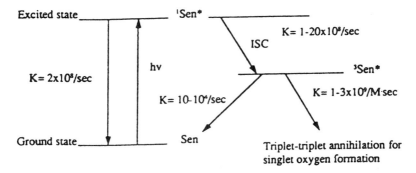

FIG. 10.8   Scheme for the quenching of triplet sensitizer and singlet oxygen. (*From Foote, 1979.*)

a y-intercept equal to $K^{-1}(1 + K_Q[Q]/k_o[^3O_2])$. The ratio of slope to the y-intercept of this plot is k_d/k_r and independent of [Q].

SINGLET OXYGEN QUENCHERS IN VEGETABLE OIL OXIDATIONS

Carotenoids, which are responsible for many of the yellow and red colors of plants and animal products, have been known to minimize singlet oxygen oxidation (Foote, 1979; Min et al., 1989). Carotenoids include a class of hydrocarbons, called carotenes, and their oxygenated derivatives, called xanthophylls.

The energy transfer quenching mechanism is responsible for the minimization of singlet oxygen oxidation of lipids by β-carotene (Foote, 1979; Neff et al., 1982, 1983). Electron excitation energy is transferred from singlet oxygen to singlet state carotenoid, producing the triplet state of carotenoid and triplet oxygen, called singlet oxygen quenching. Energy is also transferred from excited triplet state sensitizer (^{3}Sen*) to the singlet state carotenoid, called triplet sensitizer quenching. The triplet state of carotenoid is changed to the singlet state of carotenoid without any radiation.

$$^1\text{Carotenoid} + {}^1O_2 \rightarrow {}^3\text{Carotenoid} + {}^3O_2$$
$$^1\text{Carotenoid} + {}^3\text{Sen*} \rightarrow {}^3\text{Carotenoid} + {}^1\text{Sen}$$
$$^3\text{Carotenoid} \rightarrow {}^1\text{Carotenoid}$$

The energy transfer from singlet oxygen (22 kcal/mole) to carotenoids with nine or more conjugated double bonds (<22 kcal/mole) is exothermic (Foote, 1979). Foote (1979) reported that the carotenoid with seven conjugated double bonds was effective to quench triplet chlorophyll. Carotenoids with fewer than nine conjugated double bonds have energies above that of singlet oxygen and are less efficient singlet oxygen quenchers. Carotenoids with 11 or more conjugated double bonds quench at a diffusion-controlled rate of singlet oxygen.

One molecule of β-carotene can quench 250–1000 molecules of singlet oxygen (Foote, 1976). Flavor deterioration of soybean oil initiated by light can be minimized by β-carotene at levels of 5–10 ppm (Warner and Frankel, 1987). A high concentration of β-carotene produces off-flavors and facilitates oxidation by breaking down into secondary oxidation products that can initiate and promote free radicals.

Jung and Min (1991b) reported the effects of β-carotene on the headspace oxygen depletion of soybean oil in methylene chloride containing 4 ppm chlorophyll under light storage at 10°C, as shown in Figure 10.9. The quenching effectiveness of β-carotene on the chlorophyll-sensitized photo-oxidation of soybean oil was proportional to the increment of β-carotene concentration. The results show that β-carotene serves as an effective antioxidant by quenching the chlorophyll and/or singlet oxygen. The same y-intercepts of regression lines of the samples containing 0, 5, 10, and 20 ppm β-carotene suggest that β-carotene quenched the singlet oxygen to minimize the chlorophyll–photosensitized oxidation.

The rate constants for quenching singlet oxygen by carotenoids are as follows: b-apo-8′-carotenal, 3.06×10^9; β-carotene, 4.6×10^9; and canthaxanthin, 1.12×10^{10} $M^{-1}S^{-1}$ (Jung et al., 1991b). Carotenoids are excellent quenchers in singlet oxygen lipid oxidation, but they can be destroyed via free radical oxidation or prolonged irradiation and may react with singlet oxygen (Spikes and Swartz, 1978; Foote, 1979).

The decomposition of β-carotene implies three important meanings: first, the color change in the products may result in alteration of product acceptability; second, the quenching effect decreases and photosensitized oxidation increases, and finally, the vitamin A activity is lost (Francis, 1979). Fortunately, the decomposition of β-carotene can be prevented by tocopherols (Matsushita and Terao, 1980). The stability of β-carotene may be high in an oil containing large amounts of tocopherols. Min and Lee (1988) reported that the minimization of oil oxidation by β-carotene was partially attributed to the light-filtering effect.

Tocopherols are free radical scavengers and singlet oxygen quenchers (Fahrenholtz et al. 1974; Foote, 1976). Tocopherols minimize free radicals produced by singlet oxygen oxidation of free fatty acids and quench singlet oxygen (Yamauchi and Matsushita, 1977).

Foote (1979) reported that α-tocopherol quenched singlet oxygen physically and chemically, and α-tocopherol is an effective antioxidant against

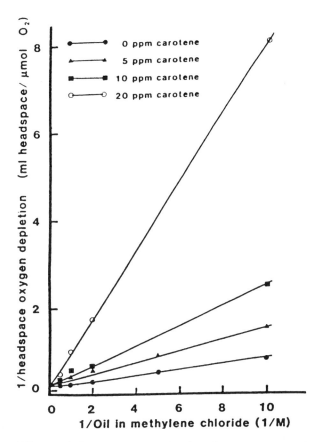

FIG. 10.9   Effects of β-carotene on the headspace oxygen depletion of soybean oil in methylene chloride containing 4 ppm chlorophyll under light storage at 10°C for 1 day. (*From Jung and Min, 1991b.*)

photosensitized singlet oxygen oxidation. The proportion of physical quenching vs. chemical quenching is structure dependent and possibly solvent system dependent. The ratio of physical quenching to chemical quenching is 13.5 in methanol (Foote, 1979) but 120 in pyridine (Fahrenholtz et al., 1974). Physical quenching is the major mechanism in the tocopherols (Foote, 1979). Tocopherols deactivate about 120 singlet oxygen molecules before they are destroyed (Spikes and Swartz, 1978). Carlsson et al. (1976) proposed that tocopherols undergo singlet oxygen oxidation to produce hydroperoxides. Yamauchi and Matsushita (1977) isolated and identified the two isomers of 8-α-hydroperoxy tocopherones as the primary products from the oxidized tocopherols in ethanol by singlet oxygen oxidation. Jung and Min (1992) proposed that the oxidized tocopherols could be prooxidants by initiating new free radical chain reactions.

Jung et al. (1991) reported the quenching effects of α-tocopherol on the headspace depletion of samples containing 3 ppm chlorophyll in soybean oil as shown in Figure 10.10. As the tocopherol amount in oil increases, the headspace depletion of samples containing chlorophyll decreases. Jung et al. (1991) reported that tocopherol quenched singlet oxygen to minimize the chlorophyll photosensitized soybean oil oxidation.

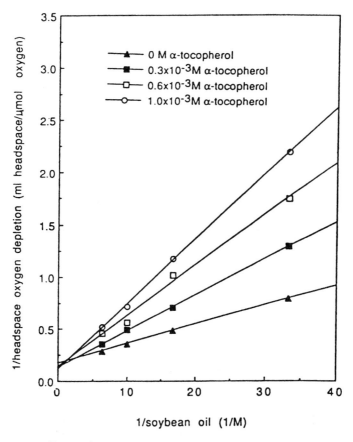

FIG. 10.10 Effects of α-tocopherol on the headspace oxygen depletion of soybean oil in methylene chloride containing 3 ppm chlorophyll under light storage at 25°C for 2 hours. (*From Jung et al., 1991.*)

Jung et al. (1991) reported that the singlet oxygen quenching rate constants of α-tocopherol where 2.7×10^7 M^{-1}sec^{-1} by peroxide value and 2.6×10^7 M^{-1}sec^{-1} by headspace oxygen and that α-tocopherol showed the highest antioxidant effect, followed by γ-tocopherol and then δ-tocopherol. The quenching ratios of α-, γ-, and δ-tocopherols were 100:26:10, respectively, in that the reactivities of α-, γ-, and δ-tocopherols with singlet oxygen were 1:0.26:0.1 (Grams and Eskins, 1972). Since the reaction rates between tocopherols and singlet oxygen are high, tocopherols may not be good antioxidants in the photosensitized oxidation of lipid foods, although in a model system δ-tocopherol acted as inhibitor in the chlorophyll-sensitized photooxidation of methyl linoleate (Terao and Matsushita, 1977). The stability of tocopherols during photosensitized oxidation showed that α-tocopherol in methyl linoeate disappeared completely after 12-hour irradiation, while γ- and δ-tocopherols remained in amounts of 34 and 48% after 48 hours, respectively (Matsushita and Terao, 1980). The higher stability of γ and δ-tocopherols to photosensitized oxidation enabled their quenching activities to last for a long period of time (Yamauchi and Matsushita, 1977).

FORMATION AND IDENTIFICATION OF SINGLET OXYGEN BY ESR SPECTROSCOPY

The detection of singlet oxygen during photosensitized oxidation is difficult to measure in that is lifetime is only a few microseconds. Electron spin resonance (ESR) spectroscopy is a highly sensitive analytical method, which detects the presence of free radicals. The use of spin trapping techniques has been developed for observing the formation of singlet oxygen by the generation of stable nitroxide radicals from sterically hindered amines. A spin trapping agent such as 2,2,6,6-tetramethyl-4-piperidone (TMPD) interacts with $^1O_2$ to form a stable nitroxide radical adduct 2,2,6,6-tetramethyl-4-piperidone-N-oxyl (TAN), which can be detected by ESR spectroscopy (Moan and Wold, 1979). Nitroxide radicals are remarkably stable because of the protective effect exerted by the four methyl groups. The TAN compound formed between the interaction of $^1O_2$ and the spin trapper TMPD has a characteristic ESR spectrum with three hyperfine lines. The three hyperfine lines are a result of the coupling of the unpaired electron with an atom of nitrogen (I = 1). The effect of illumination time on ESR spectra of TAN in water solution containing riboflavin and TMPD is shown in Figure 10.11 (Bradley et al., 1994). The spectra of Figure 10.11 after illumination for 5 and 10 minutes were identified as TAN by comparing the hyperfine coupling constant (16.1G) and spectroscopic splitting factor (2.0048 g) of

O MINUTES

5 MINUTES

15 MINUTES

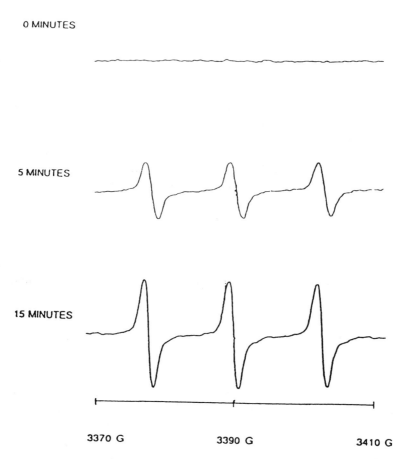

3370 G   3390 G   3410 G

FIG. 10.11   Effects of illumination on ESR spectra of TAN in water solution of riboflavin and TMPD. (*From Bradley et al., 1994.*)

the spectrum with those of the standard spectrum of TAN prepared in distilled water. As the light exposure increased, the spectrum of TAN intensity increased. The riboflavin produced singlet oxygen in the presence of light. Bradley et al. (1994) also reported that riboflavin produced singlet oxygen in milk under light and not under dark when singlet oxygen was determined by ESR spectroscopy. The ESR spectra of TAN were observed when TMPD was added to both skim and whole milk after 5 minutes of illumination. Singlet oxygen was not produced in milk under light storage when the milk was purged with nitrogen for 5 minutes.

A major limitation in radical detection by ESR is the requirement for constant radical concentrations of greater than 10^{-8} M, and reasonable spectral resolution requires 10^{-6} to 10^{-5} M. Measurement times vary from tens of seconds to hours, whereas radical lifetimes in solution are less than 1 μsec, and thus steady-state concentrations generally remain less than 10^{-7} M. Spin-trapping has been developed to overcome this problem by diminishing the rate of disappearance. Substantial development and refinement of this method is yet to come, but the initial demonstration of detecting singlet oxygen has been made.

CONCLUSION

Much evidence has been accumulated regarding the damaging effect of light and oxygen in food. Significant quantities of singlet oxygen may be generated in almost any processed foods due to the presence of photosensitizers. Rarely is the oxidation reaction exclusively perpetuated by singlet oxygen; however, lipids, proteins, and other food components can easily interact with singlet oxygen to initiate the free radical chain reaction. The information obtained in studies on model systems may not accurately reflect the complexity of the interactions that occur in foods. This chapter shows that the presence of light, oxygen, and sensitizers in vegetable oils and dairy products causes the damaging effects of singlet oxygen oxidation of foods. A better understanding of these damaging effects will provide essential information for controlling the course of singlet oxygen oxidation of foods.

REFERENCES

Aurand, L. W., Boone, N. H., and Giddings, G. G. 1977. Superoxide and singlet oxygen in milk lipid peroxidation. *J. Dairy Sci.* 60: 363.

Bader, L. W. and Orgryzlo, E. A. 1964. Reactions of oxygen ($^1\Delta_g$) and oxygen ($^1\Sigma_g$). *Discuss. Faraday Soc.* 37: 46.

Bradley, D. and Min, D. B. 1992. Singlet oxygen oxidation of foods. *CRC Crit. Rev. Food Nutr.* 31: 211–236.

Bradley, D. and Min, D. B. 1995. Riboflavin photosensitized oxidation of milk products. Presented at the Annual meeting of the Inst. of Food Technologists, Anaheim, CA.

Bradley, D. B., Ogata, T., Meinholtz, D., Berliner, L., and Min, D. B. 1994. Detection of riboflavin photosensitized singlet oxygen formation in milk by electron spin resonance. *Supramolecular Structure and Function* (Rehovot, Israel) p. 67–77.

Brekke, O. L. 1984. Bleaching. In *Handbook of Soy Oil Processing and Utiliza-*

tion, D. R. Erickson, E. H. Pyrde, O. L. Brekke, T. L. Mounts, and R. A. Falb (Ed.), p. 1080. American Oil Chemists Society, Champaign, IL.

Carlsson, D. J., Mendenhall, T., Suprunchuk, T., and Wiles, D. M. 1972. Singlet oxygen quenching in the liquid phase by metal (II) chelates. *J. Am. Chem. Soc.* 94: 8960.

Carlsson, D. J., Suprunchuk, T., and Wiles, D. W. 1976. Photooxidation of unsaturated soils: Effects of singlet oxygen quenchers. *JAOCS* 53: 656.

Chan, H. W. S. 1977. Photosensitized oxidation of unsaturated fatty acid methyl esters. The identification of different pathways. *JAOCS* 54: 100.

Clements, A. H., Van Den Engh, R. H., Frost, D. H., Hoogenhout, K., and Nooi, J. R. 1973. Participation of singlet oxygen in photosensitized oxidation of 1,4-dienoic systems and photooxidation of soybean oil. *JAOCS* 50: 325.

Deger, D. and Ashoor, S. H. 1987. Light induced changes in taste, appearance, odor, and riboflavin content of cheese. *J. Dairy Sci.* 70: 1371.

Dimick, P. S. 1976. Effect of fluorescent light on amino acid composition of serum proteins from homogenized milk. *J. Dairy Sci.* 59: 305.

Doleiden, F. H., Farenholtz, S. R., and Lamola, A. A., and Trozzolo, A. M. 1974. Reactivity of cholesterol and some fatty acids toward singlet oxygen. *Photochem. Photobiol.* 20: 519.

Endo, Y., Usuki, R., and Kaneda, T. 1984. Prooxidant activities of chlorophylls and their decomposition products on the photooxidation of methyl linoleate. *JAOCS* 61: 781.

Fahrenholtz, S. R., Doleiden, F. H., Trozzolo, A. M., and Lamola, A. A. 1974. On the quenching of singlet oxygen by α-tocopherol. *Photochem. Photobiol.* 20: 505.

Finley, J. W. and Shipe, W. F. 1968. Light induced degradation of low density lipoproteins of bovine milk. *J. Dairy Sci.* 51: 929.

Flanagan, V. P. and Feretti, A. 1974. Characterization of two steroidal olefins in nonfat dry milk. *Lipids* 9: 471.

Foote, C. S. 1976. Photosensitized oxidation and singlet oxygen: consequences in biological systems. In *Free Radicals in Biology*, Vol. 2, W. A. Pryor (Ed.). Academic Press, New York.

Foote, C. S. 1968. Photosensitized oxygenation and the role of singlet oxygen. *Acc. Chem. Res.* 1: 104.

Foote, C. S. 1979. Quenching of singlet oxygen. In *Singlet Oxygen*, H. H. Wasserman and R. W. Murray (Ed.), pp. 139–171. Academic Press, New York.

Francis, F. J. 1979. Pigments and other colorants. In *Food Chemistry*, O. R. Fennema (Ed.), pp. 546–582. Marcel Dekker, New York.

Frankel, E. N. 1980. Lipid oxidation. *Prog. Lipid Res.* 19: 1.

Frankel, E. N., Warner, K., and Moulton, K. J. Sr. 1985. Effects of hydrogenation and additives on cooking oil performance of soybean oil. *JAOCS* 62: 1354.

Gaylord, A. M., Warthensen, J. J., and Smith, D. E. 1985. Effect of fluorescent light on the isomerization of retinyl palmitate in skim milk. *J. Food Sci.* 51: 1456.

Grams, G. W. and Eskins, K. 1972. Dye sensitized photoxidation of α-tocopherol. *Biochemistry* 11: 606.

Gunstone, F. D. 1984. Reaction of oxygen and unsaturated fatty acids. *JAOCS* 61: 441.

Held, A. M., Halko, D. J., and Hurst, J. K. 1978. Mechanism of chlorine oxidation in hydrogen peroxide. *J. Am. Chem. Soc.* 100: 5732.

Jung, M. Y. and Min, D. B. 1991a. Quenching rates of carotenoids in the singlet oxygen lipid oxidation. *J. Am. Oil Chem. Soc.* 68(9): 653–658.

Jung, Y. and Min, D. B. 1991b. Effects of oxidized α-, γ-, and δ-tocopherols on the oxidative stability of soybean oil. *Food Chem.* 183–187.

Jung, Y. J., Lee, E., and Min, D. B. 1991. α-, γ-, δ-Tocopherol effects on chlorophyll photosensitized oxidation of soybean oil. *J. Food Sci.* 56: 807.

Jung, M. Y., Yoon, S. H., Lee, Hyung-Ok, and Min, D. B. 1995. Effects of ascorbic acid on the formation of light-induced off-flavor of skim milk. *J. Food Sci.* (in press).

Kearsley, M. W. and Rodriguez, N. 1981. The stability and use of natural colors in foods: Anthocyanin, β-carotene and riboflavin. *J. Food Technol.* 16: 421.

Kahn, T. M. M. and Martell, E. 1967. Metal ion and metal chelate catalyzed oxidation of ascorbic acid by molecular oxygen. I. Cupric and ferric ion catalyzed oxidation. *J. Am. Chem. Soc.* 88: 4176.

Korycka, Dahl, M. and Richardson, T. 1979. Photogeneration of superoxide anion upon illumination of bovine milk serum proteins with fluorescent light in the presence of riboflavin. *J. Dairy Sci.* 62: 183.

Korycka-Dahl, M. B. and Richardson, T. 1978. Activated oxygen species and oxidation of food constituents. *CRC Crit. Rev. Food Sci. Nutr.* 10: 209.

Kulig, M. J. and Smith, L. L. 1973. Sterol metabolism. XXV. Cholesterol oxidation by singlet molecular oxygen. *J. Org. Chem.* 38: 3639.

Labuza, T. P. 1971. Kinetics of lipid oxidation in foods. *CRC Crit. Rev. Food Sci. Nutr.* 2: 355.

Lee, E. C. and Min, D. B. 1988. Quenching mechanism of β-carotene on the chlorophyll sensitized photooxidation of soybean oil. *J. Food Sci.* 53: 1894.

Lee, S. H. and Min, D. B. 1990. Effects, quenching mechanisms, and kinetics of carotenoids in chlorophyll-sensitized photooxidation of soybean oil. *J. Agric. Food Chem.* 38: 1630.

Lee, S. H. and Min, D. B. 1991. Effects, quenching mechanisms, and kinetics of nickel chelates in singlet oxygen oxidation of soybean oil. *J. Agric. Food Chem.* 39: 642.

Livingstone, R. 1961. *Autoxidation and Antioxidants*, Vol. 1, Ch. 2. Wiley, New York.

Luby, J. M., Gray, J. I., Harte, B. R., and Ryan, T. C. 1986. Photooxidation of cholesterol in butter. *J. Food Sci.* 51: 904.

Maniere, F. Y. and Dimick, P. S. 1976. Effect of fluorescent light on repartition of riboflavin in homogenized milk. *J. Dairy Sci.* 59: 2019.

Matsushita, S. and Terao, J. 1980. Singlet oxygen-initiated photooxidation of unsaturated fatty acids and esters and inhibitory effect of tocopherols and β-carotene. In *Autoxidation in Food and Biological Systems*, M. G. Simic and M. Karel (Ed.), pp. 27–44. Plenum Press, New York.

McCord, J. M. and Fridovich, I. 1969. Superoxide dismutase. An enzymic function for erythrocuprein. *J. Biol. Chem.* 244: 6049.

Min, D. B. and Lee, E. C. 1988. Factors affecting the singlet, oxygen oxidation of soybean oil. In *Frontiers of Flavor*, G. Charalambous (Ed.), pp. 473–498. Elsevier, Amsterdam.

Min, D. B., Lee, E. C. and Lee, S. H. 1989. Singlet oxidation of vegetable oils. In *Flavor Chemistry of Lipid Foods*, D. B. Min and T. H. Smouse (Ed.), p. 57. American Oil Chemists' Society, Champaign, IL.

Moan, J. and Wold E. 1979. Detection of singlet oxygen production by ESR. *Nature* 279: 450.

Neff, W. E., Frankel, E. N., Selke, E., and Weisleder, D. 1983. Photosensitized oxidation of methyl linoleate monohydroperoxides: hydroperoxy cyclic peroxides, dihydroperoxides, keto esters, and volatile thermal decomposition products. *Lipids* 18: 868.

Neff, W. E., Frankel, E. N., and Weisledger, D. 1982. Photosensitized oxidation of methyl linoleate. Secondary products. *Lipids* 17: 780.

Neff, W. E., Frankel, E. N., Selke, E., and Weisledger, D. *Lipids* 18: 868.

Nelson, K. H. and Cathcart, W. M. 1984. Transmission of light through pigmented polyethylene milk bottles. *J. Food Protect.* 47: 346.

Patton, S. 1954. The mechanism of sunlight flavor formation in milk with special reference to methionine and riboflavin. *J. Dairy Sci.* 37: 446.

Rawls, H. R. and VanSanten, P. J. 1970. A possible role for singlet oxidation in the initiation of fatty acid autoxidation. *JAOCS* 47: 121.

Rosenthal, I. 1985. Photooxidation of foods. In *Singlet Oxygen*, Vol. IV. *Polymers and Biomolecules*, A. A. Frimer (Ed.), CRC Press, Inc., Boca Raton, FL.

Samuel, D. and Steckel, F. 1974. The physiochemical properties of molecular oxygen. In *Molecular Oxygen in Biology*, O. Hayaishi (Ed.). Elsevier, New York.

Sattar, A., DeMan, J. M., and Alexander, J. C. 1977. Light-induced degradation of vitamins. II. Kinetic studies on ascorbic acid decomposition in solution. *Can. Inst. Food Sci. Technol. J.* 10: 65.

Singleton, T. A., Aurand, L. W., and Lancaster, F. W. 1963. Sunlight flavor in milk. I. A study of components involved in the flavor development. *J. Dairy Sci.* 46: 1050.

Spikes, J. D. 1977. In *The Science of Photobiology*, K. C. Smith (Ed.), pp. 87–112. Plenum Press, New York.

Spikes, J. D. and Livingstone, R. 1969. The molecular biology of photodynamic action. *Radiat. Biol.* 3: 29.

Spikes, J. D. and Swartz, H. M. 1978. International conference on singlet oxygen and related species in chemistry and biology, a review and general discussion. *Photochem. Photobiol.* 28: 921.

Stevenson, S. G., Vaisey-Genser, M., and Eskin, N. A. M. 1984. Photooxidation of soybean oil. *J. Am. Oil Chem.* 61: 1102.

Swern, D. 1982. Cooking oils, salad oils, and salad dressings. In *Bailey's Industrial Oil and Fat Prod.*, Vol. 2, 4th ed., p. 315. John Wiley, New York.

Tada, M., Kobayashi, N., and Kobayashi, S. 1971. Studies on the photosensitized degradation of food constituents. Part II. Photosensitized degradation of methionine by riboflavin. *J. Agr. Chem. Soc.* (Japan) 45: 471.

Terao, J. and Matsushita, S. 1977. Products formed by photosensitized oxidation of unsaturated fatty acid esters. *JAOCS* 54: 234.

Umehara, T., Terao, J., and Matsushita, S. 1979. Photosensitized oxidation of oils with food colors. *J. Agric. Chem. Soc.* 53: 51.

Usuki, R., Endo, Y., and Kaneda, T. 1984. Prooxidant activities of chlorophylls, and pheophytins on the photooxidation of edible oils. *Agric. Biol. Chem.* 48: 991.

Warner, K. and Frankel, E. N. 1987. Effects of β-carotene on light stability of soybean oil. *JAOCS* 64: 213.

Warner, K., Frankel, E. N., Snyder, J. M., and Porter, W. L. 1986. Storage stability of soybean oil-based salad dressings: effect of antioxidants and hydrogenation. *J. Food Sci.* 51: 703.

Wayne, R. P. 1969. Singlet molecular oxygen. *Adv. Photochem.* 7: 311.

Yamauchi, R. and Matsushita, S. 1977. Quenching effect of tocopherols on the methyl linoleate photooxidation and their oxidation products. *Agric. Biol. Chem.* 41: 1425.

Yang, W. T. and Min, D. B. 1994. Effects of photosensitized synthetic colorants on the singlet oxygen oxidation of foods. American Oil Chemists' Society meeting, Atlanta, GA. May.

11
Significance of Lipid Oxidation to Food Processors

Thomas H. Smouse[†]

Archer Daniels Midland Company
Decatur, Illinois

INTRODUCTION

Lipid oxidation is an important process for all food processors and food products. It has a direct influence upon consumer acceptance and affects several important quality characteristics, such as color (visual perception), flavor (taste and odor perception), and texture (feel perception), as well as nutrition. In some cases, such as the crunchability of a chip, it can even affect sound, e.g., as an oil oxidizes in the fryer, the cooking time is lengthened, and if the frying time is not lengthened, the chip will not be as crisp.

The most common and important type of lipid oxidation involves chemical oxidation via a free radical mechanism. Other types critical to a food's acceptance are enzymatic, hydrolytic, and photogenic oxidation. Although most lipid oxidation causes a decrease in acceptance, in some cases enzymatic oxidation is essential for flavor development, e.g., the "green" fresh

[†]Deceased.

flavor of a tomato or cucumber or the "green bean" flavor of legumes like soybeans, lima beans, or peas. Even the flavor of fish has been attributed to the slight oxidation of unsaturated fatty acids. These flavors are caused by the enzyme lipoxygenase. For dairy products such as sour cream, cheese and yogurt, hydrolytic rancidity or the production of short-chain fatty acids such as butyric, valeric, and caproic acids are essential to develop the correct flavor profile. For coconuts and some dairy products like blue cheese, the formation of methyl ketones are important. These flavors, which are formed by hydrolytic and ketonic rancidity, can either be desirable or undesirable, depending upon the food and time of development.

Chemical oxidation of lipids with the formation of hydroperoxides that decompose into a wide range of chemical compounds such as hydrocarbons, aldehydes, alcohols, esters, ketones, acids, lactones, and even several aromatic classes cause off-flavors and poor product acceptance. For example, in a fresh salad dressing, the blend of spice flavors will yield a desirable and well-accepted product, but as the oil oxidizes and other flavors are formed, the desirable "top notes" of the salad dressing are diminished and replaced with stale oxidation flavor notes, which eventually progress to oxidative rancidity and a nonpalatable product.

LIPID OXIDATION

The previous chapter by Min and Lee covered the mechanisms of triplet and singlet oxygen and their involvement in lipid oxidation. It is a complex reaction with many chemical compounds being formed, and even after 50 years of study, new compounds are being found every day.

Some important characteristics of food that are affected by lipid oxidation are given in Table 11.1. The total flavor of a food is changed as oxidation progresses. We are all familiar with the highly desirable flavor of a fresh roasted peanut or a deep fat fried potato chip, but with time stale oxidized flavors develop, and eventually a nonpalatable, undesirable product is formed. It is interesting to note that when this stage of oxidation is reached, the nutritional value of the product is diminished and in fact will cause sickness, especially diarrhea. Animals that have been fed rancid oils dehydrate and eventually die.

The color of food can also be affected by lipid oxidation. In some cases the food becomes darker, such as the surface of butter or margarine or a bottle of corn oil. This is normally thought to result from an oxidation reaction with tocopherols or sterols. In the case of vegetable products it is the result of the formation of compounds like "toco red" and "toco purple" from the oxidation of tocopherol. However, in oils and food products with carotene as the major pigment, the product can become lighter as a

TABLE 11.1 Some Factors That Affect Stability of a Lipid

Seed storage
Oil storage
Antioxidants
Soaps
Metals
Phospholipids
Pigments
Fatty acid composition
Type of clay
Deodorization time and temperature
Sequestrants
Deodorization cool-down rates, light, and inert gas covers

result of oxidation, such as the yellow-red color of paprika or the light yellow color of soybean oil. As the double bonds in carotene are oxidized, a less conjugated system is formed, which bleaches the pigment. In soybean oil processing, this is referred to as heat bleaching and is done by heating the oil to 500°F under a vacuum and holding it at this elevated temperature for several minutes.

As lipid oxidation occurs, the emulsion characteristics of a system will change. For example, as frying fats are used, hydrolysis products and polymers are formed. These products increase the surface tension of the frying medium and entrap more air and water vapor in the fat, causing it eventually to foam. The entrapped air changes the thermal conductivity of the fat, thus changing the rate of cooking. In lecithin processing, hydrogen peroxide is used to bleach the lecithin to make a lighter color. Extensive bleaching leads to hydroxylation or the formation of a lecithin product with a more hydrophillic nature, which forms a more stable oil-in-water emulsions.

As for solubility, when a lipid oxidizes and other food components such as proteins and carbohydrates are present, cross-linking can occur, as can the Maillard reaction from the aldehydes of hydroperoxide decomposition and the amine groups of proteins. These reactions lead to less solubility or dispersibility. This can easily be seen over a period of a few weeks when one stores soy protein isolate at 110°F (43°C) and measures its nitrogen solubility index (NSI) or protein dispersibility index (PDI). For example, Jones and Gersdorff (1938) showed a decrease in the dispersibility of nitrogenous compounds of a high-fat and low-fat soybean meal after aging for 1, 2, and 3 months at different temperatures. A high-fat soybean meal at 30°F (−1°C) and 60°F (15.5°C) storage is shown in Figure 11.1. As expected, the higher

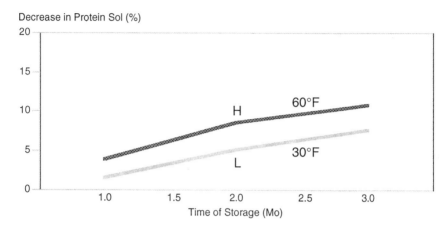

FIG. 11.1   Percent decrease in protein solubility at 30 and 60°F storage.

storage temperature shows a greater decrease in protein solubility, but note that even some decrease is observed at 30°F ($-1°C$).

This also occurs in other dried food products like soy protein isolate, sodium caseinate, and others. Although there is less fat in the low-fat meal, it is distributed over the same surface area and thus reacts with oxygen at a greater rate. One method of counteracting this is to add a small amount of highly stable fat to the low-fat powder, which acts as an oxygen barrier to prevent it from reaching the more unsaturated soy lipids in the meal. This could also be a problem in a fat-free soy isolate. Before the new labeling laws of 1993, the fat or oil in soybean protein isolate was less than 1% as defined by hexane extractables. However, if chloroform/methanol was used as the solvent, 3.5–4.5% lipid material could be extracted, which is mostly phospholipids.

It is also important to point out that lipid oxidation can affect taste and odor, which in turn affects flavor. For example, when a phospholipid oxidizes, unsaturated hydroxy fatty acids are formed, which cause a strong, bitter flavor. One example of an odor would be "rancid fat." The aldehydes and other organic compounds can be detected by the nose long before any off-tastes are detected. For this reason, when evaluating a salad oil, it should be heated to about 50°C, smelled first to detect any off-odors, and then tasted for the complete sensory test. Kathleen Warner covers sensory evaluation in detail in a later chapter.

Finally, all of these changes from lipid oxidation affect consumer acceptance. One definition of quality is that which the consumer expects and accepts. Therefore, if a product is not accepted, it does not have quality.

FACTORS AFFECTING OIL QUALITY

In a recent book by Warner and Eskin (1995), I wrote a chapter on oil quality and stability. Many of the processing steps used to process a salad oil, a frying fat, or a baking shortening have a direct influence upon the quality and stability of the product; some of these cause-and-effect relationships are reviewed in the following.

An oil seed must first be harvested by the farmer before it is sent to the oil processor for crushing and refining. The seed quality will influence the oil quality. For example, immature seeds will be high in chlorophyll, pro-oxidant for singlet oxidation. Chlorophyll not only gives a green tint to the oil, but its presence has a direct relationship to the oxidation stability. The oxygen stability of the same canola oil bleached with three different bleaching clays is shown in Figure 11.2. Initially the refined canola oil had about 15,000 ppb chlorophyll and an OSI at 110°F (43°C) of a little more than 8 hours. However, when the chlorophyll level was lowered to less than 50 ppb, the OSI time went as high as almost 10 hours. A 2-hour increase in OSI time at 110°F (43°C) is comparable to a 5-hour increase in AOM time at 208°F (97.8°C), which in the case of a canola salad oil is a significant improvement in oxidation stability and would amount to several weeks more on the grocery store shelf.

Chlorophyll would also give a green tint to the oil. For example, Figure 11.3 shows the effect that chlorophyll has upon the color of the same canola oil used above. Using the total color difference from a white plate, values of zero would be obtained for a colorless solution. On the other hand, very high values approaching 100 would be obtained from a very dark color.

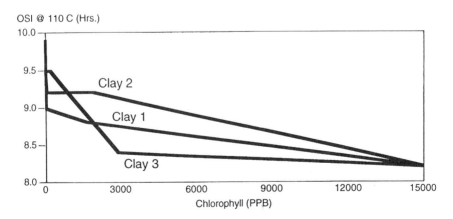

FIG. 11.2   Relationship of chlorophyll and oxidation stability.

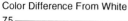

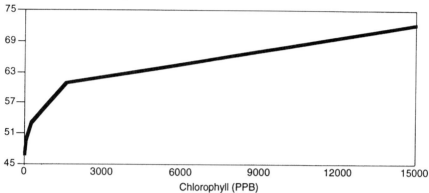

FIG. 11.3   Relationship of total color difference from a white slate and amount of chlorophyll in oil.

Using these color values, canola salad oil does shows no green tint when it has a color difference from white of <48.5. Although you cannot see it in Figure 11.3, such a value would be comparable to a chlorophyll value of 50 ppb or less.

If the seed is wet or cracked, enzymes will be released that have a direct relationship to the flavor stability of the finished oil. For example, in soybeans, lipoxygenase is present, which will oxidize the linoleic acid, forming flavor precursors. These will later develop off-flavors. Much research has been done and many patents have been issued for various processes inactivating lipoxygenase so it will not oxidize soybean oil.

Besides chlorophyll and enzymes, other compounds in the oil have a direct influence upon their performance and quality in a food product. In Table 11.1 are listed factors that may affect the stability of a fat and oil. These are covered briefly below.

Seed Storage

Earlier the effect of immature seeds high in chlorophyll or cracked seeds with active enzyme release was discussed. The storage of the seed and/or crude oil can also affect the oil quality. Storage of beans with moistures of greater than 13–14% results in spontaneous heating and the beans turn black. In some cases the beans in the center ignite and smolder, producing a nonusable product. Even with proper storage, the nonhydrable phospholipids increase, yielding a bean that has less extractable oil and an oil of poorer quality with higher refining losses because of the free fatty acids and phospholipids.

The temperature of crude oil storage also has a direct relationship to the level of oxidation. For example, in a study (Smouse, 1995) on aging crude soybean oil at five different temperatures—10, 38, 60, 77, and 93°C—the rate of oxidation could be followed by a peroxide measurement and a conjugated diene measurement. Figure 11.4 shows the effects that time and temperature have on peroxide development. Note that at 77°C or higher, crude oil can be held only several days before it oxidizes. Conjugated diene data confirm the PV data and also show a rapid increase in a few days if the storage temperature is above 77°C. The oxidation of the crude oil is important, because it can be related to the nonhydrable phospholipids. These must be removed from oil during processing to give a light-colored product with good flavor.

The data in Table 11.2 show that after 20 days of aging at 60°C, the phospholipids cannot be removed from the crude oil to a level below 51 ppm of phosphorus. This corresponds to PV and CD values of around 20 and 0.5, respectively. Chu and Lin (1993) also showed that tocopherol is oxidized to chroman-5,6-quinone and phosphatidyl ethanolamine is reduced during storage of crude soybean oil. It is interesting to note that they stored their crude oil at 60°C about 19 days before they observed significant drops in tocopherol and PE. This agrees well with the 15 days this author observed (Smouse, 1995).

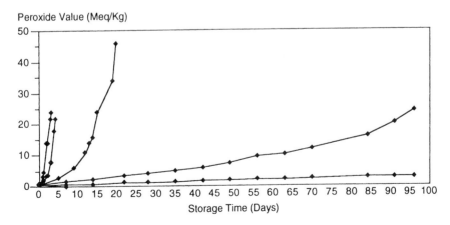

FIG. 11.4   Effect of time and temperature on peroxide value of crude soybean oil.

TABLE 11.2 Effect of Time Upon PV and CD of Crude Soybean Oil and Upon Phosphorus in Degummed Oil

Storage time (days) at 60°C	PV (mEq/kg) in crude soybean oil	CD (E @ 234) in crude soybean oil	Phosphorus (ppm) in degummed crude oil
0	0.6	0.18	47
2	1.3	0.17	44
6	2.5	0.20	47
10	3.5	0.23	38
13	4.5	0.22	44
15	6.5	0.28	44
16	8.8	0.28	34
20	22.5	0.52	38
23	38.6	0.69	51
27	61.0	0.96	103

Antioxidants

The tocopherols in vegetable oils are natural antioxidants. Gamma-tocopherol shows the greatest antioxidant activity. It has a pronounced effect upon the oxidative stability of a finished food product. Figure 11.5 shows the relationship of pressure DSC induction times to the tocopherol content of deoiled lecithin at 500 psig oxygen pressure and 120°C. As you can see from the excellent linear fit, when the tocopherols are low, the oxidative stability is poor. In addition to the tocopherols being affected by storage, the deodorization time and temperature has a direct effect upon their amount in a finished oil. Klagge and Sen Gupta (1990) showed that deodorization temperatures of 235°C and above would strip from the oil substantial amounts of tocopherols, which are collected in the deodorizer condensate. Scavone and Braun (1988) also patented a deodorization process to remove tocopherols, giving a better fry life of frying fats. Their fry life of the oil was defined spectrophotometrically as the amount of time it takes for a frying oil to darken in color to an absorbance of 1.4 at 520 nm after deep frying foods. When one oxidizes tocopherol, a chroman-5,6-quinone is formed, which has been shown to be the cause of color reversion in soybean oil, corn oil, and cottonseed oil. Therefore, by removing the tocopherol during deodorization, a frying fat with better color stability is obtained, but it will have poorer oxidative stability. This may not be a problem if long-term shelf stability is not needed.

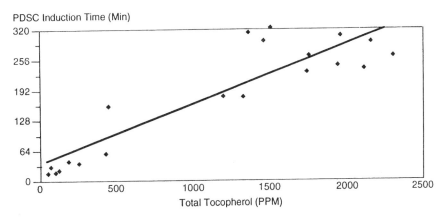

FIG. 11.5 Relationship of pressure DSC induction time and tocopherol content. Y = 30.698 + 1.129X; S = 48.669; R^2 = 0.818.

The time/temperature conditions for tocopherol removal can be determined by analyzing total tocopherols before and after deodorization. By using different times and temperatures, the three-dimensional plot shown in Figure 11.6 is achieved. When temperature is plotted on the X-axis, time on the Y-axis, and percent tocopherol reduction on the Z-axis, you can see that temperatures greater than 550°F (288°C) and times greater than 120 minutes will remove about 60% of the tocopherols. However, at 470°F (243°C) and 40 minutes, only 10% of tocopherols will be removed. The quadratic equation for this relationship is

$$\% \text{ removed} = \text{temperature squared} + 0.006186 \text{ time} \times \text{temperature} + 0.000531 \text{ time squared} + 5.130986 \text{ temperature} - 3.104911 \text{ time} - 1284.870868$$

This equation has a correlation coefficient of 0.827, which shows a fair degree of fit for the 21 data points.

Soaps

Crude oil from oil seeds contains small amounts of free fatty acids. These are normally removed by caustic refining, where the fatty acid is converted to a sodium soap, which is then removed by centrifugation and water washing. Trace amounts of soap not removed from the oil will be adsorbed by the activated clay, reducing its effectiveness. They will poison the catalyst for hydrogenation, producing more *trans* isomers, and in the case of a frying fat they will cause excessive hydrolysis during frying, producing an increased

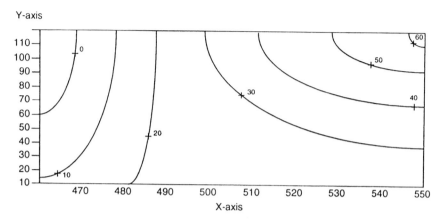

FIG. 11.6 Three-dimensional plot of percent tocopherol reduction (Z) vs. time (Y) and temperature (X) of deodorization.

rate of free fatty acid development. Soaps are usually measured in the refinery by the titration method recommended by the AOCS (1994). This method has a MDL of approximately 3 ppm soap, which is comparable to 0.2 ppm sodium. Frying fats with sodium levels higher than 0.2 ppm will have very poor hydrolysis stability.

Metals

The metals in a processed oil have a direct relationship to various chemical and physical characteristics. For example, it is well known that aluminum reacts with yellow egg pigments, forming a green color. And manganese and zinc react with cocoa to yield an off-flavor. Iron and copper are two metals in edible oils that can harm oxidative stability. For this reason, edible oils should be stored in stainless steel tanks, shipped in stainless steel containers, and transferred by stainless steel pipes. No iron, copper, or brass fittings or valves should be in contact with an edible oil.

Metals in oil are reduced in several of the unit processes. First, removal of phospholipids by degumming will reduce the metals phosphorus, calcium, magnesium, and iron. These metals are associated with phospholipids, so when the phospholipids are removed, the metals follow along. During pigment removal by acid- activated clays, metals are also adsorbed and reduced. Even a good filtration can lower metals. Typical metal values will vary from oil to oil and from one process location to another. However, some typical values found in 20 samples of soybean oil processed to different degrees are given in Table 11.3, along with the standard deviation. The

TABLE 11.3 Metals Found in Soybean Oil at Various Stages of Processing

Soybean oil	Metals from 20 Obs. (ppm $\pm$ sd)			
	Phosphorus	Calcium	Magnesium	Iron
Crude	709 $\pm$ 166	63 $\pm$ 15	65 $\pm$ 14	1 $\pm$ 0
Degummed	108 $\pm$ 58	38 $\pm$ 20	18 $\pm$ 8	0.3 $\pm$ 0.1
Refined	4.5 $\pm$ 3.9	1.1 $\pm$ 1.4	0.5 $\pm$ 0.6	<0.05
Bleached	0.7 $\pm$ 0.8	0.2 $\pm$ 0.4	0.1 $\pm$ 0.2	<0.05
RBD	<0.5	0.1	<0.05	<0.05

amount of copper is also evaluated, but it is consistently less than 0.05 so is not included in these data. Please note that metals in the refined, bleached, and deodorized oil are extremely low and many times below our detection limits using an inductively coupled argon plasma/atomic emission spectrophotometry (ICAP/AES).

In recent years, Canessa et al. (1993) showed that a sodium silicate (Britesorb, NC) could be used to reduce metals. And, Toeneboehn (1992) showed that a silica gel in modified refining would reduce metals and soap more effectively than water washing, thus yielding better oxidative and flavor stability. These silica processes are used in some refineries either with refining or bleaching and sometimes in a posthydrogenation bleach to remove all traces of the nickel catalyst.

Phospholipids

The common phospholipids phosphatidyl choline (PC), phosphatidyl ethanolamine (PE), and phosphatidyl inositol (PI) make up most of the surface active agents in soy lecithin. For good flavor and color of a RBD SBO, all of these must be removed before the deodorization step. Lecithin color is very sensitive to heat and will tend to darken from the Maillard reaction when the temperature is over 150°F (65.6°C). For example, using the total color difference from white as a color measurement, the plot in Figure 11.7 shows that the more phospholipids present in the oil to be deodorized, the darker the color of the deodorized oil. The fit is a quadratic curve, which shows a steep slope at low levels of phospholipids and a "flattening" at the higher levels. Again, a value of 65 is dark, while a value of 35 is a light yellow. For this reason, oil processors normally strive for phosphorus levels below 0.5 ppm, which is comparable to a phospholipid value of 0.0015% or a 99.97% reduction in phospholipids from the crude oil.

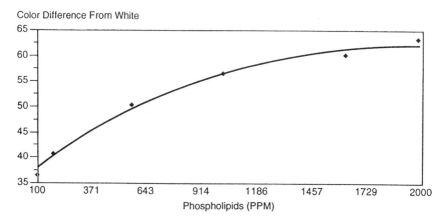

FIG. 11.7 Effect of phospholipids upon deodorized oil color. $Y = 35.039 + 0.029X - 0.7742E - 5X^2$; $S = 1.117$; $R^2 = 0.987$.

Pigments

Color pigments are removed by a process called bleaching. Adsorptive materials such as activated clay, diatomaceous earths, carbons, or various types of silicas are used to selectively absorb the color compounds and remove them with the spent adsorbent when it is filtered from the oil. A recent monograph by Patterson (1992) covers this subject in detail. Essentially, the adsorbent is added to a heated refined oil and the mixture agitated under a partial vacuum to reduce oxidation. Adsorption isotherms are exponential, and after a period of time the spent adsorbent is filtered from the oil, yielding a spent adsorbent and bleached oil. Cowan (1966) compared a bleached and unbleached soybean oil and showed that the bleached product had better initial flavor, had better aged flavor, and oxidized much more slowly than its unbleached counterpart. Therefore, in addition to reducing the color, bleaching also improves the oxidative stability. For example, in a refined canola oil, chlorophyll was reduced from 15 ppm in the refined product to <50 ppm in the bleached product. A significant improvement in oxidative stability of canola oil was observed when the bleached product was compared to the unbleached product (see Fig. 11.2). Mag (1989) states that the concentration of chlorophylloid compounds must be reduced to 50 ppb or lower to avoid rapid oxidation of the oil in the presence of light.

Since some adsorbents show different selectivities for different components, sometimes a two-stage bleaching is done. In this case, an adsorbent is used for one type of compound followed by a second adsorbent for another type of compound. Silica has been shown to be effective in reducing metals, soaps, and phospholipids. Welsh et al. (1989) showed the effectiveness of amorphous synthetic silicas in removing phospholipids, calcium, and magnesium. When followed by an activated earth, it enables the earth to be more effective in reducing the pigments.

Fatty Acid Composition

Fats and oils are a mixture of mixed triglycerides. A triglyceride is a triester of one molecule of glycerol and three molecules of fatty acids. Although all fatty acids are known to oxidize, the unsaturated fatty acids react the fastest, with a reaction order of linolenic > linoleic > oleic. For this reason, vegetable oils with high amounts of oleic acid show good oxidative stability. Examples of these include olive oil, high oleic sunflower seed oil, and high oleic safflower seed oil. However, other oils such as soybean, cottonseed, and canola have more linoleic acid than oleic acid, so they do not have as good oxidative stability. However, by selectively adding hydrogen to the linoleic acid, forming oleic acid, these oils can be improved for oxidative stability. This process, called hydrogenation, is used to make frying fats, shortenings, and cream filler fats where improved oxidative stability is necessary for the long storage times of the products made from these fats.

Type of Clay

Figure 11.2 shows the effect of three clays in reducing chlorophyll in canola oil. The type of clay can also have an effect upon the oxidative stability. Various grades (available from several suppliers) must be evaluated in order to select the clay that performs best in each application. Also, the type of acid used to activate the clay can play an important role in how well the clay adsorbs as well as if other trace metals are present that can act as prooxidants to the oil. Table 11.4 shows the effect that six different activated earths have upon the oxidative stability of a refined and bleached canola oil. The same caustic refined canola oil was bleached with various levels of six different clays. The amounts of clay used were selected to bleach to about 50 ppb chlorophyll. When these same oils were evaluated for their oxidative stability, OSI times from 6.3 to 9.45 hours were observed. A difference of 3.15 hours in OSI time at 110°C is highly significant, and in this study, clay A was selected since less of it had to be used to reach 50 ppb chlorophyll and it did not harm the oil as much as some of the others. For oxidative stability, clay B was the best, but an additional 1.0% higher use level makes it uneconomical when compared to clay A.

TABLE 11.4 Effect of Activated Clay Upon
Oxidative Stability of Refined and Bleached
Canola Oil

Clay	Amount (%)	Chlorophyll (ppb)	OSI at 110°C (hr)
A	1.5	59	9.05
B	2.0	31	7.30
C	2.0	61	7.40
D	2.5	43	9.45
E	2.5	42	9.20
F	2.5	61	6.30

Deodorizer Time and Temperature

The last major processing step given to an edible oil is deodorization. This procedure removes all the volatiles, producing an oil with a bland flavor. Normally, temperatures in the range 350–600°F (177–316°C) are used with times from a few minutes to as much as a few hours. Since steam is used to help strip the volatiles from the oil, the amount can vary from 0.5% to as much as several percent. During this process, some of the *cis* unconjugated double bonds are isomerized to the *trans* conjugated form. It is important to minimize this effect, because conjugated double bonds oxidize at a much faster rate. This is the reason why a drying oil like linseed oil is conjugated when it is used for paint so that oxidation occurs faster and the paint dries more quickly.

If the oil is abused during this process, large amounts of *trans* conjugated fatty acids can be formed, yielding a finished product with poor oxidative stability. The degree to which this will occur depends upon the oil, the processor, and the equipment. The *trans* fatty acids at these low levels must be measured by high-resolution capillary gas-liquid chromatography, which is expensive and time consuming. However, the conjugated diene content can be measured quickly and cheaply using an ultraviolet spectrophotometer at 234 nm. The relationship between these two measurements is shown in Figure 11.8. As can be seen from these data, a *trans* fatty acid value of ≤0.5% is predicted when the CD extinction value is <3.06 adsorption unit. This value is a good goal. Some older deodorizers that operate at high temperatures for several hours can generate several percent *trans* fatty acids, at the same time forming conjugated dienes, which cause poor oxidative stability. Mariani et al. (1991) showed the effect of deodorization times and temperatures on lampante olive oil. At temperatures as high as 500°F

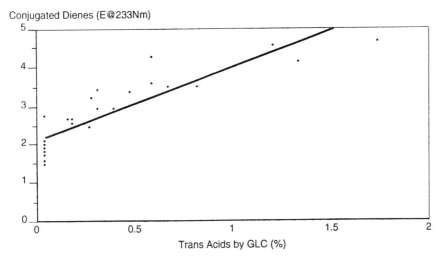

FIG. 11.8   Linear relationship between CD values of salad soybean oil samples and total *trans* fatty acid content. Y = 2.1736 + 1.7834; S = 0.4119; R^2 = 0.7744.

(260°C) for 2 hours they found as much as 2% *trans* fatty acids in their deodorized olive oil. Wolff (1993) also showed the effect of time and temperature upon the isomerization of linseed oil. At 500°F (260°C), isomerization of linolenic acid was very fast and more than 30% isomerization was found to occur in a 2-hour isomerization. Therefore, for optimum oxidative stability, the time and temperature profiles for each deodorizer and each oil must be determined to yield a finished product with optimum oxidative stability.

Once the product is deodorized, it must be cooled from temperatures of 500°F (260°C) to temperatures in the area of 150°F (65.6°C). During this cool-down period, the fat must be kept under a high vacuum with a small amount of steam sparge to keep the product bland. If this is not done, the high heat produces oxidative materials, which condense in the oil. The data in Table 11.5 show the effect that several deodorization variables have upon the oxidative stability of soybean oil. This experiment was conducted in a plant continuous deodorizer capable of oil rates as high as 50,000 pounds per hour. If the oil rate were varied between a low rate and a rate 1.7 times greater, the lower rate of throughput was found to give a 43% increase in the oxidative stability. For the outlet temperature of the oil, the lower temperature showed a 23% increase in OSI times. The temperature effect in this experiment had a 17% increase in OSI times for the lower temperature, and

TABLE 11.5   Effect of Deodorization Variables Upon Oxidative Stability

Variable	OSI at 110°C (hr)	Difference (%)
Oil rate (H vs. 1.7 L)	21 vs. 30	43
Oil outlet temp. (H vs. 1.2 L)	22 vs. 27	23
Temperature of Deod. (H vs. 1.1 L)	18 vs. 21	17
Steam rate (H vs. 2.0 L)	27 vs. 22	23

the amount of steam used showed a 23% increase in OSI time for the run where twice as much steam was used. The actual values of each of these variables could not be given because they are proprietary, but from the OSI values one can see that the manner in which a deodorizer is operated has a significant impact upon the oil's stability.

Sequestrants

A sequestrant is defined as an organic or inorganic compound capable of forming coordination complexes with metals (Furia, 1978). In food processing, sequestrants are employed as additives to limit the participation of metals in numerous deleterious reactions in food systems. Several sequestrants used in foods are listed in Table 11.6. The stability constant is a value that shows the efficiency of a sequestrant for complexing specific metals. In Table 11.6, only values for the ferric ion are shown. A complete listing of other sequestrants and metal stability constants can be found in the *Handbook of Food Additives* (Furia, 1975) or in *The Sequestration of Metals* (Smith, 1959).

For fats and oils, many of these compounds have poor solubility, which hinders their use in a nonaqueous system. Although EDTA and its salts are used in many aqueous systems such as salad dressings, the ones commonly used in fats and oils are citric acid and phosphoric acid. Even these are not very soluble, and their use level is around 30 ppm for citric and 10 ppm for phosphoric. Although they are not classified as antioxidants, they do improve oxidative stability by complexing trace amounts of iron and copper, preventing their pro-oxidant properties.

Light and Inert Gas

The detrimental affect that light has upon the stability of an edible oil has been known for many years. Coe (1938) showed that light-induced deterio-

TABLE 11.6   Some Sequestrants Commonly Used in
Foods

Compounds	Fe^{3+} stability constant
EDTA	25.7
Citric acid	11.8
Phosphoric acid	—
Gluconate	—
Phosphate salts (TSP) (SAPP)	22.2
Phospholipids	—
Lactic acid	6.4
Phytate	—
Poly phosphate (Na TPP)	—

ration is an oxidative phenomenon, and Min has shown its effectiveness at increasing the rate of singlet oxygen oxidation (Min et al., 1989). The detrimental effects are acute at wavelengths below 597 nm, which is within the spectral range of artificial light of 450–600 nm. Normally, this is not a concern in oil processing since handling, processing, and storage are all carried out within a closed system. However, when the finished product is marketed as a salad oil or the fat in a potato chip, light must be considered in obtaining maximum shelf life.

Likewise, inert gases such as nitrogen are used to displace the oxygen to remove it from the system, thus eliminating a necessary ingredient in oxidation. Once an oil is deodorized and cooled, it is common to keep the storage tanks under a positive nitrogen cover to reduce oxidation. Normally, oxygen must be reduced to less than 2%, and for effective oxygen displacement by an inert gas, the gaseous environment should be less than 0.1% O_2.

REFERENCES

Canessa, C. E., Patterson, R. E., Berg, K., and Seybold, J. C. 1993. The 84th AOCS Annual Meeting and Exposition, April 25–29, Abs. II: 1.

Chu, Y. H. and Lin, J. Y. 1993. *J. Am. Oil Chem. Soc.* 70: 1263–1267.

Coe, M. 1938. *Oil Soap* 15: 230–236.

Cowan, J. C. 1966. *J. Am. Oil Chem. Soc.* 43: 300A.

Furia, T. E. 1975. In *Handbook of Food Additives*, 2nd ed. Chemical Rubber Co., Cleveland.

Furia, T. E. 1978. Sequestrants. In *Encyclopedia of Food Science*, M. S. Peterson and A. H. Johnson (Ed.), p. 694. Avi, Westport, CT.

Jones, D. B. and Gersdorff, E. F. 1938. Changes that occur in the protein of soybeans as a result of storage, *J. Am. Chem. Soc.* 60: 723–724.

Klagge, P. and Sen Gupta, A. K. 1990. *Fat Sci. Technol.* 92: 315.

Mag, T. K. 1989. Bleaching—Theory and practice. In *Edible Fats and Oils Processing: Basic Principles and Modern Practices*, D. Erickson (Ed.), p. 108. The American Oil Chemists' Society, Champaign, IL.

Mariani, C., Bondioli, P., Venturini, S., and Fedeli, E. 1991. *La Rivista Ital. Delle Sostanze Grasse* 68: 455–459.

Min, D. B., Lee, E. C., and Lee, S. H. 1989. Singlet oxidation of vegetable oils. In *Flavor Chemistry of Lipid Foods*, D. B. Min and T. H. Smouse (Ed.), p. 57. American Oil Chemists Society, Champaign, IL.

Patterson, H. B. W. 1992. *Bleaching and Purifying Fats and Oils: Theory and Practice*, The American Oil Chemists' Society, Champaign, IL.

Scavone, T. A. and Braun, J. L. 1988. High temperature vacuum steam distillation process to purify and increase the fry life of edible oils. U.S. Patent 4,789,554.

Smith, R. L. 1959. *The Sequestration of Metals: Theoretical Considerations and Practical Applications.* Macmillan Co., New York.

Smouse, T. H. 1995. Factors affecting oil quality and stability. In *Methods to Assess Quality and Stability of Oils and Fat-Containing Foods*, p. 25. AOCS Press, American Oil Chemists' Society, Champaign, IL.

Toeneboehn, G. J. 1992. Environmental contributions of silica refining. Presented at the Fourth Latin American Meeting on Fats and Oils, Nov. 22–26, Rosario, Argentina.

Warner, K. and Eskin, M. N. A. 1995. *Methods to Assess Quality and Stability of Oils and Fat-Containing Foods.* AOCS Press, American Oil Chemists' Society, Champaign, IL.

Welsh, W. A., Bogdanor, J. M., and Toeneboehn, G. J. 1989. Silica Refining of oils and fats. In *Edible Fats and Oils Processing: Basic Principles and Modern Practices*, D. Erickson (Ed.). The American Oil Chemists' Society, Champaign, IL.

Wolff, R. L. 1993. *J. Am. Oil Chem. Soc.* 70: 425–430.

12

Contributions of Lipids to Desirable and Undesirable Flavors in Foods

Jane Love

Iowa State University
Ames, Iowa

INTRODUCTION: DEFINITION OF FLAVOR AND FACTORS AFFECTING FLAVOR PERCEPTION

Flavor is a complex psychological phenomenon that occurs when a human eats a food. Food scientists usually define flavor as the unified sensation resulting from the stimulation of taste and odor receptors. Some definitions of flavor include in addition to taste and odor other impressions perceived via the chemical senses from a product in the mouth. For example, Meilgaard et al. (1991) defined flavor to include the olfactory perceptions caused by volatiles, tastes caused by soluble substances, and chemical feeling factors that stimulate nerve endings in the membranes of the mouth and nose. Others have included as part of flavor factors such as temperature (Beauchamp and Brand, 1994), pressure and mild pain (Amerine et al., 1965), and texture and color (Van Toller, 1994). Although all of the sensations that arise when a food is eaten affect flavor, taste and odor are usually of major importance in flavor. While taste, the perception of water-soluble components sensed by the taste receptors in the oral cavity, can be a very important component of flavor in certain foods, it often is difficult to recognize specific foods based only on taste and without the additional information provided by the odor. The volatile components of foods are to a large extent responsible for the characteristic flavors of many foods. The olfactory receptors are sensitive to very low concentrations of many volatiles, and it is generally accepted that humans have the ability to discriminate among a great many more odors than tastes.

The olfactory receptors in humans are located in a recessed area of the nasal cavity remote from the main stream of inspired air. During normal breathing, only a small proportion of the inhaled volatiles reach the olfactory epithelium. When foods are chewed and swallowed, volatile compounds released from the food are transported into the exhaled air, where they are carried to the olfactory epithelium. Overbosch et al. (1991) have reviewed studies related to the release of flavor in the mouth. The volatile components in foods may be modified as the food is eaten. Water-soluble compounds may be adsorbed and held by moist tissues, while other compounds may be adsorbed and desorbed at different rates and perhaps modified by the moist tissues of the upper airways. Therefore, the time sequence and magnitude of the volatiles reaching the olfactory receptors depend on a number of variables related to the composition and breakdown of the food.

Understanding and manipulating the flavor of foods requires knowledge of both the components of food and the sensory response to these components. Heymann et al. (1993) have described the measurement of flavor by sensory descriptive techniques. Sensory analysis, combined with the knowledge of the volatile components of foods, can help elucidate which of the typically very numerous volatile components of foods are important in flavor. Much progress has been made in identifying the volatiles present in a number of foods. The role of lipid oxidation in the generation of the flavor volatiles in a number of foods is widely recognized. Although lipids in foods contribute to flavors in many ways other than serving as a source of or precursor for volatiles, the role of volatiles derived from oxidized lipids in food flavors will be emphasized in this presentation. Forss (1969) has discussed the taste contributions of lipids, as well as the way that rheological characteristics due to lipids affect the perception of flavors. The difficulties in formulating low-fat foods with flavor that is as desirable as their higher-fat counterparts has been summarized by Bennett (1992). Overbosch et al. (1991) have discussed the binding of volatiles to food ingredients and other effects of ingredients on flavor release.

The topic of this chapter is quite broad. An in-depth review of all of the areas related to the topic is not possible within the space limitations. However, a number of review articles relevant to the topic have recently been published and are cited throughout the text. Readers are encouraged to consult these reviews for additional information. The goal of this chapter is to provide an overview of the topic, as well as to present some of the most recent advances in the understanding of the flavor contributions of volatiles derived from oxidized lipids in a few specific types of foods. It is hoped that the reader will gain an appreciation of the extensive role of lipid oxidation products in food flavor and of the challenges that remain is studying this topic.

FLAVOR VOLATILES FROM OXIDIZED LIPIDS

Lipid Oxidation

Lipid oxidation is probably the chemical reaction that most commonly imparts off-flavors to stored foods. Nearly all foods contain some lipid, and in many foods this lipid is, under some conditions, susceptible to oxidation. The volatile products of oxidized unsaturated fatty acids are known to cause off-flavors in a variety of foods, including but not limited to milk and dairy products, meats and fish, and products derived from soybeans. Low levels of lipid oxidation volatiles, however, also contribute to the characteristic desirable flavors in many foods. In some foods, lipids other than those containing fatty acid residues, for example, the carotenoid pigments (Gloria et al., 1993), also can undergo oxidation and degrade to yield products having characteristic flavors.

The volatile compounds from oxidized fatty acids that impart flavors to fats and oils and fat-containing foods are, for the most part, carbonyl compounds. These carbonyl compounds arise from the breakdown of lipid hydroperoxides. The lipid hydroperoxides are odorless. They are, however, very unstable, and they break down to yield a variety of products. As shown in the simplified scheme in Figure 12.1, once the alkoxy radical is produced, the fatty acid chain adjacent to this radical can be cleaved. If the alkyl group is saturated and the chain cleaves at A, a saturated aldehyde is formed. Cleavage at B yields an alkyl radical that can result in an alkane. Reaction of the alkyl radical with oxygen yields a hydroperoxide, which can undergo further breakdown. The specific compounds that are formed will, of course, depend on the structure of the fatty acid precursor and the position of the hydroperoxide within the molecule, as well as the type of scission (position A or B) and the subsequent reactions undergone by the radical species. The domination of a particular reaction pathway will be affected by such factors as the temperature, the oxygen pressure, and the presence in the food of catalysts and antioxidants. Prediction of the volatiles that will be formed is further complicated because unsaturated products resulting from the deg-

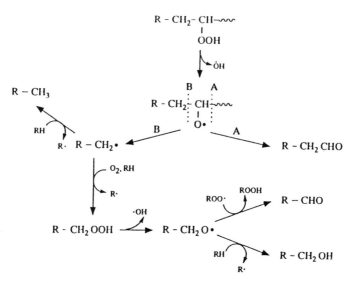

FIG. 12.1 Scheme showing the breakdown of lipid hydroperoxides to yield volatile compounds. (*From Mottram, 1994, with permission of Chapman & Hall.*)

radation of lipid hydroperoxides also can undergo further reactions. In general, the pathways for formation of volatiles from hydroperoxides are not as well elucidated as are the mechanisms for hydroperoxide formation (Allen, 1983). Additional information on the formation of volatile decomposition products can be found in recent reviews by Frankel (1985, 1991) and Kochhar (1993).

The schemes for the oxidative breakdown of unsaturated fatty acids show that a number of volatile products can result from a single fatty acid. For example, Kochhar (1993) indicated that based on the generally accepted reaction schemes, the aldehydes from oleate could include octanal, nonanal, decanal, 2-decenal, and 2-undenenal. Aldehydes from linoleate could include 3-nonenal, 2,4-decadienal, and hexanal. Linolenate could produce propanal, 3-hexenal, 2,4-heptadienal, 3,6-nonadienal, and 2,4,7-decatrienal. Arachidonate could produce hexanal, 3-nonenal, 2,4-decadienal, 3,6-dodecadienal, and 2,4,7-tridecatrienal. A number of lipid oxidation volatiles have been reported in the literature that are not accounted for by the mechanisms shown in Figure 12.1. Schemes to account for the production of many of these compounds have been elaborated. Frankel (1985) and Kochhar (1993) discuss many of these mechanisms.

In plants, an array of enzymes metabolize the hydroperoxide products produced by lipoxygenase activity to produce volatiles that are important in flavor. The occurrence, substrate specificity, and products of the plant lipoxygenases and hydroperoxide lyases have been reviewed by Gardner (1985, 1991). Hydroperoxide lyases catalyze the formation of aldehydes from fatty acid hydroperoxides by cleaving the fatty acid chain between the hydroperoxide group and the α-olefinic carbon, yielding an aldehyde and an ω-oxoacid. The lyases from the various plant sources have differing substrate specificities. The 13-hydroperoxides of linoleic and linolenic acids cleave to hexanal and (Z)-3-hexenal, respectively. The 9-hydroperoxides of linoleic acid and linolenic acid yield (Z)-3-nonenal and (Z,Z)-3,6-nonadienal, respectively. The other product from the 13-hydroperoxides is (Z)-12-oxo-9-dodecenoic acid, and from the 9-hydroperoxides, 9-oxononanoic acid. The products of hydroperoxide lyase activity can be further transformed by enzymatic (enal isomerase or alcohol dehydrogenase) or nonenzymatic reactions. Gardner (1985) has summarized the impact of isomerization of double bonds in compounds resulting from lipid oxidation in a number of plant products on the flavor of these foods. Fischer and Grosch (1991) noted that aroma effects in products such as apple and tomato juice are related to the loss of the (E)-2-hexenal and the production of breakdown products. They studied the breakdown of this compound in aqueous ethanol and triacetin at 38°C. In the aqueous ethanol, 3-ethoxy hexanal and 3-hydroxyhexanal were formed; these compounds smell fruity. In this system, (Z)-3-hexenal was a minor component but had a flavor dilution factor of about 30. In the triacetin system, butanoic acid had the highest flavor dilution factor: this compound smells musty.

Gardner (1985) summarized the results of several studies that indicated that the predominant volatiles from soy, pea, and peanut were hexanal, followed by 2-heptenal, 2,4-decadienal, 2-octenal, and pentanal. A number of other volatiles were also identified. In general, similar volatiles have been identified in a number of other oxidized foods (Kochhar, 1993), yet the flavors are different. The significance of the volatiles in a food to the flavor often is very difficult to evaluate. Part of the problem inherent in flavor chemistry is that different methods of analyzing volatiles give different results. Snyder et al. (1988) compared three frequently used gas chromatographic methods (direct injection, dynamic headspace, and static headspace) for determining volatiles in vegetable oil. The volatile profiles for oxidized soy oil produced by the different methods were not the same. To further evaluate the significance of the volatiles, weighted percentages for each volatile were calculated on the basis of 1-octen-3-ol, which had the lowest threshold value of the identified volatiles (Table 12.1). The relative orders of the volatiles were compared for the three methods. By using the direct injection or dynamic headspace methods, the isomers of 2,4-decadienal were first and second in the relative order, while n-propanal was first when the static headspace technique was used. The order of impor-

TABLE 12.1 Flavor Significance of Volatiles in Soybean Oil

Major volatiles	TH values	Rel %			Weighted %[a]			Relative order		
		DI	DHS	SHS	DI	DHS	SHS	DI	DHS	SHS
t,t-2,4-Decadienal	0.10	46.9	40.5	0.3	4.7	4.1	0.03	2	2	7
t,c-2,4-Decadienal	0.02	23.8	21.5	1.0	11.9	10.8	0.5	1	1	3
t,t-2,4-Heptadienal	0.04	6.5	13.3	2.0	1.6	3.3	0.5	3	3	3
t-2-Heptenal	0.20	3.1	6.7	8.3	0.16	0.33	0.4	7	7	5
t,c-2,4-Heptadienal	0.10	3.1	5.4	2.5	0.31	0.54	0.25	6	6	6
n-Hexanal	0.08	6.9	5.4	24.7	0.86	0.68	3.1	5	5	2
n-Pentane	340	4.8	3.7	38.6	0.14[b]	0.11[b]	1.1[b]	11	10	10
t-2-Pentenal	1.00	1.9	1.4	1.2	0.02	0.01	0.01	9	8	8
1-Octen-3-ol	0.01	1.4	1.1	0.3	1.4	1.1	0.3	4	4	4
2-Pentylfuran	2.00	1.2	1.0	0.5	6.0[b]	6.0[b]	2.5[b]	10	9	9
n-Propanal	0.06	0.5	—	20.6	0.08	—	3.4	8	—	1

TH = threshold values (Forss, 1972); DI = direct injection; DHS = dynamic headspace; SHS = static headspace; t,t- = trans,trans-; t,c = trans,cis-.

[a]Calculated on the basis of 1-octen-3-ol, which has the lowest threshold value.

[b]$\times 10^{-3}$.

Source: Frankel, 1991.

tance also varied for other compounds depending on the technique used. Reineccius (1993) recently discussed the biases in analytical flavor profiles introduced by the isolation method.

Considerable general knowledge of the likely contribution of volatiles to flavors in foods has been gained based on knowledge of the flavor potency of the compounds, the concentrations of the components in the food, and the flavor quality associated with the components. The different types of volatiles produced from oxidized lipids have different odor threshold values. Wide ranges of thresholds have been reported for a single compound or classes of compounds, but some generalizations can be made about comparative threshold values for lipid oxidation products. The hydrocarbons have relatively high threshold values (Table 12.2), and, of the typical lipid oxidation volatiles, they as a group are generally presumed to have minor impact on flavor. The substituted furans, vinyl alcohols, and 1-alkenes also have relatively high thresholds. Ranges for threshold values for these compounds also are shown in Table 12.2. Compounds such as the 2-alkenals, alkanals, 2,4-dienals, and vinyl ketones generally have lower thresholds (Table 12.2) and could reasonably be expected to be important contributors to flavors. Thresholds for a number of the compounds that have been associated with characteristic flavors from oxidized fats in various foods are shown in Table 12.3.

Aldehydes

Aldehydes are often considered to be of major importance in contributing characteristic off-flavors from oxidized fats to foods. Low levels of the same aldehydes that have been implicated in off-flavors may impart desirable flavor characteristics. The formation of hexanal and 2,4-decadienal (two of the major lipid oxidation aldehydes) can be explained by the thermal decomposition of linoleate 9- and 13-hydroperoxides. Frankel (1985) and Kochhar (1993) have reviewed schemes proposed to account for a number of the aldehydes that have been associated with lipid oxidation off-flavors in foods.

Some of the unsaturated aldehydes have quite low threshold values and are potent flavorants. The off-flavor aldehyde compounds that result from the deterioration of linolenate or other n-3 fatty acids have particularly low thresholds. These compounds include (Z)-3-hexanal (0.09–0.11 mg/kg), (Z)-4-heptenal (0.0005–0.0016 mg/kg), (E,Z)-2,4-heptadienal (0.04–0.06 mg/kg), (E,Z)-2,6-nonadienal (0.002 mg/kg), and (E,Z,Z)-2,4,7–decatrienal (0.024 mg/kg) (Kochhar, 1993).

According to Kochhar (1993), the lower saturated aldehydes generally

TABLE 12.2 Threshold Values of Different
Types of Volatile Compounds

Hydrocarbons	90–2150 ppm
Substituted furans	2–27
Vinyl alcohols	0.5–3
1-Alkenes	0.02–9
2-Alkenals	0.04–2.5
Alkanals	0.04–1.0
trans,trans-2,4-Alkadienals	0.04–0.3
Isolated alkadienals	0.002–0.3
Isolated cis-alkenals	0.0003–0.1
trans,cis-2,4-Alkadienals	0.002–0.006
Vinyl ketones	0.00002–0.007

Source: Frankel, 1985.

TABLE 12.3 Characteristic Odors and Threshold Values for Some Lipid
Oxidation Products

Compound	Odor character	Threshold in oil (ppb)
Hexanal	Green	80
Heptanal	Oily, putty	55
Octanal	Fatty	40
Nonanal	Tallowy	200
trans-2-Hexenal	Green	600
trans-2-Heptenal	Putty, fatty	500
trans-2-Octenal	Fatty	150
trans-2-Nonenal	Tallowy, cucumbers	40
cis-2-Heptenal	Creamy, putty	0.5
trans-2,trans-4-Hexadienal	Fatty, green	40
trans-2,trans-4-Heptadienal	Fatty, oily	100
trans-2,trans-4-Decadienal	Deep-fried	20
trans-2,cis-6-Nonadienal	Fresh cucumbers	1.5
1-Penten-3-ol	Sharp, irritating	4200
1-Octen-3-ol	Mushroom	7.5
1-Penten-3-one	Fishy, oily	3
1-Octen-3-one	Metallic	0.1
3.5-Octadien-2-one	Fruity, fatty	300

Source: Mottram, 1987.

give rise to sharp and irritating off-flavors, those in the intermediate range (C6–C9) have fatty, tallowy, bitter, soapy-fruity, and green flavors, and the higher members of the series have citrus peel flavors. The 2,4-decadienals are said to have odors characteristic of deep-fat fried foods. The flavors of the (Z)-2-alkenals with 5 to 7 carbons were described by Kochhar as being green, painty, or puttylike, while the C8 and C9 members of this series are said to have nutty and tallowy/cucumber flavors, respectively. The odor quality of a compound may depend on concentration. There does not seem to be a general, easily explained relationship between the molecular structure of aldehydes and their flavor intensity.

Ketones

Aliphatic ketones formed by autoxidation of unsaturated fatty acids also contribute to undesirable flavors in oxidized fats and foods. For example, 1-octen-3-one has long been known to be related to the metallic off-flavor in oxidized dairy products (Stark and Forss, 1962). The odor thresholds of the vinyl ketones are similar to those of the most potent aldehydes. The methyl ketones, however, have thresholds higher than those of their isomeric aldehydes. Kochhar (1993) reported several mechanisms for the formation of the methyl ketones observed in the volatiles from foods and discussed their flavor impact.

Alcohols

The alcohols produced in lipid oxidation generally have higher thresholds than the aldehydes and as a group are presumed to be of less importance in off-flavors. Many of the saturated and unsaturated alcohols have desirable flavor characteristics, and some are commercially important in flavor compounds. Hamilton (1983) described the flavor of the C3 saturated alcohol as solventy and nondescript, while the C6 alcohol was said to be grassy and green. The C9 alcohol was said to have a fatty and green flavor. The C8–C12 2-alken-1-ols have fatty odors (Forss, 1972). 1-Octen-3-ol has a low odor threshold, and its role in flavors has been summarized by Kochhar (1993).

Other Volatiles

Other volatiles, including furans, fatty acids, and hydrocarbons, are found in oxidized fats and foods and make contributions to flavor. General aspects of the formation and significance of these compounds are covered in several reviews (Grosch, 1982; Hamilton, 1983; Kochhar, 1993).

MEASURING THE FLAVOR IMPACT OF VOLATILE COMPONENTS IN FOODS

Advances in analytical methodologies and instrumentation have made it possible to isolate, identify, and quantitate large numbers of compounds in foods. More difficult, however, is the task of determining how these different chemical compounds influence the flavor of a food. In some foods, a chemical or small number of chemicals give the characteristic odor; more generally the odor results from a large number of chemicals. Several approaches to establishing the flavor significance of volatiles have been utilized.

Odor Units

One technique that has been used to determine the relative importance of volatile components is that of calculating "odor units" for particular compounds. With this method, the concentration of a component in food is determined and compared to the odor threshold value for that component. If a component is present in a food at a concentration that greatly exceeds its threshold concentration, this component is considered to contribute to the flavor of the food. However, if a component is present at a concentration below its threshold, it is not considered to contribute to the flavor (Buttery, 1993).

Gas Chromatography-Olfactometry

The technique most commonly used to determine the effect that individual chemical compounds have on aroma is to have human subjects smell the compounds eluting from a gas chromatograph column. In this technique, which is termed gas chromatography-olfactometry, a flavor sample is injected into a gas chromatograph and the effluent from the column split with part continuing to a chromatographic detector and part being routed to a "sniffing port" (Acree et al., 1984; Acree, 1993a,b). Alternatively, traditional chromatographic runs and separate runs using a human subject to detect eluted odors could be conducted. The elution time and description of any odors noted by the subject are recorded and later correlated to the peaks on the chromatogram to produce an "aromagram." This technique has become very popular among flavor analysts and can be used with serially diluted aroma isolates to determine the relative aroma potency of the constituents. Two specific approaches to dilution analysis have been described—aroma extract dilution analysis and CharmAnalysis™.

Aroma Extract Dilution Analysis.   One specific adaptation of gas chromatography-olfactometry is called aroma extract dilution analysis (AEDA). In
the AEDA method (Grosch, 1993), serial dilutions are prepared from a
flavor sample. These dilutions are then injected into a gas chromatograph
(GC) and the effluent passed both through a detector and to a human
subject. The highest dilution at which the subject can still detect a component is called the flavor dilution (FD) value for that component. These
dilution values can then be plotted against elution time or retention index
to create an aroma chromatogram.

CharmAnalysis™.   The CharmAnalysis™ (Acree, 1984, 1993a,b) is similar
to the AEDA method in that several dilutions of the extract are analyzed
using human subjects. The subjects record the times for when they first
detect an odor and when they can no longer detect it. The information
obtained during the GC runs with the different dilutions is then compiled
to form a Charm chromatogram with flavor dilution value plotted versus
retention index. Further details of the procedure are described by Acree
(1993a, b).

Limitations of Current Methods

While odor units and methods based on gas chromatography-olfactometry
can provide useful information about the relative contribution of odor
components, there are some limitations to these approaches. The most
fundamental limitation is probably that these methods do not account for
the way that the perceived intensity of a compound changes with concentration. The premise that the compounds with the lowest thresholds are the
most important for flavor may not always be true. Another limitation in
analyzing odor components individually is that there is no consideration of
the effects due to the interaction of odor components with each other or
with other components in the food. While there are instances in which a
single odor component or a few components impart a characteristic flavor
to a food, in most foods the characteristic flavor is due to a mixture of many
volatiles. The perception of these mixtures of flavor compounds is very
complicated. Studies in which the components presumed to be important
to the overall flavor are combined and compared to the flavor of interest are
useful in verifying the results of the flavor potency assays.

It would seem, at least to the author, that considerable training is needed
to enable subjects to be able to describe the aromas of compounds as they
elute from a capillary GC column. Compounds elute rapidly, especially at
the beginning of the run, and judgments must be made quickly. Translation
of sensory impressions into specific descriptors often is difficult unless the

subject has considerable experience. It also is important to conduct all sensory evaluations in a way that minimizes the possibility of subject bias. Careful attention to the details of experimental design (sample order, replication, etc.) would seem to be as necessary for aroma dilution assays as for other types of sensory testing. Christensen and Reineccius (1995) reported that in order to minimize bias in AEDA runs, cheese extracts were analyzed starting with the most dilute and working toward the less diluted samples. These authors also only reported odors that could be detected in two separate trials, and extracts were evaluated by two subjects. Figure 12.2 shows the flavor dilution values for components of aged cheddar cheese evaluated independently by the two subjects. The two subjects used in this study seemed to differ considerably in their sensitivity to certain compounds. The subjective nature of spontaneous odor descriptors is also apparent from the descriptions provided by the two subjects utilized in this study (Table 12.4), both of whom were experienced. The difficulty in

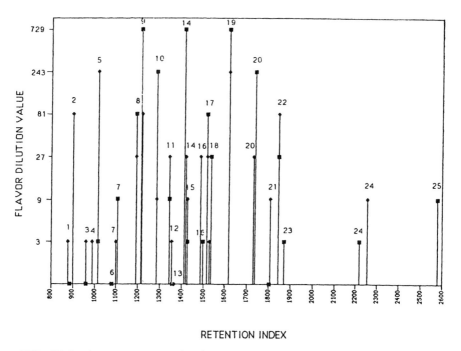

RETENTION INDEX

FIG. 12.2   Aromagram results for two subjects. The height of the lines corresponds to highest flavor dilution values reached by subject 1 (■) and subject 2 (♦). In peaks 6 and 13, results for the two judges were identical, so only results of subject 1 are visible. (*From Christensen and Reineccius, 1995.*)

TABLE 12.4 Descriptors Given by Two Subjects to Peaks That Could be Reliably Sniffed in GC Effluent

No.	Judge 1	Judge 2
1	Juicy Fruit gum	Apples
2	Tootsie Rolls	
3	Butter	Butter, mild cheddar
4	Pine, green	
5	Sweet, fruity	Apple blossom
6	Plastic	Glue
7	Cooked milk	Oxidized, glue
8	Sulfur	Potato, cardboard
9	Fruit, melon	Sour fruit
10	Mushroom, smoky	Mushroom, metallic
11	Burnt sugar or garlic	Garlic, "sickly sweet"
12	Oxidized, glue	
13	Green, floral	Geraniums
14	Peppers, green	Green, fruity, floral
15	Cooked milk, acrid	Sulfur, oil, onions
16	Green	Pungent, green, cereal
17	Gas, burnt, sulfur	Sulfur, cloves, solvent
18	Green, wood, vegetable	Green, cardboard, glue
19	Nacho cheese	Cheese, toasted cheese
20	Rain, wood, vegetable	Spicy, nutty, grain
21	Acrid	Toasted, cardboard
22	Bad breath, popcorn	Goaty, free fatty acid
23	Peppers, green and red	
24	Warm, stale butter	Sour fruit
25	Soapy	

Source: Christensen and Reineccius, 1995.

describing odors out of context was suggested as a possible explanation for the unexpected descriptors provided for some of the peaks.

Other approaches to understanding how mixtures of volatiles cause flavor involve the determination of mathematical relationships between the variables in data sets collected on food samples with different flavors. Several methods have been proposed to correlate data from the chemical analysis of food volatiles with descriptive data obtained using sensory analysis (Chien and Peppard, 1993; Bett and Grimm, 1994). Factor analysis, cluster analysis, regression and correlation, and neural networks are among the approaches suggested for exploring relationships between chemical or physical and sensory data. The continued development and application of multiple approaches is probably most likely to advance the knowledge of the volatile components most important in food flavors. Piggott (1990) suggested that the major barrier to progress in relating chemical and sensory data was the lack of sufficient understanding of the chemical senses. He further suggested that substantial progress in relating chemical and sensory data is unlikely until this understanding is gained.

LIPID-DERIVED FLAVORS IN SPECIFIC FOODS

Dairy Products

The contributions of milk fats to the characteristic flavors in milk and dairy products are well established. Badings (1991) has reviewed this topic. Several types of compounds derived from milk lipids are known to contribute to the flavor of dairy products.

Fatty Acids

Lipolyzed flavor is a common and important off-flavor in milk and dairy products. The lipase that liberates fatty acids may be native to milk or produced by psychrotropic microorganisms. In some dairy products, free fatty acids at a certain level may provide desirable "background" flavor notes. Excessive levels of free fatty acids in milk, however, give an undesirable flavor that is generally termed hydrolytic, rancid, or lipolyzed. Allen (1983) described lipolyzed milk as having a soapy taste and a sharp aroma, while lipolyzed butter and similar products are said to have more distinctive off-flavors. Duncan et al. (1991) examined the relationship between free fatty acids and the sensory perception of rancidity in milk. The relationship between concentration of fatty acids and rancid flavor was difficult to explain. They suggested that as the concentration of long-chain fatty acids increased, a greater concentration of short-chain fatty acids may have been needed to impart rancid flavor. Woo and Lindsay (1983) and Lin and Jeon (1987) are among the researchers who have examined the relationship of free fatty acids to rancidity in butter and cheese, respectively. The contributions of fatty acids to flavors of dairy products do not seem to be particularly simple or straightforward.

Hamilton (1983) noted that the aliphatic acids have flavors that are "sour," "fruity," "cheesy," or "animal-like." According to Hamilton, the C2 acids are "vinegary;" the C3 "sour" or "Swiss-cheesy;" the C4 "sweaty-cheesy;" the C8 "goat-cheesy;" while the C9 acids are "paraffinic." The C14 to C18 fatty acids have very little odor. The C4 and C6 acids are said to impart "rancid" flavors, while the C10 and C12 acids give "unclean" and "soapy" flavors.

Certain low molecular weight branched-chain fatty acids may contribute to the flavor of some cheeses. Vangtal and Hammond (1986) noted that some *iso-* and aromatic acids seemed to be related to flavor notes in Swiss cheese. Brennand et al. (1989) noted that fatty acids with branches at the 4-position had "goaty/muttony/sheepy" aroma notes. In particular, 4-ethyl-octanoic acid was found to have a low threshold of 6 ppb and a potent "goatlike" odor. "Cheeselike" aromas were noted in a number of dilute solutions of fatty acids, especially shorter, branched-chain acids. For example, at 5 ppm, 2-methylpentanoic acid exhibited a "Swiss cheese–like" aroma.

Compounds Formed from Fatty Acids

Grosch (1982), Hamilton (1983), and Bakker and Law (1994) have summarized the research related to the production of methyl ketones and lactones from fatty acids. The research papers cited by these authors suggest the following mechanisms for the production of methyl ketones or lactones: heating can promote the decarboxylation of oxo-acids, minor constituents of milk fats, yielding methyl ketones. Alkanoic acids released from milk fat can undergo β-oxidation to β-ketoacids, followed by decarboxylation to methyl ketones (the latter reaction is important in producing characteristic flavors in cheese matured with actively growing molds). Milk fat contains small quantities of δ-hydroxyacids, which, if released by lipases, under certain conditions lactonize to form the corresponding δ-lactones. Unsaturated C18 fatty acids can, via hydration, produce hydroxy acids, which, via β-oxidation can lead to γ-lactones. Another possible mechanism reported to exist in yeasts and molds involves the reduction of δ-keto acids, followed by ring closure.

Aldehydes, Ketones, and Other Oxidation Products

Jeon (1993) has summarized the results of studies in which volatiles in oxidized dairy products have been isolated and their flavor properties identified. Most of these compounds are *n*-alkanals, *n*-alk-2-enals, *n*-alk-2,4-enals, and alk-2-ones.

Even a slight degree of lipid oxidation in milk and other dairy products results in off-flavors that have been associated with the formation of several carbonyl compounds. Terms used to describe these flavors include "cardboard," "metallic," "oily," "stale," "tallowy," "painty," and "fishy." The off-flavor varies in character and intensity among different dairy products and at different stages of oxidation. For example, in fluid milk, the terms "cardboard" and "papery" are often used to describe the off-flavor at early stages of metal-induced lipid oxidation. In ice cream, the term "flat" is often used to describe the early stages of oxidation. At moderate stages of oxidation, the flavor may be described as "metallic" as well as "cardboardy" or "papery." At intense stages of oxidation, the descriptors "painty," "fishy," "oily," or "tallowy" are often applied (Jeon, 1993).

Fish and Seafood

Fish flavor has been reviewed by Lindsay (1990) and Josephson (1991). Many studies have been conducted to elucidate the role played by lipid-derived volatile compounds in the flavor of seafoods. Certain of the characteristic desirable aromas and flavors of freshly harvested fish seem to be due to a number of 6-, 8-, and 9-carbon aldehydes, ketones, and alcohols derived from long-chain polyunsaturated fatty acids. These compounds result from the specific activity of lipoxygenases (Josephson, 1991). Information in the reviews cited above indicates that differences in the lipoxygenases in fresh and salt water species result in distinct volatile profiles and thus different flavors. Eight-carbon volatile alcohols and ketones have been found to occur in most seafoods, where they contribute distinct "fresh" or "plantlike" or "metallic" aromas, even though individually they may exhibit somewhat different odors. Although the 8-carbon alcohols are present in higher concentrations, the low threshold value for the vinyl ketones accounts for their greater flavor impact. Six-carbon volatile compounds (aldehydes and alcohols) have been identified in some species of seafood. Compounds with 9 carbon atoms are found mainly in freshwater fish and contribute to the "melonlike" flavor impression. Hexanal and unsaturated alcohols with 8 carbon atoms contribute "green" and "heavy" character to the flavor of fresh and salt water fish.

Kobayashi et al. (1989) reported that 5Z,8Z,11Z-, and 5E-, 8Z-, and 11Z-tetradecatrien-2-one had an aroma similar to cooked shrimp and crab and suggested that these components were probably derived from lipid. Kuo and Pan (1991) found that adding soybean lipoxygense increased these ketone components in the volatiles from shrimp.

The role of autoxidation in producing undesirable flavors in fish has long been recognized. Lindsay (1990) has reviewed the major volatiles derived from the autoxidation of polyunsaturated fatty acids in seafoods. In fish oil, green aromas are due to (E)-2-hexenal, (Z)-3-hexen-1-ol, and (E,Z)2,6-nonadienal. At greater degrees of oxidation, stronger fishy aromas are due to (E,Z,Z)-2,4,7-decatrienal and (E,E,Z)-2,4,7-decatrienal from C20:5 ω3 and C22:6 ω6. Lindsay reviews the evidence, suggesting that (Z)-4-heptenal from the water-mediated retro-aldol degradation of (E,Z)-2,6-nonadienal has a low odor threshold (0.04 ppb) and potentiates the fishy flavors.

The development of characteristic flavors as a result of cooking fish has not been studied extensively, although it has been suggested that the oxidation of polyunsaturated lipids is involved in producing some of these flavors. Josephson et al. (1991) found that to obtain the characteristic salmon loaf note, both the carotenoid fraction and a fish oil fraction were required. Typically (E)-2, (Z)-4-, and (E)-2, (E)-4-heptadienals are the most abundant oxidatively derived carbonyl compounds in oxidized fish; next most abundant are (E)-3, (Z)-5- and (E)-3, (E)-5-octadien-2-ol. But when carotenoid-rich salmon oils were oxidized, the 3,5-octadien-2-ones exceeded the 2-4 heptadienals. This phenomenon was not true when the salmon oil was devoid of carotenoid. Although both compounds are derived from the n-7 hydroperoxide of a n-3 polyunsaturated fatty acid, the carotenoids seem to favor the formation of certain types of products.

Meat

The characteristic flavor of meat is, to a large extent, developed during cooking. The desirable attribute termed "meat flavor" cannot be attributed to a single group of compounds. Lipid degradation during cooking is generally considered to be important in generating "fatty" aromas and species-characteristic flavors. According to Bailey (1983), about 90% of the flavor volatiles in cooked meat arise due to lipid reactions. Several hundred volatile compounds derived from lipids occur in cooked meat, including aliphatic hydrocarbons, aldehydes, ketones, alcohols, carboxylic acids, and esters. Because many meat volatiles are present in the ppm or ppb range, only those compounds with low odor thresholds are likely to contribute to meat flavor (Mottram, 1994). Saturated and unsaturated aldehydes with 6–10 carbon atoms are major volatile components of all cooked meat. These compounds have relatively low odor thresholds and are likely contributors to meaty aromas. Reviews of meat flavor include those by Shahidi et al. (1986), Mottram (1991, 1994), and Reineccius (1994).

Desirable and Species-Specific Flavors

When meat lipids are heated, aroma compounds are released and contribute to the species-specific flavors. Bailey and Eining (1989) have reviewed the lipid degradation reactions leading to meat flavor. When meat is heated, lipids contribute volatiles via thermally induced oxidative reactions. Thermally induced oxidation produces somewhat different volatiles products than does low temperature oxidation (Nawar, 1989).

Some of the compounds produced when lipids oxidize may also react with other meat components to produce volatiles. Products of lipid autoxidation are known to be involved in Maillard-type reactions (Mottram and

Salter, 1989). According to Farmer and Mottram (1990), the most likely pathways for these reactions are as follows: the reaction of carbonyl compounds from lipids with the amino groups of cysteine and ammonia produced by Strecker degradation; the reaction of the amino group in phosphatidylethanolamine with sugar-derived carbonyl compounds; the interaction of free radicals from oxidized lipids in the Maillard reaction; and the reaction of hydroxy and carbonyl lipid oxidation products with free hydrogen sulfide.

Thiophenes with long alkyl chains probably are formed when hydrogen sulfide reacts with unsaturated fatty acids or oxidation products derived from unsaturated fatty acids. Long-chain 2-alkylthiophenes were formed when phospholipids were included in a heated cysteine/ribose model system (Farmer et al., 1989). Farmer and Mottram (1990) noted that inclusion of lipid in this type of model system reduced the formation of some of the compounds formed at 140°C. Other components were formed only in the presence of lipid and Maillard reactants. In general, the phospholipid from beef or egg had more effect than did the triglycerides.

Werkhoff et al. (1992) have discussed the flavor properties of dihydro-1,3,4-dithiazines. These compounds are formed during cooking or roasting from the degradation products of lipids and amino acids. Pork contains a higher concentration of these compounds than does beef. Pork (also roasted peanuts) contain dithiazines, which are partially formed from fatty aldehydes (pentanal, hexanal, heptanal, octanal, and nonanal). Ho et al. (1989) also discuss the role of lipid degradation products in pyrazine formation. The trialkylthiazoles with long-chain 2-alkyl substituents could be formed when hydrogen sulfide and ammonia act on mixtures of aliphatic aldehydes.

Volatile free fatty acids are important flavor compounds in some types of meat. Meat from sheep contains certain methyl-branched fatty acids not reported in other types of meat. According to Wong et al. (1975), branched-chain fatty acids having 8–10 carbon atoms contribute to the undesirable flavor of cooked mutton. The compounds 4-methyloctanoic acid and 4-methylnonanoic acid were thought to be especially important causes of this flavor.

Ha and Lindsay (1990) found 4-ethyloctanoic acid in male goat, ram, ewe, and lamb depot fats but not in beef, pork, veal, or horse depot fats. This compound has a "goatlike" aroma (Brennand and Lindsay, 1992a) and a low odor threshold of 0.006 ppm (Brennand et al., 1989). Brennand and Lindsay (1992a,b) reported that certain volatile free fatty acids (4-methyloctanoic, 4-ethyloctanoic, and 4-methylnonaoic) were present in various fractions from mutton during cooking in quantities that would be adequate to provide the species-characteristic flavor.

A steroid, androstenone (5-α-androst-16-en-3-one), found in the fat of uncastrated male pigs is responsible for the flavor defect known as boar taint or boar odor (Patterson, 1968). People who detect the odor that is released when the fat is heated typically describe it as sweaty or urinous. Four other steroids having slightly different structures and possessing similar odors were later isolated from the fat of mature boars (Berry and Sink, 1971; Berry et al., 1971; Thompson et al., 1972).

Guth and Grosch (1993) screened the volatile fraction from stewed beef by AEDA for potent odorants. Thirty compounds had FD values in the range of 1 to 1024. They found that 12-methyltridecanal smelled "tallowy" and "beeflike." The lipid fraction was then isolated from meat from several species, then hydrolyzed. Greater amounts of 12-methyltridecanal were present in beef than in lamb, pork, turkey, or chicken. These researchers suggested that plasmalogens may be the precursors for this compound.

Gasser and Grosch (1990) used AEDA to study the odorants in broths from chicken, cow, and ox. The flavor dilution factor for 2(E), 4(E)-decadienal was much higher in chicken broth than in the other samples. This difference may indicate that lipid oxidation products are important in imparting the unique chicken meat flavor. More unsaturated aldehydes are found in the volatiles of chicken than of other species (Mottram, 1994).

Lipid Oxidation and Warmed-over Flavor

Lipid oxidation is one of the major causes of the deterioration of quality in meat and meat products. The flavor of cooked meat deteriorates very rapidly during refrigerated storage. The off-flavors developed on storage or when meat is reheated have been termed "warmed-over flavor." Some compounds known to be oxidation products of unsaturated fatty acids increase during the storage and reheating of meat. Hexanal, one of the major secondary products formed during the oxidation of linoleic acid, is one of the major volatiles in stored meat. Ajuyah et al. (1993) reported that hexanal was the most abundant volatile in the volatiles from stored chicken meat. Ramarathnam et al. (1993) reported that hexanal was the major constituent of the volatiles of uncured beef (4.63 mg/kg), chicken (7.25 mg/kg), and pork (7.39 mg/kg), while hexanal was present only in trace amounts in cured meats from these three species. Other compounds found only in uncured meat were (E)-2-octenal, decanal, dodecanal, tridecenal, tetradecanal, decane, 1,1-dimethylcyclopentane, nonylcyclopropane, and 5-propyl decane. Other recent studies of volatiles in cured meat include those of Barbieri et al. (1992) and Shahidi et al. (1987). The latter suggested that hexanal is a useful indicator of lipid oxidation in uncured meat. St. Angelo et al. (1987) recommended that hexanal, pentanal, and 2,3-octanedione plus the total volatile content be used as a marker for warmed-over flavor in meat. Brewer et al. (1992) reported that hexanal and 2,4-decadienal increased in ground pork during 13 weeks of frozen storage but decreased at 26 and 39 weeks of storage.

Konapka and Grosch (1991) used AEDA to study the odorants causing warmed-over flavor in boiled beef. They concluded that the principal components responsible for warmed-over flavor were hexanal, 1-octen-3-one, (E)- and (Z)-2-octenal, (Z)-2-nonenal, (EE)-2,4-nonadienal, and trans-4,5-epoxy-(E)-2-decenal. The epoxydecenal had the highest FD value and may be responsible for the metallic note in warmed-over flavor.

Fruits and Vegetables

Flavors in fruits and vegetables are often classified as primary or secondary, with the difference between categories being the way the flavors are formed. Primary flavors are formed by metabolic processes in the living plant, and the flavor is largely retained after harvesting. Secondary flavors are produced by enzymes when the plant tissue is disrupted during cutting, cleaning, and processing. Lipids serve as precursors for some of the primary and secondary flavor components in certain fruits and vegetables. Schreier (1986) reviewed the role of lipid degradation reactions in the biogeneration of plant aromas, and O'Connor and O'Brien (1991) reviewed the significance of lipoxygenase in fruits and vegetables. Although lipid-derived volatiles are involved in aromas in a number of fruits and vegetables, only a few examples will be discussed in this chapter.

Cucumber and Melons.   The flavor of raw cucumber results mainly from C9 unsaturated carbonyls formed by enzymatic action when the tissue is disrupted. A major flavor component is (E,Z)-2,6-nonadienal (Whitfield and Last, 1991). This component, which has a characteristic cucumber aroma, is formed when linolenic acid is acted upon by lipoxygenase, and the reaction products are further modified by hydroperoxide lyase and an enol isomerase.

Other saturated and unsaturated aldehydes also may contribute to cucumber flavor. Schieberle et al. (1990) used aroma extract dilution analysis to study the odorants in cucumber. (E,Z)-2,6-nonadienal followed by (Z)-2-nonenal and (E)-2-nonenal were the most significant odorants. The flavor dilution factor for the (E,Z)-2,6-nonadienal was 64 times larger than that for (Z)-2-nonenal, which was the second highest.

In muskmelons, (Z)-6-nonenal (Kemp et al., 1972) and some volatile esters (Yuabumoto et al., 1977) have been reported to be most responsible for the melonlike and fruity notes, respectively. The use of AEDA (Schieberle et al., 1990) showed that the flavor of muskmelons was more complex than that of cucumber. Methyl 2-methylbutanoate, (Z)-3-hexenal, (E)-2-hexenal, and ethyl 2-methylpropanoate were the primary odorants of the melon flavor. The compounds most important in cucumber were less important in melon. The volatile esters contributed "sweet," "fruity" notes, while the hexenal isomers had "green," "applelike" odors. (Z)-6-nonenal was absent in the aromagram.

Mushrooms.   In mushrooms, 1-octen-3-ol and 1-octen-3-one are generally considered to be important volatiles. According to Fischer and Grosch (1987), 1-octen-3-one is the more important flavor volatile in *Psalliota bispora* mushroom, although 1-octen-3-ol is present in greater quantities. Mau et al. (1992) found that the enzymatic activity and 1-octen-3-ol content of cultivated mushroom, *Agaricus bisporus*, decreased dramatically during 10 days of storage at 12°C.

Tomato.   Although hundreds of volatile have been identified in tomatoes, their relative importance for flavor is not clearly understood. According to Buttery (1993), the most important aroma compound in fresh tomatoes is (Z)-3-hexenal. When fresh ripe tomato is blended, the concentration of this compound increases rapidly, peaks at about 3 minutes, then decreases gradually. Baldwin et al. (1993) reported about 5–10 ppm of (E)-2-hexenal and <5 ppm of (Z)-3-hexenal in Florida cultivars of ripened tomatoes.

Buttery et al. (1987) attempted to evaluate the contributions of the major volatiles to tomato flavor by determining the ratio of their concentrations in fresh tomatoes to the odor threshold values. Sixteen compounds had odor unit values that indicated that they probably contributed to tomato odor. The major volatile compounds in fresh tomatoes were (Z)-3-hexenal, hexanal, 2- and 3-methylbutanols, (E)-2-hexenal, and 1-pentene-3-one. Compounds considered most important to aroma were (Z)-3-hexenal, 3-methylbutenal, β-ionone, 1-penten-3-one, hexanal, (Z)-3-hexenal, (E)-2-hexenal, 2- and 3-methylbutanal, 2-(2-methylpropyl) thiazole, eugenol, and 6-methyl-5-hepten-2-one.

Lipid oxidation is important in generating flavors in a number of other fruit and vegetable products. For example, Maga (1994) has documented the many ways that volatiles from oxidized lipids are presumed to affect the flavor of raw and cooked potatoes and a variety of processed potato products.

Soybeans and Other Legumes.   Off-flavor production (beaniness, bitterness, and astringency) is a particular problem in soybeans and other legumes. Flavor problems occur in soy oil as well as in soy protein products and in certain soy foods, for example, soy milk. The undesirable "green" and "beany" notes are generally believed to be caused by aldehydes such as hexanal, *cis*-3-hexenal and *trans*-2-hexenal. MacLeod and Ames (1988) have published a comprehensive review of soy flavor. They report that bitterness in soybeans and soy products may be due to the action of lipoxygenase. Various nonvolatile oxygenated derivatives of fatty acids have been implicated in causing bitterness in soy foods, especially certain trihydroxy unsaturated acids. Fatty acid dimers formed from hydroperoxides and Schiff bases formed by the reaction of aldehydes with soy phosphatidyl ethanolamine also have been implicated. The review by MacLeod and Ames includes a table listing the volatiles isolated from soy beans, flours, concentrates, and isolates. Straight-chain alcohol and carbonyl compounds are the major classes of volatiles present in soybeans. Although lipooxygenase-generated compounds are generally believed to be the major cause of off-flavors in products derived from soybeans, both enzymatic and nonenzymatic lipid oxidation mechanisms also are believed to be involved in producing off-flavors in soy products.

In summary, considerable knowledge of the volatiles from oxidized lipids that occur in foods has been gained. Some of these volatiles impart a characteristic flavor, while others may contribute to background flavors or combine to produce flavors. The understanding of the contributions of lipids to the complex flavors of food products is, however, far from complete. Further advances in relating chemical composition to flavor will probably require a better understanding of the olfactory perception of complex mixtures. Methods that measure the volatiles present in the mouth or nose have been developed (Overbosch et al., 1991; Linforth and Taylor, 1993). Further development and application of these methods should benefit our understanding of the contributions of products from oxidized lipids to food flavors.

REFERENCES

Acree, T. E. 1993a. Bioassays for flavor. In *Flavor Science. Sensible Principles and Techniques*, T. E. Acree and R. Teranishi (Ed.), pp. 1–20. American Chemical Society, Washington, DC.

Acree, T. E. 1993b. Gas chromatography-olfactometry. In *Flavor Measurement*, C-T. Ho and C. H. Manley (Ed.), pp. 77–94. Marcel Dekker, Inc., New York.

Acree, T. E., Barnard, J., and Cunningham, D. G. 1984. The analysis of odor-active volatiles in gas chromatographic effluents. In *Analysis of Volatiles. Methods. Applications*, P. Schreier (Ed.), pp. 251–267. Walter de Gruyter & Co., Berlin.

Ajuyah, A. O., Fenton, T. W., Hardin, R. T., and Sim, J. S. 1993. Measuring lipid oxidation volatiles in meats. *J. Food Sci.* 58: 270–273, 277.

Allen, J. C. 1983. Rancidity in dairy products. In *Rancidity in Foods*, J. C. Allen and R. J. Hamilton (Ed.), pp. 169–178. Applied Science Publishers, London.

Amerine, M. A., Pangborn, R. M., and Roessler, E. B. 1965. *Principles of the Sensory Evaluation of Foods*, p. 549. Academic Press, New York.

Badings, H. T. 1991. Milk. In *Volatile Compounds in Foods and Beverages*, H. Maarse (Ed.), pp. 91–106. Marcel Dekker, Inc., New York.

Bailey, M. E. 1983. The Maillard reaction and meat flavor. In *The Maillard Reaction in Foods and Nutrition*. G. R. Waller and M. S. Feather (Ed.), pp. 169–183. American Chemical Society, Washington, DC.

Bailey, M. E. and Einig, R. G. 1989. Reaction flavors of meat. In *Thermal Generation of Aromas*. T. H. Parliment, R. J. McGorrin, and C-T. Ho. (Ed.), pp. 421–432. American Chemical Society, Washington, DC.

Bakker, J. and Law, B. A. 1994. Cheese flavour. In *Understanding Natural Flavors*, J. R. Piggott and A. Paterson (Ed.), pp. 281–297. Blackie Academic and Professional, Glasgow, United Kingdom.

Baldwin, E. A., Nisperos-Carriedo, M. O., Baker, R., and Scott, J. W. 1991. Quantitative analysis of flavor parameters in six Florida tomato cultivars (*Lycopersican esculentum*). *J. Agric. Food Chem.* 39: 1135–1140.

Barbieri, G., Bolzoni, L., Parolari, G., Virgili, R., Buttini, R., Careri, M., and Margia, A. 1992. Flavor compounds of dry-cured hams. *J. Agric. Food Chem.* 40: 2389–2394.

Beauchamp, G. K. and Brand, J. G. 1994. The chemical senses. In *Quality Attributes and Their Measurement in Meat, Poultry and Fish Products*, A. M. Pearson and T. R. Dutson (Ed.), pp. 162–183. Blackie Academic and Professional, Glasgow, United Kingdom.

Bennett, C. J. 1992. Formulating low-fat foods with good taste. *Cereal Foods World* 37: 430–432.

Berry, K. E. and Sink, J. D. 1971. Isolation and identification of 3α-hydroxy-5α-androst-16-ene and 5α-androst-16-en-3-one from porcine tissue. *J. Endocrinol.* 51: 223–224.

Berry, K. E., Sink, J. D., Patton, S., and Ziegler, J. H. 1971. Characterization of the swine sex odor (SSO) components of boar fat volatiles. *J. Food Sci.* 36: 1086–1090.

Bett, K. L. and Grimm, C. C. 1994. Flavor and aroma—its measurement. In *Quality Attributes and Their Measurement in Meat, Poultry and Fish Products*, A. M. Pearson and T. R. Dutson (Ed.), pp. 202–221. Blackie Academic and Professional, Glasgow, United Kingdom.

Brennand, C. P. and Lindsay, R. C. 1992a. Distribution of volatile branched-chain fatty acids in various lamb tissues. *Meat Sci.* 31: 411–421.

Brennand, C. P. and Lindsay, R. C. 1992b. Influence of cooking on the species-related flavor compounds in mutton. *Lebensm. Wiss. Technol.* 25: 357–364.

Brennand, C. P., Ha, J. K., and Lindsay, R. C. 1989. Aroma properties and thresholds of some branched-chain and other minor volatile fatty acids occurring in milkfat and meat lipids. *J. Sensory Studies* 4: 105–120.

Brewer, M. S., Ikins, W. G., and Harbers, C. A. Z. 1992. TBA values, sensory characteristics, and volatiles in ground pork during long-term frozen storage: Effects of packaging. *J. Food Sci.* 57: 558–563, 580.

Buttery, R. G. 1993. Quantitative and sensory aspects of flavor of tomato and other vegetables and fruits. In *Flavor Science, Sensible Principles and Techniques*, T. E. Acree and R. Teranishi (Ed.), pp. 259. American Chemical Society, Washington, DC.

Buttery, R. G., Teranishi, R., and Ling, L. C., 1987. Fresh tomato aroma volatiles: A quantitative study. *J. Agric. Food Chem.* 35: 540–544.

Chien, M. and Peppard, T. 1993. Use of statistical methods to better understand gas chromatographic data obtained from complex flavor systems. In *Flavor Measurement*, C-T. Ho and C. H. Manley (Ed.), pp. 1–36. Marcel Dekker, Inc., New York.

Christensen, K. R. and Reineccius, G. A. 1995. Aroma extract dilution analysis of aged cheddar cheese. *J. Food Sci.* 60: 218–220.

Duncan, S. E., Christen, G. L., and Penfield, M. P. 1991. Rancid flavor of milk: Relationship of acid degree value, free fatty acids, and sensory perception. *J. Food Sci.* 56: 394–397.

Farmer, L. J. and Mottram, D. S. 1990. Recent studies on the formation of meat-like aroma compounds. In *Flavour Science and Technology*, Y. Bessiere and A. F. Thomas (Ed.), pp. 113–116. John Wiley and Sons, Chichester, United Kingdom.

Farmer, L. J., Mottram, D. S., and Whitfield, F. B. 1989. Volatile compounds produced in Maillard reactions involving cysteine, ribose and phospholipid. *J. Sci. Food Agric.* 49: 347–368.

Fischer, K.-H. and Grosch, W. 1987. Volatile compounds of importance in the aroma of mushrooms (*Psalliota bispora*). *Lebensm. Wiss. Technol.* 20: 233–236.

Fisher, U. and Grosch, W. 1991. Breakdown of the flavour compound 2 (E)-hexenal in different solvents. *Food Chem.* 39: 59–72.

Forss, D. A. 1969. Role of lipids in flavors. *J. Agr. Food Chem.* 17: 681–685.

Forss, D. A. 1972. Odour and flavour compounds from lipids. In *Progress in Chemistry of Fats and Other Lipids*, Vol. XIII, Part 4, R. T. Holman (Ed.). Pergamon Press, Oxford.

Frankel, E. N. 1985. Chemistry of autoxidation: Mechanism, products and flavor significance. In *Flavor Chemistry of Fats and Oils*, D. B. Min and T. H. Smouse (Ed.), pp. 1–37. American Oil Chemists' Society, Champaign, IL.

Frankel, E. N. 1991. Review. Recent advances in lipid oxidation. *J. Sci. Food Agric.* 42: 495–511.

Gardner, H. W. 1985. Flavors and bitter tastes from oxidation of lipids by enzymes. In *Flavor Chemistry of Fats and Oils*, D. B. Min and T. H. Smouse (Ed.), pp. 189–206. American Oil Chemists' Society, Champaign, IL.

Gardner, H. W. 1991. Recent investigations into the lipoxygenase pathways of plants. *Biochim. Biophys. Acta* 1084: 221–239.

Gasser, U. and Grosch, W. 1990. Primary odorants of chicken broth: A comparative study with meat broths from cow and ox. *Z. Lebens. Unters. Forsch.* 190: 3–7

Gloria, M. B. A., Grulke, E. A., and Gray, J. I. 1993. Effect of type of oxidation on beta-carotene loss and volatile products formation in model systems. *Food Chem.* 46: 401–406.

Grosch, W. 1982. Lipid degradation products and flavour. In *Developments in Food Science 3A. Food Flavours. Part A. Introduction*, D. Morton and A. J. MacLeod (Ed.), pp. 325–398. Elsevier Press, New York.

Grosch, W. 1993. Detection of potent odorants in foods by aroma extract dilution analysis. *Trends Food Sci. Technol.* 4: 68–73.

Guth, H. and Grosch, W. 1993. 12-Methyltridecanal, a species-specific odorant of stewed beef. *Lebensm. Wiss. Technol.* 26: 171–177.

Ha, J. K. and Lindsay, R. C. 1990. Distribution of volatile branched-chain fatty acids in perinephric fats of various red meat species. *Lebensm. Wiss. Technol.* 23: 433–440.

Hamilton, R. J. 1983. The chemistry of rancidity in foods. In *Rancidity in Foods*, J. C. Allen and R. J. Hamilton (Ed.), pp. 1–20. Applied Science Publishers, London.

Heymann, H., Holt, D. L. and Cliff, M. A. 1993. Measurement of flavor by descriptive techniques. In *Flavor Measurement*, C-T. Ho and C. H. Manley (Ed.), pp. 113–132. Marcel Dekker, Inc., New York.

Ho, C. T., Bruechert, L. J., Zhang, Y., and Chiu, E. M. 1989. Contributions of lipids to the formation of heterocyclic compounds in model systems. In *Thermal Generation of Aromas*, T. H. Parliment, R. J. McGorrin, and C-T. Ho (Ed.). American Chemical Society, Washington, DC.

Jeon, I. J. 1993. Undesirable flavors in dairy products. In *Food Taints and Off-Flavors*, M. J. Saxby (Ed.), pp. 122–149. Blackie Academic and Professional, Glasgow.

Josephson, D. B. 1991. Seafood. In *Volatile Compounds in Foods and Beverages*, H. Maarse (Ed.), pp. 179–202. Marcel Dekker, Inc., New York.

Josephson, D. B., Lindsay, R. C., and Stubier, P. A. 1991. Volatile carotenoid-related oxidation compounds contributing to cooked salmon flavor. *Lebensm. Wiss. Technol.* 24: 424–432.

Kemp, T. R., Knavel, D. E., and Stoltz, L. P. 1972. cis-6-Nonenal: A flavor component of muskmelon fruit. *Phytochemistry* 11: 3321–3322.

Kobayashi, A., Kubiota, K., Swamoto, M., and Tamura, H. 1989. Syntheses and sensory characterization of 5,8,11-tetradecatrien-2-one isomers. *J. Agric. Food Chem.* 37: 151–154.

Kochhar, S. P. 1993. Oxidative pathways to the formation of off-flavours. In *Food Taints and Off-Flavours*, M. J. Saxby (Ed.), pp. 150–201. Blackie Academic and Professional, Glasgow.

Konopka, U. C. and Grosch, W. 1991. Potent odorants causing the warmed-over flavor in boiled beef. *Lebensm. Unters. Forsch.* 193: 123–125.

Kuo, J. and Pan, B. S. 1991. *Note.* Effects of lipoxygenase on formation of the cooked shrimp flavor component 5,8,11-tetradecatrien-2-one. *Agric. Biol. Chem.* 55: 847–848.

Lin, J. C. C. and Jeon, I. J. 1987. Effects of commercial food grade enzymes on free fatty acid profiles in granular cheddar cheese. *J. Food Sci.* 52: 78–83, 87.

Lindsay, R. C. 1990. Fish flavors. *Food Rev. Int.* 6: 437–455.

Linforth, R. S. T. and Taylor, A. J. 1993. Measurement of volatile release in the mouth. *Food Chem.* 48: 115–120.

MacLeod, G. and Ames, J. 1988. Soy flavor and its improvement. *CRC Crit. Rev. Food Sci. Nutr.* 27: 219–400.

Maga, J. A. 1994. Potato flavor. *Food Rev. Int.* 10: 1–48.

Mau, J.-L., Beelman, R. B., and Ziegler, G. R. 1992. 1-Octen-3-ol in the cultivated mushroom, *Agaricus bisporus. J. Food Sci.* 57: 704–706.

Meilgaard, M., Civille, G. V., and Carr, B. T. 1991. *Sensory Evaluation Techniques*, 2nd ed., p. 10. CRC Press, Inc. Boca Raton, FL.

Mottram, D. S. 1987. Lipid oxidation and flavour in meat products. *Food Sci. Technol. Today* 1(3): 159–162.

Mottram, D. 1991. Meat. In *Volatile Compounds in Foods and Beverages*, H. Maarse (Ed.), pp. 107–178. Marcel Dekker, Inc., New York.

Mottram, D. 1994. Meat flavour. In *Understanding Natural Flavors*, J. R. Piggott and A. Paterson (Ed.), pp. 140–163. Blackie Academic and Professional, Glasgow.

Mottram, D. S. and Salter, L. J. 1989. Flavor formation in meat-related systems containing phospholipids. In *Thermal Generation of Aromas*, T. H. Parliment, R. J. McGorrin, and C-T. Ho (Ed.), pp. 442–451. American Chemical Society, Washington, DC.

Nawar, Y. 1989. Thermal decomposition of lipids: An overview. In *Thermal Generation of Aromas*, T. H. Parliment, R. J. McGowan, and C-T. Ho (Ed.), pp. 94–101. American Chemical Society, Washington, DC.

O'Connor, T. P. and O'Brien, N. M. 1991. Significance of lipoxygenase in fruits and vegetables. In *Food Enzymology*, Vol. 1, P. F. Fox (Ed.), p. 337. Elsevier Applied Science, New York.

Overbosch, P., Afterof, W. G. M., and Haring, P. G. M. 1991. Flavor release in the mouth. *Food Rev. Int.* 7(2): 137–184.

Patterson, R. L. S. 1968. 5-Androst-16-ene-3-one: Compound responsible for taint in boar fat. *J. Sci. Food Agric.* 19: 31–38.

Piggott, J. R. 1990. Relating sensory and chemical data to understand flavor. *J. Sensory Studies* 4: 261–272.

Ramarathnam, N., Rubin, L. J., and Diosady, L. L. 1993. Studies on meat flavor. 4. Fractionation, characterization and quantitation of volatiles from uncured and cured beef and chicken. *J. Agric. Food Chem.* 41: 939–945.

Reineccius, G. 1993. Biases in analytical flavor profiles introduced by isolation method. In *Flavor Measurement*, C-T. Ho and C. H. Manely (Ed.), pp. 61–76. Marcel Dekker, Inc., New York.

Reineccius, G. 1994. Flavor and aroma chemistry. In *Quality Attributes and Their Measurement in Meat, Poultry and Fish Products*, A. M. Pearson and T. R. Dutson (Ed.), pp. 184–201. Blackie Academic & Professional, Glasgow.

Schieberle, P., Ofner, S., and Grosch, W. 1990. Evaluation of potent odorants in cucumber (*Cucumis sativus*) and muskmelon (*Cucumis melo*) by aroma extract dilution analysis. *J. Food Sci.* 55: 193–195.

Schrier, P. 1986. Biogeneration of plant aromas. In *Developments in Food Flavors*, G. G. Birch and M. G. Lindley (Ed.), pp. 89–106. Elsevier Applied Science, London.

Shahidi, F., Rubin, L. J., and D'Souza, L. A. 1986. Meat flavor volatiles: A review of the composition, techniques of analysis, and sensory evaluation. *CRC Crit. Rev. Food Tech.* 24: 141–243.

Shahidi, F., Yun, J., Rubin, L. J., and Wood, P. F. 1987. The hexanal content as an indicator of oxidative stability and flavor acceptability in cooked ground pork. *Can. Inst. Food Sci. Technol. J.* 20: 104–106.

Snyder, J. M., Frankel, E. N., Selke, E., and Warner, K. 1988. Comparison of gas chromatographic methods for volatile lipid oxidation products in soybean oil. *J. Am. Oil Chem. Soc.* 65: 1617–1620.

Stark, W. and Forss, D. A. 1962. A compound responsible for the metallic flavour in dairy products. *J. Dairy Res.* 29: 173–180.

St. Angelo, A. J., Vercelloti, J. R., Legendre, M. G., Vinnett, C. H., Kuan, J. W., James, C., Jr., and Dupuy, H. P. 1987. Chemical and instrumental analysis of warmed-over flavor in beef. *J. Food Sci.* 52: 1163–1168.

Thompson, R. H., Jr., Pearson, A. M., and Banks, K. A. 1972. Identification of some C19-Δ^{16} steroids contributing to sex odor in pork. *J. Agric. Food Chem.* 20: 185.

Vangtal, A. and Hammond, E. G. 1986. Correlation of the flavor characteristics of Swiss-type cheeses with chemical properties. *J. Dairy Sci.* 69: 2982–2993.

Van Toller, S. 1994. Psychology and psychophysiological measurements of flavor. In *Understanding Natural Flavors.* J. R. Piggott and A. Paterson (Ed.), pp. 46–59. Blackie Academic and Professional, Glasgow.

Werkhoff, P., Guntert, M., and Hopp, R. 1992. Dihydro-1,3,5-dithiazines: Unusual flavor compounds with remarkable organoleptic properties. *Food Rev. Int.* 8: 391–442.

Whitfield, F. B. and Last, J. H. 1991. Vegetables. In *Volatile Compounds in Foods and Beverages,* H. Maarse (Ed.), p. 257. Marcel Dekker, Inc., New York.

Wong, E., Nixon, L. N., and Johnson, C. B. 1975. Volatile medium chain fatty acids and mutton flavor. *J. Agric. Food Chem.* 23: 495–498.

Woo, A. H. and Lindsay, R. C. 1983. Statistical correlation of qualitative flavor intensity assessments and individual free fatty acid measurements for routine detection and prediction of hydrolytic rancidity off-flavor in butter. *J. Food Sci.* 48: 1761–1764.

Yabumoto, K., Jennings, W. G., and Yamaguchi, M. 1977. Volatile constituents of cantaloupe, *Cucumis melo,* and their biogenesis. *J. Food Sci.* 42: 32–37.

13

Natural Antioxidants: From Radical Mechanisms to Food Stabilization

Jürg Löliger, Pierre Lambelet, Robert Aeschbach, and Elizabeth M. Prior

Nestec Ltd.
Nestlé Research Centre
Lausanne, Switzerland

INTRODUCTION

A food antioxidant is a substance capable of delaying, retarding, or preventing the development in food of rancidity or other flavor deterioration due to oxidation. Application of an antioxidant extends the shelf life of a food, reduces waste and customer complaints, reduces nutritional losses (e.g., vitamins and essential fatty acids), and widens the range of fats and oils that can be used. A number of efficient and relatively cheap synthetic antioxidants such as butylated hydroxy anisole (BHA), butylated hydroxy toluene (BHT) and *tert*-butylhydroquinone (TBHQ) exist. However, their use is increasingly contested for a variety of reasons (health concerns, legal issues), and there is considerable commercial interest in the use of natural antioxidants.

The great importance that the scientific community attaches to research into new natural antioxidants can be seen from the large number of research papers and patents published in this field. An analysis of these publications reveals certain tendencies, which can be summarized as follows:

Evaluation of traditionally used ethnic food components in test systems

Antioxidant effect of crude plant and animal extracts

Structural analysis of specific molecules of fractions exhibiting antioxidant activity

Evaluation of antioxidant preparations in models, rarely in foods

Many plant and animal tissues contain fractions that show some antioxidant activity in model systems. Often the added stability is minimal, i.e., a few percentage points. Natural antioxidants relevant to the food industry are quite another picture. Extracts must show a good antioxidant efficiency and must be commercially available in large quantities at a competitive price. Very few preparations meet these criteria: ascorbic acid (vitamin C), tocopherols (vitamin E), lecithins, spice extracts (principally rosemary), and mixtures of these ingredients.

This contribution will concentrate on the most promising natural antioxidants and will discuss the radical basis for their antioxidant activity. Use of these antioxidants in model systems and particularly in foods will be illustrated by examples.

ANTIOXIDANTS

Antioxidants can be divided into two broad classes, referred to as chain-breaking antioxidants, which interfere with one or more of the propagation steps, and preventive antioxidants, which reduce the rate of initiation.

Chain-Breaking Antioxidants

Lipid autoxidation is a radical chain reaction catalyzed by the peroxy radical $ROO\cdot$:

Initiation:

$$R-H \rightarrow R\cdot + H\cdot$$

Propagation:

$$R\cdot + O_2 \rightarrow ROO\cdot$$
$$ROO\cdot + R'-H \rightarrow ROOH + R'\cdot$$
$$ROOH \rightarrow RO\cdot + \cdot OH$$
$$2\,ROOH \rightarrow ROO\cdot + RO\cdot + H_2O$$
$$RO\cdot + R'-H \rightarrow ROH + R'\cdot$$

Termination:

> Reactions leading to stable products.

Chain-breaking antioxidants are hydrogen atom donors. They transform chain-propagating radicals into much less reactive species via a hydrogen atom transfer.

$$ROO\cdot + AH \rightarrow ROOH + A\cdot \tag{1}$$

Chain-breaking antioxidants are only effective when the concentration of peroxy radicals is low, i.e., in the initiation phase. As soon as peroxy radicals are present at high concentrations (propagation phase), the antioxidants are rapidly decomposed.

By conducting experiments under a very low concentration of oxygen (Zhu et al., 1990), it has been shown that antioxidants are also able to react directly with alkyl radicals.

$$R\cdot + AH \rightarrow RH + A\cdot \tag{2}$$

From the mechanistic point of view, a chain-breaking antioxidant is a compound that can easily give one or more hydrogen atoms and form an unreactive radical species, which does not participate in radical reactions involved in the lipid oxidation process. For example, dl-α-tocopherol, vitamin E (Fig. 13.1), has been shown to be an excellent chain-breaking antioxidant, being more effective than other synthetic o- or p-substituted phenols (Burton and Ingold, 1986). The radical, which is formed during the reaction of the vitamin E, the tocopheroxy radical, is stabilized by delocalization of the unpaired electron over the aromatic ring and also over the oxygen atom in the heterocyclic ring (Burton and Ingold, 1986). This is particularly useful because electron delocalization is expected to correlate with antioxidant activity, i.e., the greater the electron delocalization, the greater the stability of the phenoxy radical relative to the parent phenol. Hence reactions (1) and (2) are favored. Tocopheroxy radicals do not, in general, continue the oxidation chain but are destroyed by reaction with a second peroxy radical.

Some chain-breaking antioxidants can react in cascade with lipid radicals. Under certain circumstances, tocopherols can form dimers during their reaction with peroxidizing lipids (Gottstein and Grosh, 1990). These dimers, which still possess a phenolic hydrogen atom, can in turn react with a lipid radial, i.e., they are also effective as antioxidants.

A combination of two or more antioxidants may work better than the equivalent quantity of any one antioxidant. For example, the synergistic antioxidant effect between vitamin E and vitamin C is very well known and abundantly documented (Tappel, 1968; Packer et al., 1979; Niki et al., 1982;

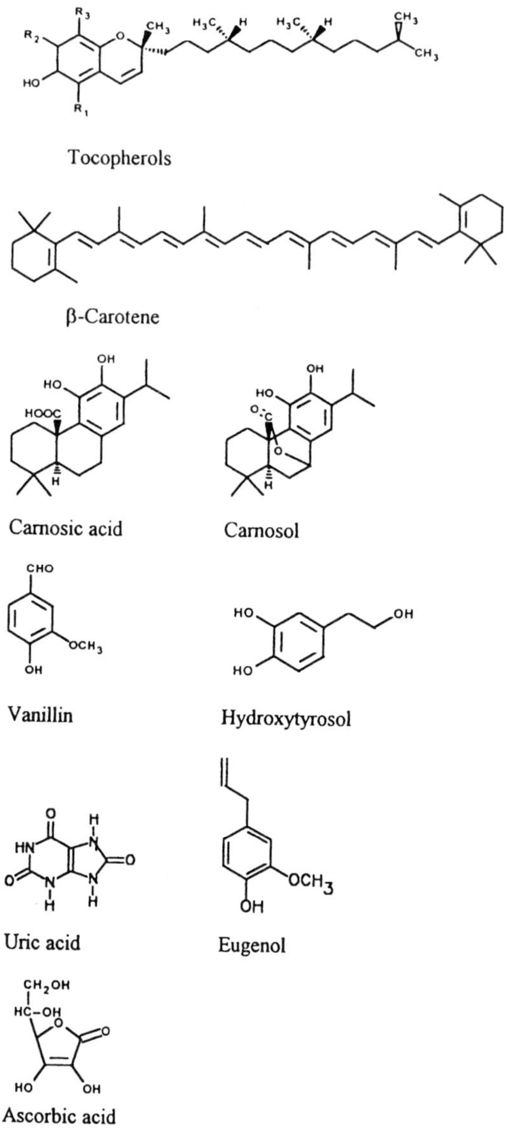

Tocopherols

β-Carotene

Carnosic acid   Carnosol

Vanillin   Hydroxytyrosol

Uric acid   Eugenol

Ascorbic acid

FIG. 13.1   Structures of some natural antioxidants.

Lambelet et al., 1987). A regeneration schema between vitamin E and vitamin C has been shown to take place (Fig. 13.2). In the beginning vitamin E reacts with peroxy radicals to form tocopheroxy radicals. These tocopheroxy radicals are then scavenged by vitamin C, which in turn is transformed into the ascorbyl radical by a hydrogen atom transfer reaction.

Mechanistic studies on the functionality of phenolic-type antioxidants such as tocopherols and common synthetic antioxidants (e.g., BHT, BHA, TBHQ) appearing in the literature have generally been performed in nonfood systems. In these studies the radicals were generated conventionally by chemical oxidation with, for example, PbO_2, by reaction with radicals such as 2,2-diphenyl-1-picrylhydrazyl (DPPH) or those formed by thermal decomposition of azo compounds. Radicals can also be generated by irradiation with UV light, by radiolysis, and by electrolysis. It has rarely been demonstrated that these radicals are formed during the reaction of antioxidants with fats or oils.

Radicals from antioxidants can, however, be formed by reaction with oxidizing lipids and observed by ESR spectroscopy directly in the lipid medium (Lambelet et al., 1987). The ESR spectrum of the dl-α-tocopheroxy radical recorded in a lipid medium is given in Figure 13.3. Since lipid autoxidation is by definition oxygen dependent, it is not surprising that the intensity of this ESR spectrum decreases dramatically under oxygen-limiting conditions (Saucy et al., 1990). It can, therefore, be assumed that the radicals observed are transient: they are continuously formed but also

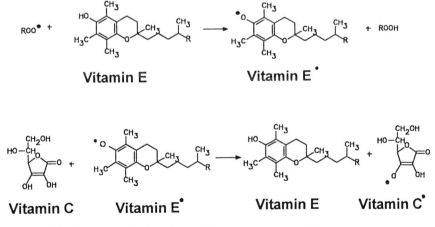

FIG. 13.2   Schema of vitamin E, vitamin C regeneration.

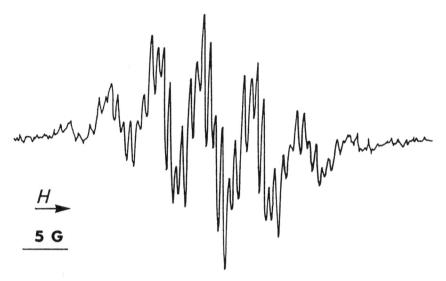

FIG. 13.3   ESR spectrum of dl-α-tocopheroxy radical in a lipid medium.

continuously decomposed. The use of oxidizing lipids is a simple method for generating radicals from antioxidants and allows observation of these radicals under conditions similar to those encountered during lipid autoxidation. Interactions between antioxidants, e.g., tocopherol and ascorbic acid, can also be investigated with this technique.

Preventive Antioxidants

These antioxidants prevent or delay lipid oxidation by decreasing oxygen active compounds in the medium. Some of them decrease the concentration of oxygen (triplet oxygen, $^3O_2$) through a direct reaction. A much more active oxygen species is singlet oxygen ($^1O_2$). It is known that singlet oxygen reacts with unsaturated lipids more than 1000 times faster than triplet oxygen (Dawson and Gartner, 1983). Some compounds can convert singlet oxygen into the more stable triplet oxygen and are therefore called singlet oxygen quenchers. A number of compounds help to increase the shelf life of a lipid by complexing with trace quantities of metals, which would otherwise promote the oxidative reactions. These chelating agents are not true antioxidants because they do not exhibit any antioxidant activity in a fat from which all traces of metal have been removed.

TYPES OF NATURAL ANTIOXIDANTS

Natural antioxidants acting as radical scavengers (Fig. 13.1) are generally phenols and to a lesser extent compounds with an amino group. Among the monophenols are the tocopherols, tocotrienols, vanillin and eugenol, the antioxidant of cloves (Sandmeier and Ziegleder, 1982). Tocopherols are widely distributed throughout the vegetable kingdom (Müller-Mulot, 1976; Carpenter, 1979). However, most tocopherols used as antioxidants are synthetic compounds. For this reason they have been called "nature identical antioxidants." Examples of polyphenols are carnosic acid and carnosol, the active principles of rosemary and sage (Schwarz and Ternes, 1992a); hydroxytyrosol, an antioxidant found in olive (Perrin, 1992); and the catechins of tea (Lunder, 1992). Examples of natural antioxidants having an amino group are uric acid (Farr et al., 1986) and carnosine (Decker and Crum, 1991). Vitamin C is the natural compound most commonly used as an oxygen scavenger, carotenoids are the most common singlet oxygen quenchers, and vitamin E is the most widely used chain-breaking antioxidant.

PREPARATION OF NATURAL ANTIOXIDANTS

Extracts of herbs and spices, in particular rosemary, are usually produced from plant materials using organic solvents and are sold in the form of powders, pastes, or liquids of different viscosities. A procedure for extracting antioxidant principles from spices, especially rosemary and sage, with organic solvents is schematically represented in Figure 13.4. A beige, nearly tasteless powder is obtained from rosemary using procedure A (Aeschbach and Philippossian, 1988), whereas procedure B gives an orange-colored, fluid oil (Aeschbach and Wille, 1992). A purely mechanical process for extracting the antioxidant principles from plant material has been elaborated. The aim was to simplify extraction of natural antioxidants by avoiding use of organic solvents and to produce a liquid extract with a high antioxidant content for direct incorporation into foods (Aeschbach et al., 1994a).

The mechanical process uses a piston press and liquid carriers as extraction media. The flow sheet is illustrated in Figure 13.5. Liquid and limpid oils are obtained by contacting the plant materials with a carrier followed by pressing on a piston press. Two carriers are predominantly used: medium chain triglycerides (MCT) for liposoluble antioxidants (Aeschbach and Wille, 1993) and propylene glycol (PG) for water-soluble antioxidants (Aeschbach and Rossi, 1995). These extracts can easily be incorporated into

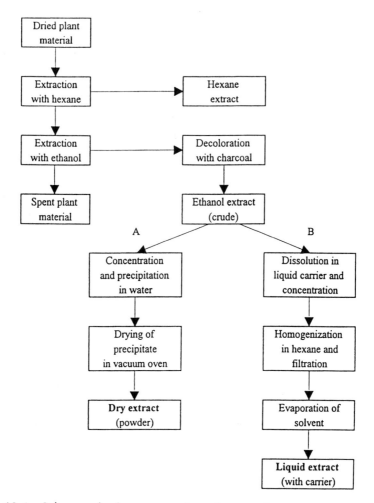

FIG. 13.4   Schema of solvent extraction of antioxidants.

oils or emulsions, respectively. This procedure may also be used to extract antioxidants directly into oils and fats. The plant material is contacted with the fat or oil, e.g., chicken fat, palm oil, or pork fat, and pressed as previously described. The resulting extract, added at 0.2% (w/w) to the corresponding nontreated oil, prolonged its stability up to sixfold (rosemary in chicken fat) (Aeschbach et al., 1994a).

Carnosic acid and carnosol (the antioxidants of rosemary) are colorless, odorless, and almost tasteless. It is possible to obtain an organoleptically

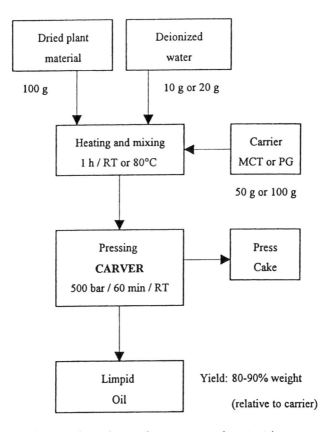

FIG. 13.5   Schema of mechanical extraction of antioxidants.

neutral antioxidant preparation from rosemary after deodorization. In other plant materials the antioxidant activity is inherent to specific properties, e.g., spicy odor in oregano, pungency in chili, and intense color in turmeric. These properties can be exploited to produce antioxidant "cocktails," e.g., provençal or oriental type for specific applications. Antioxidant activity of extracts obtained by the mechanical procedure are given in another section.

TECHNIQUES FOR EVALUATION OF ANTIOXIDANTS

As outlined previously, lipid autoxidation is a three-phase process. In the first phase, *initiation*, radicals are gradually formed. During this stage, changes in the composition of the lipid are hardly detectable. In the second phase, *propagation*, a relatively rapid chain reaction sets in. This phase is characterized by a rapid absorption of oxygen and a simultaneous generation of peroxides. The third phase, *termination*, comprises the recombination of various radicals. The induction period (IP) corresponds to the onset of the rapid absorption of oxygen and usually to an important flavor deterioration due to production of secondary degradation products.

The activity of an antioxidant, or antioxidant index (AI), is calculated by dividing the IP measured with an oil containing the antioxidant by the corresponding value obtained with an unstabilized oil:

$$AI = \frac{IP \text{ of oil containing the antioxidant}}{IP \text{ of unstabilized oil}}$$

As IPs can be very long under normal conditions, they are frequently measured under accelerating conditions. IPs are usually determined by the following techniques: a modified active oxygen method (AOM) test for lipid samples, the oxygen electrode test for emulsions, and the induction time graph (ITG) test for food products. To these continuous methods can be added measurement of changes in headspace gas composition. This last technique is particularly useful for foods that have a long shelf life and where a continuous measurement cannot realistically be made.

Modified Active Oxygen Method (AOM)

The AOM or Swift Test operates on the principle of bubbling air through the oil at ~100°C. Originally the peroxide value was determined at intervals, plotted, and the curve interpreted. Automated versions of this method are available based on the development of Zürcher and Hadorn (1979) and commercialized by Metrohm as the Rancimat and by Omnion as the Oxidative Stability Instrument (OSI) (Rossel, 1994). Air is bubbled through the heated oil (80–120°C) sweeping the volatiles into a recipient containing distilled water. The electrical conductivity of the water is determined with an electrode. The increase in conductivity recorded at the end of the IP is caused by the presence of fatty acids of low molecular weight such as formic acid (de Man et al., 1987).

The Rancimat is almost exclusively used for determining the IP in oils and fats. It has, nevertheless, been applied to high-fat foods such as potato chips (Barrera-Arellano and Esteves, 1992), but normally extraction of the fat is required. This can be successful but introduces another preparation step and impurities.

Because of the high temperatures used and the flow of air, the Rancimat cannot be used to evaluate volatile antioxidants, such as BHT and BHA.

Also, it cannot be used for oils containing large amounts of volatiles, such as essential oils.

Oxygen Electrode Method

The method is based on the determination of oxygen consumption by an oil-in-water emulsion. The analysis is carried out at relatively low temperatures (30–40°C), and oxidation is initiated by addition of heme as catalyst (Farr et al., 1986). The decrease in oxygen concentration in the emulsion (5% oil in an air-saturated phosphate buffer containing an emulsifier) is recorded as a function of time using an oxygen electrode. The curve exhibits a typical IP as with the other techniques. The great interest of this method is the possibility of measuring the effect of antioxidants in an emulsion, since many foods are emulsions, e.g., mayonnaise.

Induction Time Graph (ITG)

This method operates on the principle of measuring the decrease of pressure in a closed system caused by consumption of oxygen by oxidation. It is based on the Sylvester Test and developed by the FIRA Astell test (Rossel, 1994). The pressure changes in the vessel containing the sample are monitored using a differential pressure sensor as a function of time (Wille et al., 1994) (Fig. 13.6).

Certain foods and fatty products are altered or damaged (or even burned) by high temperatures, i.e., 40–50°C: structural changes occur and artefacts are produced. To perform accelerated tests on these delicate products at lower temperatures, oxidation is accelerated by adding a catalyst, e.g., a hydroperoxide. To increase the sharpness of the onset of oxidation (end of IP), a pure oxygen atmosphere is used.

This test can be applied to fats and oils as well as to emulsions and to whole food products. Because it is a closed system, the ITG can be used for evaluating volatile antioxidants and volatile oils (see Rancimat above). The apparatus is commercialized by Omnion (Rockland, MA) as the Food Stability Analyzer (FSA).

Headspace Gases

This method is necessarily carried out in sealed containers. The decrease in the concentration of oxygen in the headspace caused by oxidation is measured with an oxygen analyzer (Servomex). The production of selected secondary oxidation products (in this case, ethane and pentane from oxidation of linolenic and linoleic acids, respectively) is monitored by injection of an aliquot of the headspace gas onto a gas chromatograph. The relevant

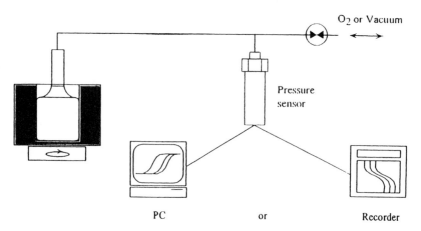

O$_2$ or Vacuum

Pressure
sensor

PC   or   Recorder

FIG. 13.6   Schema of working principle of ITG.

compounds are chromatographed and quantified as previously described (Löliger, 1990; Prior and Löliger, 1994). Measurements are made periodically on a new container each time, making this a discontinuous technique.

Although this method has been principally applied to foods, it can also be used for oils. The size and type of container (cans or glass jars), storage temperature, and sampling frequency are chosen according to the product to be analyzed.

ELECTRON SPIN RESONANCE (ESR) STUDIES OF NATURAL ANTIOXIDANTS

Research on the mode of action of natural antioxidants has been pursued. Investigations were focused on reactions involving antioxidants from rosemary and those resulting from the mixture of vitamin E, vitamin C, and phospholipid (also known as the ternary mix).

Rosemary Antioxidants

Carnosic acid and carnosol (Fig. 13.1) probably account for over 90% of the antioxidant properties of rosemary (*Rosmarinus officinalis* L) extract (Aruoma et al., 1992). Carnosic acid and carnosol have been shown to react fairly quickly with trichloromethyl peroxy radical ($CCl_3O_2^{\cdot}$), a reactive radical frequently used to assess the ability of a compound to react with peroxy radicals (Aruoma et al., 1992). The calculated rate constants were 2.7×10^7

$M^{-1}s^{-1}$ and $1\text{–}3 \times 10^6$ $M^{-1}s^{-1}$ for carnosic acid and carnosol, respectively. The rate constant of the reaction of propyl gallate with $CCl_3O_2^\bullet$ is 2×10^7 $M^{-1}s^{-1}$ (Aruoma et al., 1992). Thus, carnosic acid and carnosol appear to be reasonably good scavengers of peroxy radicals, carnosic acid being about 10 times more effective than carnosol.

This radical-scavenging activity of carnosic acid and carnosol has been verified by ESR spectroscopy in a lipid medium (Geoffroy et al., 1994). Reacting carnosic acid with methyl oleate in the temperature range of 60–100°C led to the observation of several ESR lines whose number and relative intensities were reversibly dependent on temperature (Fig. 13.7a). This spectrum was shown to be associated with two paramagnetic species. One could a priori think that the two radicals formed by abstracting the two hydrogen atoms belonging to the two hydroxyl groups could explain this spectrum. However, this ESR spectrum does not result from these two radicals: only the hydrogen atom belonging to the hydroxyl next to the isopropyl group is removed during the reaction of carnosic acid with lipids. This is probably because of the carboxyl group, which interacts with the other hydroxyl group. The primary radical observed during the reaction of carnosic acid with autoxidizing lipids is, therefore, the *o*-semiquinone radi-

1

cal **1**. The two species associated with the ESR spectrum correspond to two slightly different conformations of the cyclohexene ring in radical **1**.

Above 110°C and up to 160°C a new ESR spectrum could be observed (Fig. 13.7b) attesting to the presence of secondary radicals formed during the reaction of carnosic acid with autoxidizing lipids. This spectrum, although of poorer resolution and lower intensity, is similar to that observed during the reaction of carnosol with autoxidizing lipids at 130°C (Fig. 13.8). In contrast to the spectrum depicted in Figure 13.7a the spectra in Figure 13.7b and Figure 13.8 are not influenced by deuteration with MeOD. This indicates that one of the hydroxyl groups is no longer present in the secondary radicals. Furthermore, the ESR spectrum in Figure 13.8 exhibits coupling with a large number of protons, indicating a wide-ranging delocalization of the unpaired electron in the secondary radicals. This suggests that the secondary radicals contain several conjugated double bonds. Oxidation

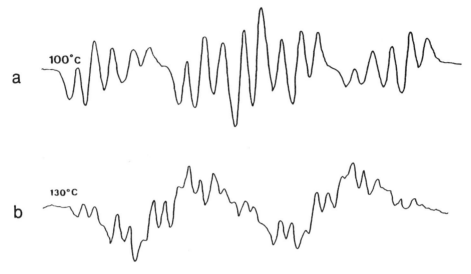

FIG. 13.7   (a) ESR spectrum from reaction of carnosic acid in a lipid medium at 100°C. (b) ESR spectrum from reaction of carnosic acid in a lipid medium at 130°C.

reactions of carnosic acid that leave the carboxyl group untouched do not increase the number of conjugated double bonds. It can be assumed that the secondary radicals observed during the reaction of carnosic acid with autoxidizing lipids have lost their carboxyl groups. The structure of a reasonable candidate for radical **2** is as follows:

2

Radical reactions of carnosic acid in an autoxidizing lipid medium can be rationalized by the following schema:

$$\text{Carnosic acid} \xrightarrow{50°C < T < 130°C} \text{primary radical}$$

$$\xrightarrow{100°C < T < 160°C} \text{diamagnetic compounds} \rightarrow \text{secondary radicals} \quad {}^{100°C < T < 160°C}$$

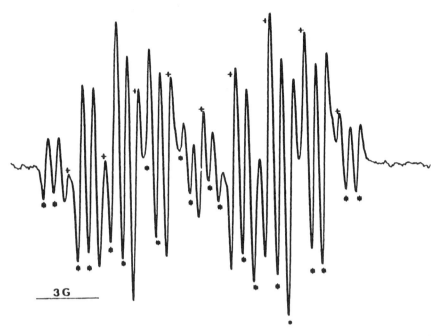

FIG. 13.8   ESR spectrum recorded during reaction of carnosol in a lipid medium at 130°C.

This interpretation is consistent with previous studies that showed that oxidation of carnosic acid results in the formation of carnosol (Schwarz and Ternes, 1992b). This succession of reactions occurring between carnosic acid and lipids at high temperatures is certainly at the basis of the high antioxidant activity of carnosic acid observed at elevated temperatures (Aeschbach et al., 1994b).

Vitamin E, Vitamin C, Phospholipid Mixture (Ternary Mix)

It has been found that a mixture of vitamin E, vitamin C, and phospholipids, the so-called ternary mix, very efficiently protects polyunsaturated lipids from oxidation (Löliger and Saucy, 1989). Trials were, therefore, undertaken to improve our understanding of the role of the phospholipids in such a mixture, i.e., whether they are only emulsifiers allowing the two vitamins (one liposoluble and the other hydrosoluble) to be in contact or whether they actively participate in the antioxidant process. Reactions between lipids and mixtures of vitamin E, vitamin C, and various phospholipids were studied at 90°C. Radicals were observed by ESR, and concentrations of antioxidants were monitored by differential pulse polarography (DPP) (Lambelet et al., 1994).

Responses recorded during this reaction varied according to the phospholipid present in the mixture. In the presence of phosphatidyl choline, i.e., a phospholipid containing a tertiary amino group, a successive consumption of vitamin C followed by vitamin E was observed (Fig. 13.9A). Accordingly, the vitamin C radical could be observed during the first part of the reaction, whereas the vitamin E radical was observed during the second part of the reaction (Fig. 13.9B). These observations are similar to those reported for analogous systems (Lambelet et al., 1987): during the induction period the vitamin C radical and then the vitamin E radical are sequentially observed while a successive disappearance of these two vitamins is recorded. Comparable results were obtained in the presence of phosphatidyl inositol, i.e., a phospholipid that does not contain an amino group.

Different observations were made during the reaction of vitamin E, vitamin C, and soya lecithin (contains a mixture of phospholipids). Although vitamin C was consumed during the first stage of the reaction, the amount of vitamin E did not decrease when all the vitamin C was depleted. The consumption of vitamin E was delayed for a while (Fig. 13.10A). Moreover, the ESR signals observed were different from those recorded in the presence of either phosphatidyl choline or phosphatidyl inositol. In the first stage of the reaction, a mixture of ESR signals was recorded (Fig. 13.10b, left). The signal marked with an *, which slowly decreased with time, was shown to be associated with the vitamin C radical. During the second stage of the reaction, ESR signals from only one radical were observed (Fig. 13.10B, center). They correspond to a strongly immobilized nitroxide radical. Hydrating the sample increased the mobility of the radical (Fig. 13.11). The ESR spectra in Figure 13.10B (center) and 13.11 are consistent with an acyl aminoxy radical (Forrester et al., 1968). These signals, which were identical to those observed when soya lecithin was replaced by phosphatidyl serine (i.e., a phospholipid containing a primary amino group), were tentatively ascribed to radical **3**.

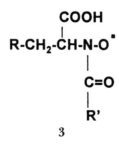

3

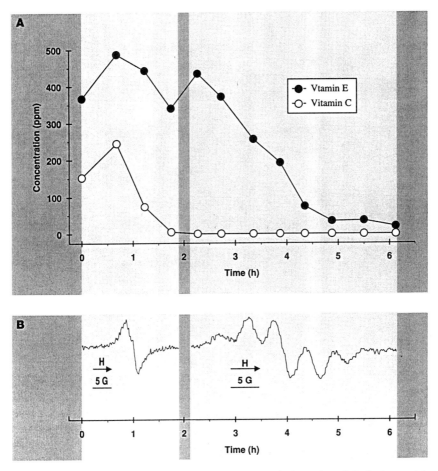

FIG. 13.9 Reaction of vitamin E, vitamin C, and phosphatidyl choline with methyl linolenate at 90°C. (A) Concentration time-course of vitamin E and vitamin C. (B) ESR spectra recorded during the reaction.

This radical was probably formed by the reaction of phosphatidyl serine with the triglyceride followed by oxidation. In the last stage of the reaction, the vitamin E was consumed while the tocopheroxy radical alone was observed in the reaction mixture (Fig. 13.10B, right).

These results show that vitamin E is spared when the nitroxide radical is formed. This finding is supported by the previously reported antioxidant properties of nitroxide radicals (Takahashi et al., 1989). Thus, the protective effect of the mixture, corresponding to the IP, is prolonged by the

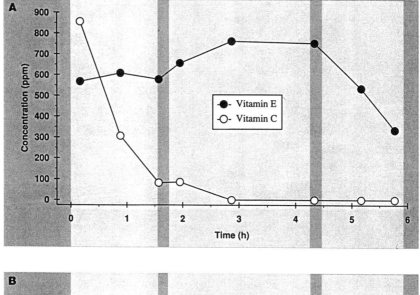

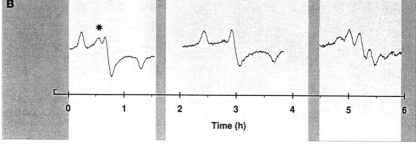

FIG. 13.10   Reaction of vitamin E, vitamin C, and soya lecithin with methyl linolenate at 90°C. (A) Concentration time-course of vitamin E and vitamin C. (B) ESR spectra recorded during the reaction.

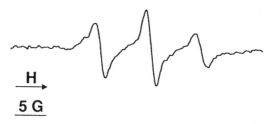

FIG. 13.11   ESR spectrum recorded during the reaction of vitamin E, vitamin C, and soya lecithin with methyl linoleate at 90°C after hydration.

participation of phospholipids in the antioxidant process. This may account for the good performance of the ternary mix (Löliger and Saucy, 1989).

APPLICATIONS OF NATURAL ANTIOXIDANTS FOR STABILIZING FOODS

Ternary Mix (TM)

The ternary mix (TM) antioxidant has been shown to be particularly effective in stabilizing highly unsaturated oils. Its composition is 500 ppm vitamin C, 1000 ppm vitamin E, and 1% phospholipid on a fat basis (Löliger and Saucy, 1989). An AI of more than 40 has been found in fish oil (Löliger, 1989) and an AI of more than 20 in calendula and chia oils (nonpublished results). Many highly unsaturated oils contain nutritionally important fatty acids, e.g., fish oil, which contains EPA and DHA and has a variety of applications in chronic disease therapy (e.g., ischemic heart disease, arthritis). Other oils have specific applications, for example, in cosmetics. These oils deteriorate readily and can be difficult to protect adequately. The TM has been shown to be of interest in these specific applications. The reason for the high efficiency of TM in unsaturated oils has not yet been elucidated.

Trials for antioxidant activity of TM have been performed in a wide variety of foods (Table 13.1). Effectiveness ranged from bad in milk powder to good in dehydrated chicken and essential oils. It could be expected from its high antioxidant activity in fish oils that the TM would be effective in fish. However, trials with frozen cod and saithe (both lean fish) were stopped because of strong off-flavors at time zero. These off-flavors probably came from the phospholipid component. Another consideration is the mode of application, as a dip and as a glaze, and it is possible that the antioxidants were not in contact with the lipids to be stabilized. Also in this application in frozen fish, the TM was added in large quantities. It can be seen from some of the other application listed in Table 13.1 that poor results were obtained with higher concentrations. The pro-oxidant effect of α-tocopherol at high concentrations is well known, and this could explain the greater development of rancidity in the malted chocolate drink and cheese filling with more elevated additions of TM. In frozen ham an interaction of the ascorbic acid component of the TM with curing substances, which normally exert an antioxidant effect, could be responsible for the pro-oxidant effect at the higher concentration. Trials in an infant formula containing corn oil showed no advantage in using the TM compared to gassing of the cans. It should also be remarked that in particularly bland products, such as dried milk and infant formula, any off-flavors would be easily detected as there is no masking effect from inherent food flavors.

TABLE 13.1 Efficiency of Ternary Mix Antioxidant in Variety of Food Applications

Food (storage temperature)	Amount of TM[a]	Effectiveness[d]	Comments
Cod and saithe[b] (−20°C)	0.4% E + 0.1% C	− − −	Strong off-flavors at time zero
Milk powder (30°C)	0.2%	− − −	Rancid after 3 months
Ham[c] (−20°C)	0.24% C + 0.1% E	+++	Acceptable after 14 months
	0.5°C + 0.25% E	− −	Rancid after 14 months
Malted chocolate drink (37°C)	0.1%, 0.2%, and 0.3%	++	Lowest concentration still acceptable after 6 months
Cheese filling for cannelloni (−18°C)	0.1%	+	Lower concentration better and higher concentration worse than reference
	0.15%	−	
Infant formula (27°C)	0.25%	+/−	No favorable effect after 12 months
Roasted hazelnuts (30°C)	0.1%, 0.25%, and 0.5%	++	Higher concentrations better than propyl gallate
Dehydrated chicken (40°C)	0.001% and 0.002% on a wet meat basis	+++	Preferred antioxidant
Essential oils (RT)	0.2%	+++	Preferred antioxidant

[a]TM, ternary mix (contains vitamin E, vitamin C and phospholipid); E, vitamin E; C, vitamin C.
[b]TM added in dip.
[c]TM added in brine.
[d]Judgments range from − − − (bad) to +++ (good).

The TM was effective in roasted hazelnuts, the two higher concentrations being more efficient than the synthetic antioxidant propyl gallate. In this case the TM was sprayed onto the surface of the hazelnuts, and it is possible that it acted by stabilizing the free oil on the surface, which is most sensitive to oxidation. A good antioxidant activity was obtained in dehydrated chicken and in essential oils, e.g., peppermint, for use in confectionery. Both of these applications are exploited industrially and represent a commercial success for natural antioxidants.

Rosemary and Other Plant Extracts

As discussed in the introduction, while extracts with some antioxidant activity can be obtained from many plants, only a very limited number have an industrial application. This is because of the cost of the raw material and extraction of the antioxidant fraction, a too low antioxidant activity, and strong accompanying flavors. Rosemary extracts are one of the few natural antioxidants with a wide commercial use (about a dozen suppliers). Spice extracts, in particular rosemary, have been proven to be very effective in stabilizing a variety of oils and foods. The antioxidant activity of mechanical extracts from a diversity of plant materials prepared in either MCT or in PG are shown in Table 13.2. Rosemary extract was the most effective, although other extracts, in particular sage and thyme, were also good antioxidants. These antioxidant activity results, together with availability of the raw mate-

TABLE 13.2   Antioxidant Index of Plant Extracts (1%) Obtained by Mechanical Extraction (Rancimat at 110°C)

	MCT as carrier		PG as carrier
	Chicken fat	Lard	Chicken fat
Rosemary	12.6	11.4	8.9
Sage	8.4	8.5	6.8
Thyme	5.7	4.8	5.2
Oregano	3.4	2.9	2.8
Spice Cocktail P[a]	8.3	9.1	7.2
Ginger	2.4	2.9	3.7
Turmeric	1.8	1.6	2.2
Cloves	2.3	1.5	2.0
Bay leaves	1.5	1.1	—[b]

[a]Composition: 2/5 rosemary, 1/5 sage, 1/5 thyme, 1/5 oregano.
[b]Not determined.

rial at a reasonable price, demonstrate why more effort has been put into commercialization of rosemary. Sage and thyme are most expensive and are less effective, resulting in a cost that is too elevated for industrial use. The antioxidant indexes of the other extracts are too low to be of commercial interest. The good performance of Spice Cocktail P is noteworthy.

The antioxidant activity of rosemary extracts vary according to the test lipid (Table 13.3). They are most effective in animal fats (e.g., AI > 8 in pork fat), but have a negligible activity in marine oils and in both saturated and unsaturated vegetable oils. This is the opposite of the TM (see above). It is interesting to note from Table 13.3 that ascorbyl-palmitate has a limited efficiency over the whole range of the fats and oils tested and that α-tocopherol is also most active in animal fats, although less so than rosemary extracts. A possible partial explanation lies in the natural antioxidant content of the various oils and fats, in particular their tocopherol content. Animal fats contain very low levels of tocopherols, whereas vegetable oils naturally contain levels near optimum for oxidative stability. Therefore, in

TABLE 13.3 Antioxidant Index of Several Antioxidants (0.05%) in a Variety of Fats and Oils (Rancimat at 100°C)

Fat or oil	Antioxidant		
	Ascorbyl palmitate	Alpha-tocopherol	Rosemary extract[a]
Animal fats			
Chicken fat	1.6	5.8	7.2
Pork fat	0.6	4.2	8.2
Beef fat	0.4	3.1	6.9
Butter fat	2.1	2.0	4.7
Marine oil			
Fish oil	1.0	1.1	1.4
Vegetable oils			
Palm oil	1.4	0.9	1.5
Coconut oil	1.0	1.1	>1.5
Soya oil	2.0	0.9	1.5
Rapeseed oil	1.9	0.9	1.4
Corn oil	1.7	1.0	1.2
Peanut oil	2.2	1.1	1.8
Sunflower seed oil	1.6	1.1	1.3

[a]Obtained by solvent extraction.

vegetable oils a further addition of antioxidant will not dramatically increase the IP (and may in fact be prooxidant). However, in animal fats the addition of an antioxidant can be highly effective as the fat is naturally poorly protected. Marine oils also contain low levels of tocopherols, but the lack of antioxidant activity of rosemary extracts (and α-tocopherol) may be due to the oil's highly unsaturated fatty acid composition. Animal fats are relatively saturated, and the different efficiency of rosemary antioxidants could also be related to the different fatty acid compositions. A further interesting point from Table 13.3 is that rosemary extract is more effective than α-tocopherol on a weight basis (both added at 0.05%). However, α-tocopherol is a pure substance, and rosemary extract contains at most 10–20% of active compounds. Therefore, the active compounds of rosemary, carnosic acid and carnosol, are highly efficient antioxidants.

Antioxidant indexes in bulk corn oil and in a corn oil emulsion are given in Table 13.4. It is extremely interesting to note the very high activity (antioxidant index up to 32) of the plant extracts in an emulsion compared to their almost nonexistent activity in the same bulk oil. Different activities of individual rosemary components in bulk oil and emulsion have also been observed (Frankel et al., 1996). Carnosic acid (more hydrophilic) was more

TABLE 13.4 Comparison of Antioxidant Index of Plant Extracts (1%) Obtained by Mechanical Extraction in Bulk Corn Oil and in a Corn Oil Emulsion

	MCT as carrier		PG as carrier	
	Bulk corn oil[a]	Corn oil emulsion[b]	Bulk corn oil[a]	Corn oil emulsion
Rosemary	1.7	12.0	1.7	32.0
Sage	1.5	4.0	1.5	19.0
Thyme	1.1	1.3	1.2	8.4
Oregano	1.0	1.2	1.1	7.0
Spice Cocktail P[c]	1.5	2.5	1.4	27.0
Ginger	1.0	1.6	1.0	2.0
Turmeric	1.0	1.0	1.0	1.6
Cloves	1.0	8.9	1.0	13.0
Bay leaves	1.0	1.1	1.0	1.1

[a]Rancimat at 110°C.
[b]Oxygen electrode at 30°C with heme catalyst.
[c]Composition: 2/5 rosemary, 1/5 sage, 1/5 thyme, 1/5 oregano.

effective in the bulk oil, whereas carnosol (more lipophilic) was more performant in the emulsion. The pH of the emulsion was also found to be important. The so-called "polar paradox" has been advanced to explain this phenomenon, i.e., that polar antioxidants are more effective in nonpolar lipids and nonpolar antioxidants are more active in polar lipid emulsions (Porter et al., 1989). The higher activity of extracts with PG as carrier compared to extracts with MCT as carrier can be attributed to additional polar substances, such as rosmarinic acid and flavonoids, which are extracted by PG (Aeschbach and Rossi, 1995). These observations have important implications for application of antioxidants in foods.

Rosemary extracts are especially efficient at high temperatures, leading to their application in frying oils. Not only do these extracts protect the oil during frying, but because of their carry-over effect they have an antioxidant activity in the fried foods. Figure 13.12 shows the IP and Totox values (anisidine value + 2 × peroxide value) of peanut oil stabilized with either TBHQ or rosemary extract plus citric acid in which French fries had been fried (180°C). The rosemary preparation behaves better than TBHQ under these conditions. In another trial with oriental noodles fried (130°C) in palm oil stabilized with TBHQ and rosemary extract plus citric acid (Fig. 13.13), the noodles fried in both stabilized oils were still acceptable after 6 months of storage at room temperature, while the control noodles (fried in palm oil containing no added antioxidant) were oxidized. This efficiency of rosemary extracts at high temperatures can be related to the different

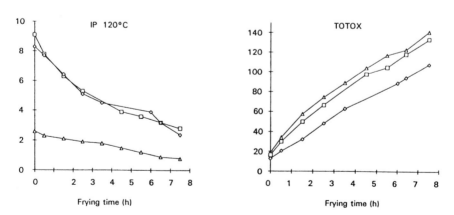

FIG. 13.12   Activity of deodorized rosemary extract with added citric acid compared to TBHQ in frying oil (peanut at 180°C) in which French fries had been fried. △, No addition; □, TBHQ 0.02%; ◇, rosemary extract 0.4% and citric acid 0.04%.

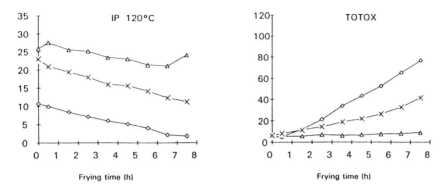

FIG. 13.13 Activity of deodorized rosemary extract with added citric acid compared to TBHQ in frying oil (palm at 130°C) in which oriental noodles had been fried. ◇, No addition; △, TBHQ 0.02%; X, rosemary extract 0.4% and citric acid 0.04%.

TABLE 13.5 Amount of Pentane Formed in the Headspace of Various Foods after 3 Months Storage at 30°C (arbitrary units)

	Rosemary extract (0.05%)	BHA (0.015%)	Ref. (no addition)
Rice flakes	10	5	55
Wheat flakes	2	1	3
Oat flakes	6	2	13
Potato flakes	1.5	1	5
Frozen pork patties	6	2	≫10

Source: Löliger, 1989.

TABLE 13.6 Amount of Pentane Formed in the Headspace of Millet Dried by Various Techniques after 3 Months Storage at 30°C (pmol/liter)

	Rosemary crude extract (0.05%)	Rosemary purified extract (0.05%)	Propyl gallate (0.02%)	Ref. (no addition)
Drum-dried	29.5	12.2	9.0	44.2
Vacuum-dried	1.9	1.4	1.2	10.9
Freeze-dried	4.8	4.5	2.7	4.4
Extruded	3.8	4.5	3.3	4.5

Source: Percheron and Löliger, 1990.

TABLE 13.7 Efficiency of Rosemary Extracts in a Variety of Food Applications

Food (storage temperature)	Amount of extract	Effectiveness[a]	Comments
Dried oats (30°C)	0.02%, 0.04%, and 0.08%	+++	Equal to propyl gallate after 12 months
Ham (−25°C)	0.01% and 0.02%	+++	No oxidation after 14 months
Dehydrated meat dumplings (30°C)	0.06%	+++	Good after 6 months
Roasted hazelnuts (30°C)	0.05%	+++	Most effective antioxidant
Dehydrated bacon (30°C)	0.05%	++	Acceptable after 18 months
Dehydrated salmon (30°C)	0.05%	++	Acceptable after 18 months
Dehydrated cream (20°C)	0.1%	+	Acceptable after 12 months
Dried milk (30°C)	0.02%, 0.04%, and 0.08%	+/−	No favorable effect, rosemary off-taste

[a]Judgments range from − − − (bad) to +++ (good).

radical species observed by ESR spectroscopy and discussed in the preceding section.

The effectiveness of rosemary extracts in various foods compared to that of the synthetic antioxidant BHA is shown in Table 13.5 (Löliger, 1989). While slightly less active than BHA, rosemary extracts showed good results in these foods compared to the unprotected reference. In another study stabilization of millet flakes prepared by several procedures was investigated (Table 13.6) (Percheron and Löliger, 1990). Both rosemary extracts inhibited oxidation and were only slightly less effective than propyl gallate.

A summary of different food applications in which activity of rosemary extracts has been evaluated is given in Table 13.7. As can be expected from their activity in animal fats (Table 13.3), rosemary extracts were particularly effective in meat products. The good results in dried oats and dehydrated salmon, both containing highly unsaturated fatty acids, are therefore somewhat surprising. This shows how difficult it is to extrapolate from activity of an antioxidant in oils obtained by accelerated tests to real food applications. Relatively unfavorable results obtained in bland products such as dehydrated cream and dried milk also show the possible negative effect of the carry-over of rosemary flavor compounds in the antioxidant extract. As mentioned above, there is little masking of the spicy flavors in bland products.

CONCLUSIONS

Results obtained from the application trials discussed above, both positive and negative, indicate that suitability of an individual antioxidant for a particular application has, at present, to be determined on a case-by-case basis, as it is difficult to predict the efficiency of a particular antioxidant in a given food. Recommendations for choice of antioxidant, dose levels, and method of incorporation are often based on the food technologist's past experience. A fundamental understanding of the mechanism of antioxidant activity, obtained from, for example, ESR studies, could be the first step in determining the optimum use of antioxidants. The cascade of radicals from carnosic acid formed at high temperatures observed by ESR and the good antioxidant activity of rosemary extracts during frying is an example.

REFERENCES

Aeschbach, R., Baechler, R., Rossi, P., Sandoz, L., and Wille, H.-J. 1994a. Mechanical extraction of plant antioxidants by means of oils. *Fat Sci. Technol.* 96: 441–443.

Aeschbach, R., Lambelet, P., and Löliger, J. 1994b. Mechanistic studies on lipid antioxidant action and their application to food. Royal Society of Chemistry Symposium, London, December 2.

Aeschbach, R. and Philppossian, G. 1988. Procédé d'obtention d'un extrait antioxydant d'épices. European patent 307,626.

Aeschbach, R. and Rossi, P. 1995. Procédé d'extraction d'antioxydants de matière végétale. European patent A-95, 102, 439.7.

Aeschbach, R. and Wille, H.-J. 1992. Procédé d'obtention d'un extrait liquide d'antioxydant d'épices. European patent 507,064.

Aeschbach, R. and Wille, H.-J. 1993. Procédé d'extraction d'antioxydant d'origine végétale sous forme liquide. European patent 639,336.

Aruoma, O. I., Halliwell, B., Aeschbach, R., and Löliger, J. 1992. Antioxidant and pro-oxidant properties of active rosemary constituents: Carnosol and carnosic acid. *Xenobiotica* 22: 257–268.

Barrera-Arellano, B. and Esteves, W. 1992. Oxidative stability of potato chips determined by Rancimat. *J. Am. Oil Chem. Soc.* 69: 335–337.

Burton, G. W. and Ingold, K. U. 1986. Vitamin E: Application of the principles of physical organic chemistry to the exploration of its structure and function. *Acc. Chem. Res.* 19: 194–201.

Carpenter, A. P. 1979. Determination of tocopherols in vegetable oils. *J. Am. Oil Chem. Soc.* 56: 668–671.

Dawson, L. E. and Gartner, R. 1983. Lipid oxidation in mechanically deboned poultry. *Food Technol.* 37: 112–116.

Decker, E. A. and Crum, A. D. 1991. Inhibition of oxidative rancidity in salted ground pork by carnosine. *J. Food Sci.* 56: 1179–1181.

deMan, J. M., Tie, F., and deMan, L. 1987. Formation of short chain volatile organic acids in the automated AOM method. *J. Am. Oil Chem. Soc.* 64: 993–996.

Farr, D. R., Löliger, J., and Savoy, M.-C. 1986. Foods protected by the important biological antioxidant: Uric acid. *J. Sci. Food Agric.* 37: 804–810.

Forrester, A. R., Hay, J. M., and Thomson, R. H. 1968. Nitroxides. In *Organic Chemistry of Stable Free Radicals*, pp. 180–246. Academic Press, London.

Frankel, E., Huang, S.-W., Aeschbach, R., and Prior, E. 1996. Antioxidant activity of a rosemary extract and its constituents, carnosic acid, carnosol and rosmarinic acid in bulk oil and oil-in-water emulsion. *J. Agr. Food Chem.* 44.

Geoffroy, M., Lambelet, P., and Richert, P. 1994. Radical intermediates and antioxidants: An ESR study of radicals formed on carnosic acid in the presence of oxidized lipids. *Free Rad. Res.* 21: 247–258.

Gottstein, T. and Grosch, W. 1990. Model study of different antioxidant properties of alpha- and gamma-tocopherol in fats. *Fat Sci. Technol.* 92: 139–144.

Kramer, R. E. 1985. Antioxidants in cloves. *J. Am. Oil Chem. Soc.* 62: 111–113.

Lambelet, P., Ducret, F., Saucy, F., Savoy, M.-C., and Löliger, J. 1987. Generation of radicals from antioxidant-type molecules by polyunsaturated lipids. *J. Chem. Soc. Faraday Trans. 1* 83: 141–149.

Lambelet, P., Saucy, F., and Löliger, J. 1985. Chemical evidence for interactions between vitamin E and vitamin. *Experientia* 41: 1384–1388.

Lambelet, P., Saucy, F., and Löliger, J. 1994. Radical exchange reactions between vitamin E, vitamin C and phospholipids in autoxidizing polyunsaturated lipids. *Free Rad. Res.* 20: 1–10.

Löliger, J. 1989. Natural antioxidants for the stabilization of foods. In *Flavor Chemistry*, D. B. Min and T. Smouse (Ed.), pp. 302–325. American Oil Chemists' Society, Champaign, IL.

Löliger, J. 1990. Headspace gas analysis of volatile hydrocarbons as a tool for the determination of the state of oxidation of foods. *J. Sci. Food Agric.* 52: 119–128.

Löliger, J. and Saucy, F. 1989. A synergistic antioxidant mixture. European patent 0326829.

Lunder, T. L. 1992. Catechins of green tea. Antioxidant activity. In *Phenolic Compounds in Food and Their Effects on Health II. Antioxidants and Cancer Prevention*, M.-T. Huang, C.-T. Ho, and C. Y. Lee (Ed.), pp. 114–120. American Chemical Society, Washington, DC.

Müller-Mulot, W. 1976. Rapid method for the quantitative determination of individual tocopherols in oils and fats. *J. Am. Oil Chem. Soc.* 53: 732–736.

Niki, E., Tsuchiya, J., Tanimura, R., and Kamiya, Y. 1982. Regeneration of vitamin E from alpha-chromanoxyl radical by glutathione and vitamin C. *Chem. Lett.* 6: 789–792.

Packer, J. E., Slater, T. F., and Wilson, R. L. 1979. Direct observation of a free radical interaction between vitamin E and vitamin C. *Nature* 278: 737–738.

Percheron, E. and Löliger, J. 1990. Influence of drying technology on precooked cereal autoxidation. *Lebensm. Wiss. Technol.* 23: 400–403.

Perrin, J.-L. 1992. Les composés mineurs et les antioxygènes naturels de l'olive et de son huile. *Rev. Fr. Corps Gras* 39: 25–32.

Porter, W. L., Black, E. D., and Drolet, A. M. 1989. Use of polyamide oxidative fluorescence test on lipid emulsions. Contrast in relative effectiveness of antioxidants in bulk versus dispersed systems. *J. Agric. Food Chem.* 37: 615–624.

Prior, E. and Löliger, J. 1994. Spectrophotometric and chromatographic assays. In *Rancidity in Foods*, 3rd ed., J. C. Allen and R. J. Hamilton (Ed.), pp. 104–127. Blackie Academic and Professional, Glasgow.

Rossel, J. B. 1994. Measurement of rancidity. In *Rancidity in Foods*, 3rd ed., J. C. Allen and R. J. Hamilton (Ed.), pp. 22–53. Blackie Academic and Professional, Glasgow.

Sandmeier and Ziegleder. 1982.

Saucy, F., Ducret, F., Lambelet, P., and Löliger, J. 1990. The fate of antioxidant radicals during lipid autoxidation. II. The influence of oxygen supply on lipid autoxidation. *Chem. Phys. Lipids* 55: 215–221.

Schwarz, K. and Ternes, W. 1992a. Antioxidative constituents of *Rosmarinus officinalis* and *Salvia officinalis*. I. Determination of phenolic diterpenes with antioxidative activity amongst tocochromanols using HPLC. *Z. Lebensm. Unters. Forsch.* 195: 95–98.

Schwarz, K. and Ternes, W. 1992b. Antioxidative constituents of *Rosmarinus officinalis* and *Salvia officinalis*. II. Isolation of carnosic acid and formation of other phenolic diterpenes. *Z. Lebensm. Unters. Forsch.* 195: 99–103.

Takahashi, M., Tsuchiya, J., and Niki, E. 1989. Oxidation of lipids. XVI. Inhibition of autoxidation of methyl linoleate by diarylamines. *Bull. Chem. Soc. Jpn.* 62: 1880–1884.

Tappel, A. L. 1968. Will antioxidant nutrients slow ageing processes? *Geriatrics* 23: 97–105.

Wille H.-J., Löliger, J., Gonus, P., Prior, E., and Studer, M. 1994. Lipid stability measurements by monitoring pressure changes. *American Oil Chemists Society Annual Meeting*, Atlanta, GA, May 8–12.

Zhu, J., Johnson, J., Sevilla, C. L., Herrington, J. W., and Sevilla, M. D. 1990. An electron spin resonance study of the reactions of lipid peroxyl radicals with antioxidants. *J. Phys. Chem.* 94: 7185–7190.

Zürcher, K. and Hadorn, H. 1979. Erfahrungen mit der Bestimmung der Induktionzeit von Speiseölen. *Gordian* 79: 182–185.

14

Evaluation of Lipid Quality and Stability

Kathleen Warner

National Center for Agricultural Utilization Research
Agricultural Research Service
U.S. Department of Agriculture
Peoria, Illinois

INTRODUCTION

Lipid oxidation is the major cause of flavor deterioration in fats, oils, and fat-containing foods. Although there are many methods to measure oxidation, the original method used to determine oxidation was probably the most sensitive instrument and is still in use today—the human nose. Human sensory perception is the optimum assessment of the oxidative state of a food product, and we frequently judge the suitability of instrumental and chemical analyses of oxidation by their ability to correlate with sensory evaluations. However, we still would like to have a test that can effectively duplicate sensory perceptions—a test that is more reliable, quicker, and less expensive. Unfortunately, no instrument or chemical analysis can yet fully replace the nose in detecting oxidized lipids.

Today, the scientist conducting lipid oxidation analyses has a long list of methods to choose from. Almost 100 years ago, when Kreis developed a qualitative test to measure oxidation, no instrumental or chemical tests existed to either qualitatively or quantitatively analyze lipids for oxidation.

In the 1930s, Joyner and McIntyre (1938) developed an oven test for measuring stability, which became known as the Schaal Oven Test. Lea (1931) and Wheeler (1932) published quantitative methods for peroxide determination to serve as an indices for oxidized fats. These methods were followed by the accelerated method known as the Swift Test or the Active Oxygen Method (AOM) developed by King and coworkers (1948). Research on the stability of fats and oils was enhanced by the development of standardized sensory tests, specifically for oils in the 1940s (Moser et al., 1947). Until this development, progress on the stability of soybean oil was limited by the lack of a suitable method to analyze the quality aspects of oil. From the 1940s through the 1960s, sensory evaluation played a significant role in determining the effects of processing research on oil stability (Cowan, 1965). The next major advance in oxidation methods came in the 1960s when gas chromatographic analysis of volatile compounds of lipids was initiated. Evans (1967) and coworkers (Evans et al., 1967) developed a direct injection technique for volatiles, which was refined by Dupuy et al. (1974). Researchers found that pentane, a breakdown product of linoleic acid, served as a marker for development of rancid flavor, as measured by a sensory panel (Evans et al., 1969). Later, static and dynamic headspace techniques were adopted and, together with the use of capillary columns, improved the science of analyzing volatile compounds (Snyder et al., 1988).

Selecting appropriate methods to measure oxidation and stability can be a problem for scientists because of the many tests available and lack of knowledge of what they measure. Several excellent papers reviewing oxidation measurement methods have been written by Frankel (1993), Gray (1978), and Melton (1983). The purpose of this chapter is to present the principal methods for measuring lipid oxidation and stability in foods that are available today and to discuss what products these methods measure and the advantages and limitations of the methods. In addition, suggested criteria for choosing oxidation procedures are included, as well as recommended protocols for evaluating food lipid oxidation and stability. Methods for measuring heated oil stability, such as in frying applications, are included in another chapter.

CRITERIA FOR SELECTING OXIDATION METHODS

The correlation or relationship of instrumental or chemical analyses to the sensory characteristics of a food is the ultimate goal of most oxidation measurements. We want to know how oxidation has affected the flavor of food lipids. In some instances, analytical sensory panels are used to assess the extent of oxidative deterioration. Many chemical and physical methods have been developed to assess the extent of oxidative deterioration of oil with the object of correlating the data with the development of off-flavors. What criteria should be used to determine whether a particular procedure is used to measure oxidation? According to Gray (1978), the following questions must be asked in making this determination:

What property is the method measuring?

Does the property arise from circumstances other than oxidation?

Is the method specific for that property?

Does the property adequately represent the extent to which oxidation has occurred?

Some procedures, such as the thiobarbituric acid (TBA) test, measure a wide range of nonspecific compounds; so using only one chemical test may not give much information about flavor stability.

SELECTION OF METHODS

According to Erickson and Bowers (1976), the lipid researcher should be aware of the following before choosing oxidation methods:

Dynamic character and complexity of the reactions involved in lipid oxidation

Low levels of peroxide decomposition products causing significant off-flavors

Realistic correlation with sensory evaluation

Judicious selection and interpretation of accelerated storage techniques as they relate to the normal situation in foods

The first two aspects, proposed by Erickson and Bowers (1976), are based on the fact that lipid oxidation is a complex process, involving many reactions and resulting in many changes over a period of time (Frankel, 1980, 1982, 1984b; Paquette et al., 1985a,b). For example, in the early stages of oxidation, peroxides, develop, conjugated dienes form, and oxygen uptake occurs. As the initial products accumulate and decompose, secondary oxidation products, such as carbonyls, form. Therefore, the times for sampling during the oxidation process are critical in producing valid analyses of oxidation. One data point by itself is of little value unless the history of the sample is known. The degree of oxidation should be determined at approximate time intervals by more than one method and by measuring different types of products, including initial and decomposition products of lipid oxidation (Frankel, 1993). Generally, the methods to measure oxidation are based on measuring primary (initial oxidation products) or secondary (decomposition) oxidation products; however, the primary products are only precursors to the secondary products, some of which produce off-flavors. Initial products of oxidation, such as hydroperoxides, are considered precursors of flavor compounds and can be estimated by determining the peroxide value or level of conjugated dienes. Decomposition products of oxidation can be measured, for example, by analyses of carbonyl compounds or volatiles by gas chromatography, and the effect of these products on the flavor quality and stability can be measured by sensory analysis. However, whatever approach to lipid oxidation analysis is chosen, it should be noted that no method is as sensitive as sensory evaluations done by a well-trained, experienced, analytical panel. Instrumental or chemical analysis is capable of verifying what is determined by the sensory panel, provided the analytical procedures are used and interpreted correctly. The ultimate criterion or the suitability of any oxidation measurement test is its agreement with sensory perception of flavors and odors (Gray, 1985). A thorough understanding of the mechanisms and products of lipid oxidation is needed when determining which oxidation tests to use (Frankel, 1993).

METHODS TO MEASURE LIPID OXIDATION

A wide variety of methods for measuring lipid oxidation have been reported in the literature (Table 14.1). Peroxide value and conjugated diene—methods that measure primary oxidation—will be discussed first, followed by carbonyl value, anisidine value, thiobarbituric acid–reactive substances (TBARS), volatile compounds, and sensory methods that measure second-

TABLE 14.1 Methods to Measure Oxidation in Oils and Fat-Containing Foods

Method	Parameter assessed
Sensory	Odors/Flavors
Peroxide value	Peroxides
TBARS	Malonaldehyde + unknown compounds
Carbonyl value	All carbonyl functions
Anisidine value	Gamma- and beta-unsaturated carbonyls
Kreis test	Epoxyaldehydes
Ultraviolet absorption	Conjugated dienes/trienes
Gas chromatography	Volatile compounds

ary oxidation products. However, the first method, the Kreis test, is included in this discussion not because it is a recommended procedure, but for historical interest, because it was one of the first tests used to evaluate the oxidation of fats. All methods will be discussed in terms of what characteristics, or properties, they measure and to what extent those properties represent the oxidative state of the lipid. In addition, we will discuss how well these methods correlate with sensory evaluation and the effects of elevated temperatures on the analyses.

The Kreis Test

The Kreis test, which was first published in 1902, measures the production of a red color as phloroglucinol reacts with oxidized fat in an acid solution (Dugan, 1955). Epoxy aldehydes, or their acetals, are thought to be the compounds responsible for the Kreis color reaction of oxidized fats; however, the development of color does not necessarily parallel the development of rancid flavor (Dugan, 1955). Unaged oil samples can show some color when they are reacted with the Kreis reagent. In addition, it is sometimes difficult to obtain comparable results in different laboratories. Although the Kreis test can indicate slight changes in the oxidation of a fat under various circumstances, it does not provide a satisfactory index of rancidity (Gray, 1978). Very few lipid scientists use the Kreis test today because of these problems and because many other methods exist that measure more specific oxidation products.

Peroxide Value

Hydroperoxides—often called peroxides—are major initial reaction products of lipid oxidation and are formed as oxygen reacts with unsaturated fatty acids. Hydroperoxides accumulate to a maximum point, then decompose to form compounds, such as carbonyls, that are responsible, in part, for the typical oxidation flavors, such as rancid or painty. Peroxides can be determined either spectrophotometrically (Chapman and MacKay, 1949) or by iodometric titration, the American Oil Chemists' Society recommended practice Cd 8-53 (1994), which is applicable to most fats and oils. The highly empirical AOCS method determines all substances—peroxides or similar fat oxidation products—in terms of milliequivalents of peroxide per 1000 g of sample that oxidize potassium iodide under the test conditions. The calculation for the PV is expressed as:

$$mEq/kg = \frac{(\text{Titration of sample, mL}) - (\text{Titration of blank, mL})}{(\text{Normality of Na thiosulfate solution})(1000)\text{g of oil}}$$

Since the peroxide value measures products produced in the initial period of oxidation, which are susceptible to decomposition, it is important to monitor the oxidation process over time to know what phase of oxidation the oil system is in. Peroxides do not have any odor or flavor themselves, so they do not have a cause-and-effect relationship with flavor evaluation. However, peroxide values correlate highly with sensory scores for such oils as soybean, sunflower, and canola (Warner et al., 1989). Liu and White (1992) calculated significant correlation coefficients between peroxide values and flavor quality scores of aged soybean oils. Frankel and Huang (1994) reported significant differences in oxidative stability of soybean oil, high oleic sunflower oil, and blends of these two oils based on the spectrophotometric method of determining peroxides (Fig. 14.1). White and Miller (1988) measured the effect of oxidation temperature on the levels of peroxides found in normal and modified soybean oils. They reported that similar total peroxide levels were reached in 6–8 days at 60°C compared to 46–67 days at 28°C. In addition, fewer significant differences in peroxide

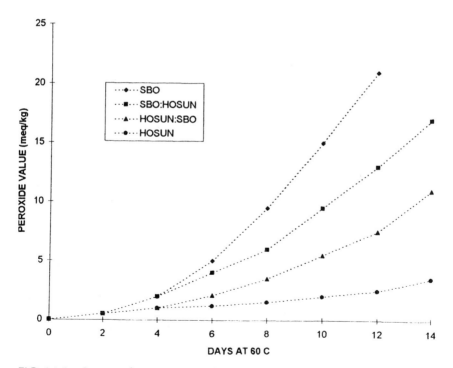

FIG. 14.1   Spectrophotometric analysis of peroxide content of aged soybean (SBO) and high oleic sunflower (HOSUN) oils and blends. (*From Frankel and Huang, 1994.*)

levels were noted between oil types at 60°C than at 28°C. Fat-containing foods can also be analyzed for peroxides by first extracting the oil from the food and conducting the peroxide analysis. Other advantages of the AOCS peroxide value method include low cost and ease of testing. Two main limitations of the peroxide value method are that the method only measures primary oxidation products and that any variation in procedure may result in variation in results.

Conjugated Dienes

Oxidation can cause double bond position shifts in polyunsaturated fatty acids that can be measured by increased ultraviolet absorption. In the process, conjugated diene structures are then formed and are an indication of primary oxidation products. Fatty acids with conjugated unsaturation absorb in the region of 230–375 nm, diene unsaturation at 234 nm, and triene unsaturation at 268 nm. Changes in the ultraviolet spectrum of an oil can be used as a relative measurement of oxidation (Gray, 1978). The conjugated diene value is expressed as a percentage of conjugated dienoic acid in the oil. The AOCS method Ti 1a-64 is a spectrophotometric determination of conjugated dienoic acid in oils. According to White (1995), conjugated diene values generally range from 0–6%, depending upon the oil type, and will increase with increasing unsaturation. Both conjugated dienes and peroxide values increase with increasing storage time, plateau, and then decrease as further oxidation and decomposition occur. This is illustrated by the work of Tautorus and McCurdy (1990) in using conjugated diene measurements to compare the oxidative stability of native and randomized soybean oils (Fig. 14.2). Conjugated diene values for samples aged at 55°C increased rapidly, then plateaued, whereas, the values for oils aged at ambient temperature increased slowly with time and showed significant

TABLE 14.2 Changes During Oxidation of Fatty Acids

Primary Changes
Oxygen uptake
Loss of polyunsaturated fatty acids
Formation of hydroperoxides
Secondary Changes
Formation of carbonyls
Formation of malonaldehyde
Formation of hydrocarbons

Source: Gray and Monahan, 1992.

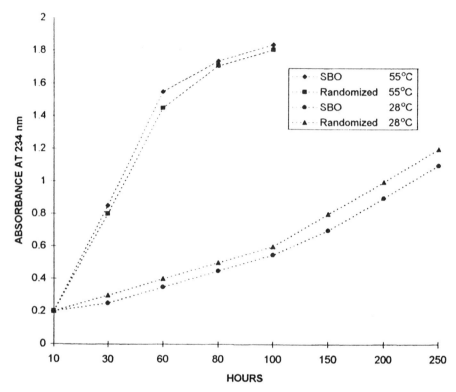

FIG. 14.2   Conjugated diene analysis of randomized and unrandomized soybean oils aged at 55°C and 28°C. (*From Tautorus and McCurdy, 1990.*)

differences at 28°C, but not at 55°C. White and Miller (1988) also found that storage temperature during oxidation affected the amount of difference between soybean oils with 3.7 and 9.1% linolenic acid. At 28°C, significant differences exist in the percentage of conjugated dienes between the two oils after 18 days of storage; however, no differences were noted between samples aged at 60°C. The conjugated diene analysis has good accuracy and reproducibility and can be used for edible vegetable oils with high polyunsaturated fatty acid levels. The usefulness of this test is limited since it only measures primary oxidation products.

Carbonyl Value

Carbonyl compounds are formed as hydroperoxides decompose to low molecular weight volatile compounds—secondary oxidation products—that include aldehydes and ketones (carbonyls), hydrocarbons, alcohols, ethers, lactones, furans, and acids. Volatile carbonyls are responsible, in part, for flavors typical of oxidized oils. The carbonyl analysis proposed by Henick et al. (1954) is widely used and is based on the formation of 2,4-dinitrophenylhydrazones of the carbonyl compounds in the presence of a trichloroacetic acid catalyst. Henick reported maximum absorption of the 2,4-dinitrophenylhydrazones of saturated aldehydes at 432 nm and of saturated aldehydes at 458 nm. The Japanese Oil Chemists' Society has an official method for measuring carbonyl content (No. 2.4.22-73) in which colored hydrazones can be measured spectrophotometrically at 440 nm, which is expressed as μmol hexanal/g fat. In a well-refined oil, the carbonyl value should be in the range of 0.5–2.0 μmol/g fat (White, 1995). Boki et al. (1991) used carbonyl analysis to compare the oxidative stabilities of oxidized soybean oils before and after filtering through activated carbon (Fig. 14.3). The treated soybean oil had significantly greater stability after treatment for up to 75 days. Carbonyl analyses are sensitive and measure secondary oxidation products that relate directly to off-flavors. The method is

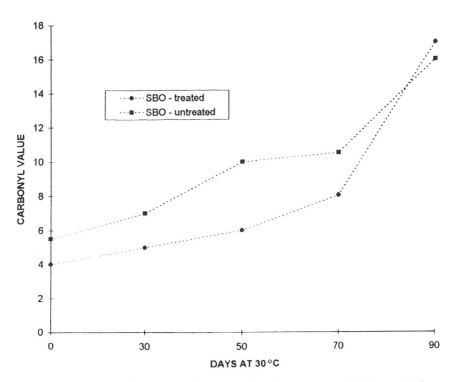

FIG. 14.3   Carbonyl value analysis of oxidized soybean oil before and after filtering through activated carbon. (*From Boki et al., 1991.*)

limited by findings that the analysis is also sensitive to carbonyls found in the test solvents and that the procedure can cause hydroperoxide decomposition, which may give misleading results (Gray, 1978). In addition, the method only measures carbonyls and not other flavor-producing compounds, such as alcohols or hydrocarbons.

Anisidine Value

Aldehydes that decompose from hydroperoxides are responsible for many of the off-flavors in oxidized oils. Some of these aldehydes—2 alkenals and 2,4-dienals—react with p-anisidine to create a yellow color measured at an absorbance of 350 nm. The intensity of the yellow color depends on the level of aldehydic compounds and on their structure. The absorbance is increased four to five times when the double bond in the carbon chain is conjugated with the carbonyl double bond (AOCS, 1994). Holm et al. (1957) developed a test reacting aldehydes with benzidine acetate, which was adopted as standard method 2.504 of the International Union of Pure and Applied Chemistry (IUPAC, 1987).

The AOCS (1990) has an Official Method Cd 18-90 for the p-anisidine value for oxidized animal and vegetable fats and oils. Well-refined oils generally have anisidine values between 1.0 and 10.0 mmol/kg fat (White, 1995), and the anisidine value for an unaged soybean oil should be less than 2.0 to indicate good stability (AOCS, 1994). List et al. (1974) found that the anisidine values were lower during all processing stages for soybean oil from sound beans compared to oil from damaged beans (Fig. 14.4). The peroxide value (PV) and anisidine value (AV) can be expressed as a total of some of the primary and secondary oxidation products in an oxidized oil. The standard equation, often referred to as TOTOX for total oxidation (OV) is OV = AV + 2 (PV). The simple anisidine value method is useful for monitoring changes during oil processing, but the method is limited by the fact that only higher molecular weight compounds are measured.

TBA-Reactive Substances

To conduct a TBARS analysis, the sample is heated at low pH with TBA, and the resulting pink chromogen is measured by absorbance at 532 nm or by fluorescence at 553 nm. Most of the aldehydes that react with TBA are derived from peroxides and unsaturated fatty acids during the test procedure. The TBARS test is widely used in meats (Melton, 1983) and in biological samples (Gutteridge and Halliwell, 1994) because it is simple and sensitive; however, TBARS is also a nonspecific assay for lipid oxidation and other radical reaction products, therefore, results can be overestimated. Browning reaction products and aldehydes from nonoxidative sources can

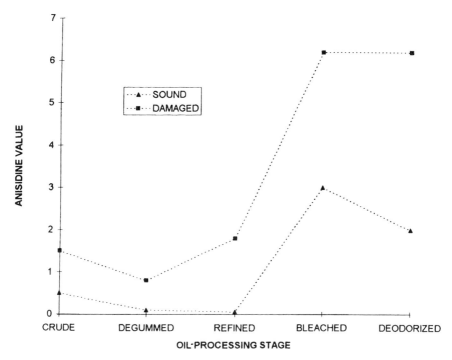

FIG. 14.4   Anisidine values for oils from sound soybeans and damaged soybeans at each oil-processing stage. (*From List et al., 1974.*)

interfere with the TBARS color reaction and give misleading results and poor correlations with flavor (Gray, 1978). The test is not recommended for oils with less than three double bonds (Frankel, 1993). Melton (1983) extensively discussed limitations of the TBA test and the precautions that should be taken in conducting the analysis and interpreting the results. Because of the nonspecific nature of the TBARS analysis, other measurements of oxidation that have superior chemical specificity should be used (Gray and Monahan, 1992).

Gas Chromatographic Volatiles Analyses

Before the 1960s, researchers had to use complicated collection procedures, such as distillation, to obtain volatile compounds from oils and fat-containing foods for analysis. In 1966, Scholz and Ptak (1966) published a procedure for easily determining pentane in oil and correlating the results with sensory evaluation. Evans (1967) developed a specially designed glass tube that was placed in the inlet of a heated gas chromatograph for analyzing hydrocarbons in oxidized soybean oil. Evans et al. (1967, 1969) also reported that the pentane formed during the decomposition of oxidized soybean oil correlated with flavor scores. Pentane also correlated significantly with rancid flavor development in potato chips (Warner et al., 1974). Dupuy et al. (1971) expanded on this prior work on direct injection techniques by placing vegetable oils on glass wool in the heated inlet liner of a gas chromatograph. The volatile compounds were eluted onto the packed column for peak separation. Dynamic headspace (purge and trap) and static headspace methods have gained attention since commercial instrumentation was developed during the 1970s. The AOCS recommended practice Cg 4-94 (1994) on volatile organic compounds in fats and oils by gas chromatography describes the three methods—direct injection, static headspace, and dynamic headspace—for measuring volatile compounds related to flavor quality and oxidative stability in oils and fats. Gas chromatographic conditions are given for conducting each type of test.

Volatile compounds are secondary breakdown products of fatty acid oxidation and are therefore direct measures of decomposition products that contribute to off-flavors. Some compounds contribute more to off-flavor development than others. For example, pentane, which is a good marker for monitoring the extent of oxidation, has a relatively high odor threshold and therefore does not contribute much to flavor. On the other hand, compounds such as hexanal and 2,4-decadienal are more directly related to flavor. Even though some volatile compounds, such as pentane, may not have a cause-and-effect relationship with flavor, most compounds show high correlations with flavor (Warner et al., 1974, 1989; Williams and Applewhite, 1977; Morrison et al., 1981; Pongracz, 1986; Raghavan et al., 1989). Chromatographers must keep in mind that the volatiles analysis methods and the temperatures used in the analyses will affect the amounts and types of peaks detected. In comparing the headspace and direct injection methods, Snyder et al. (1988) found that low molecular weight compounds, such as hydrocarbons with fewer than five carbons, were favored by static headspace techniques (Fig. 14.5). Hexanal was uniformly detected by all methods; however, 2,4-decadienal was noted at high amounts by direct injection and at moderate levels by purge and trap. Selke and Frankel (1987) found that the analysis temperature for dynamic headspace significantly affected the amounts and types of volatile compounds detected. For example, soybean oils oxidized to a peroxide value of 5.3 and heated in the purge and trap apparatus at 60°C had low levels of pentane, pentanal, and hexanal. Increasing the purge and trap temperature to 90°C increased the amounts of these compounds; however, many other compounds, including higher molecular weight products such as 2,4-decadienal, were detected

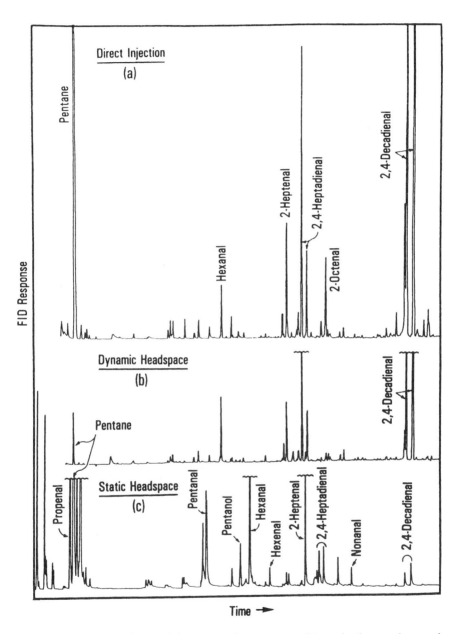

FIG. 14.5   Comparison of three gas chromatographic volatiles analyses of oxidized soybean oils heated to 180°C. (*From Snyder et al., 1988.*)

after heating the oils to 180°C. Przybylski and Eskin (1995) and Snyder (1995) have extensively discussed the procedures as well as advantages and limitations of gas chromatographic volatile analysis.

Sensory Analysis

Sensory evaluation is a scientific discipline for qualitative and quantitative analysis in which testers use their senses of smell, taste, and/or touch to identify odors, tastes, or flavors. In the food industry, sensory evaluation can be used for quality control or in a research laboratory. Testers can range from a technician trained to taste samples from production (quality control) to a group of highly trained and experienced judges identifying types and intensities of sensory characteristics of oils or fat-containing foods.

Sensory evaluation is the ultimate method to assess the quality and stability of fats, oils, and fat-containing foods. Instrumental and chemical methods measure various decomposition products—primary or secondary—that result from oxidation. Only sensory analysis can detect the flavors produced by the decomposition products from oxidation as well as other flavors from nonoxidative processes. Warner et al. (1974) reported that pentane development and rancid flavor intensity were significantly correlated in aged potato chips. However, not all off-flavors and odors are detectable by instrumental and chemical analyses; for example, the compounds responsible for the flavors characteristic of hydrogenation, such as waxy, sweet, and fruity, are not detected by standard instrumental and chemical analyses, but are readily identified by sensory analysis.

The AOCS has a recommended practice, Cg 2-83 (1994), for the flavor panel evaluation of vegetable oils, including information on sample preparation and presentation. In addition, the American Society for Testing and Materials (ASTM) has a standard practice for bulk sampling, handling, and preparing edible vegetable oils for sensory evaluation (ASTM, 1990). Details on setting up and training a sensory panel for oils and fats have been documented by Malcolmson (1995). Information on methods for analyzing oils and fat-containing foods for sensory characteristics has been published by Warner (1995).

When sensory tests are properly conducted by trained, experienced panels, results can provide information as to the type and level of oxidation of the sample. For example, many oils, including soybean, sunflower, and canola, have very little flavor when evaluated immediately after processing. Slight oxidation in the dark will produce nutty and buttery flavors detected at slight intensities. Moderate oxidation in the dark will produce flavors that are characteristic of each oil type. Soybean oil will have flavors such as green grassy and beany, whereas canola and sunflower oil will have sulfur/

cabbagelike flavors and pinelike flavors, respectively. Higher levels of oxidation will produce rancid flavors in all oils and painty flavors in oils containing linolenic acid such as soybean and canola. Finally, oils aged in the light will produce other flavors characteristic of this storage condition. For example, light-exposed soybean oil has grassy, sour, metallic flavors. Sunflower oil, which is not light-sensitive, will not produce flavors characteristic of light exposure as soybean oil does.

Williams and Applewhite (1977) justified the use of gas chromatographic volatile analysis by stating that sensory evaluation does not provide information as to the cause of an inferior taste or to the reason for variation in quality from various refining treatments of different batches of the same raw materials. On the contrary, sensory analysis can detect not only flavors produced by oxidation, but also flavors and odors that may occur due to the nature of the fat, improper processing, or contamination during processing. For example, oils processed using phosphoric acid will sometimes have a characteristic melon flavor. Soybean oils oxidized prior to deodorization will have off-flavors such as grassy and/or beany; however, no indicators of primary oxidation can be detected.

Disadvantages of sensory analysis include lack of reproducibility and sensitivity; however, these problems are usually more common when panelists do not have enough training and/or experience. Trained, experienced sensory testers, operating under controlled conditions, can provide accurate, reliable data.

METHODS TO MEASURE STABILITY

Since the days that scientists waited 2, 4, 6, or more months for an ambient storage test result, researchers have been developing a wide variety of methods to accelerate the oxidation process. Ambient storage remains an ideal test because it duplicates the conditions found during the actual shelf-life process. The accelerated methods use factors such as elevated temperatures, oxygen, metals, and/or light to promote oxidation and reduce the oxidation time from several months to a few days or even hours. It has been estimated that for every 10°C rise in temperature in the range of 97–110°C, the rate of peroxide formation in a fat or oil is approximately doubled (Dugan, 1955). The accelerating effects of heat and oxygen on the oxidative process are the factors most commonly used for speeding up tests to obtain estimates of the stability of fats and oils more quickly. Some of these methods combine accelerated storage with measurement of oxidation. The more commonly used acceleration techniques are presented along with their advantages and limitations.

TABLE 14.3   Methods to Determine Stability

Test	Conditions (°C)	Measurements
Ambient storage	25	Flavors, peroxides, conjugated dienes, carbonyl value, gas chromatographic volatiles
Schaal oven test	45–65	Flavors, peroxides, conjugated dienes, carbonyl value, gas chromatographic volatiles
Active oxygen method	97.8	Peroxides
Rancimat	100–140	Volatile organic acids
Oxidative stability index analysis	100–130	Volatile organic acids
Oxygen uptake	80–100	Headspace oxygen depletion

Source: Adapted from Frankel, 1993.

Oven Storage Test

Oven tests are conducted at elevated temperatures (usually 55–65°C) with periodic evaluation of the samples to determine the point at which rancid flavor develops or some other specific endpoint, such as peroxide value or volatiles content, is reached. Oven storage methods for evaluating fat or oil stability are sometimes referred to as Schaal oven tests, and sensory evaluations are commonly used to determine endpoints. The original oven method, developed in the baking industry in the early 1920s, to provide relative ratings to the shortenings used in crackers, was described by Joyner and McIntyre (1938) as follows: place 50-g samples in 250-mL beakers with a watchglass on top and maintain temperature about 63°C.; smell samples daily until a rancid odor develops. Lea (1962) suggested that a peroxide value endpoint be used to monitor oxidation and the use of 0.2-mL samples in small glass cups, the oil forming about a 2-mm layer on the bottom. The American Oil Chemists' Society has used a modified oven test method, in a collaborative study, that consisted of placing oil in an 8 oz, narrow-mouth glass bottle (2/3 oil; 1/3 headspace-air), and loosely sealing the bottle with a cellophane-covered cork. The sample was aged at 60°C in the dark in a forced-draft oven, and the endpoint was determined by periodically sampling the oil for sensory evaluation, peroxide value, and gas chromatographic volatiles.

The 63°C temperature in the oven method is much lower than the 100°C+ temperatures in many accelerated procedures. Hartman et al. (1975) reported that the oven method gave a better correlation with an actual shelf-life test than did the Active Oxygen Method (AOM). Since the oven test is run at temperatures only moderately greater than those found in ambient storage conditions, results can often be similar to the quality and stability found in consumer markets; however, this effect must be determined for each product. Advantages of the method include the need for minimal equipment and few technical skills to conduct the test. Precautions for the oven test include cleanliness of the glassware and selection of proper endpoint determination. The method is further limited by the time necessary to achieve an induction period for the endpoint of most analyses— usually 4–8 days.

Active Oxygen Method

The AOM, or the Swift Stability Test, was originally proposed by King et al. (1933) as follows: place 20 mL of lipid in 1 in. × 8 in. glass tubes and bubble clean, dry, air at 2.33 cm^3/sec through with temperature maintained at 97.8°C; periodically withdraw about 0.2-mL samples and measure the peroxide value until it reaches 120 mEq/kg. Originally the AOM test was used to measure the resistance of a lard to rancidity. The oil industry enthusiastically accepted this method because it gave rapid analysis and correlated with rancid flavor in lard. The usefulness of this test is questionable today because of the lack of applicability of this method to polyunsaturated oils and the fact that lipid oxidation rates are sensitive to affects of temperature (Ragnarsson and Labuza, 1977; Frankel, 1993). Temperatures of 100°C and above change the mechanisms of lipid oxidation and can give misleading results when compared to ambient temperature storage.

The oil industry frequently used AOM specifications in the past when buying and selling fats and oil, partly because it was an AOCS method (Cd 12-57) and because no suitable substitute had been found to quickly estimate the stability of an oil or fat. The AOCS has designated this AOM method as obsolete (AOCS, 1994) and replaced it with the oxygen stability index (OSI) method. The AOM test is still used by some oil processors and purchasers, although this labor-intensive method is highly empirical and reproducibility is difficult unless close attention is given to controlling such details, such as temperature, air flow, and cleanliness of glassware. The AOCS method specifies at least three titrations during each test, but decreasing the sampling times decreases the reproducibility of the method. The AOM method is suitable for fats and oils—except as noted above—but not fat-containing solid foods. Ragnarsson and Labuza (1977) also reported two other problems with the AOM test. First, the air-bubbling rate for the AOM test is arbitrary rather than oxygen-independent, as with samples aged under ambient conditions. Using higher oxygen pressures than atmospheric is the only way to maintain oxygen independence. Second, volatile antioxidants, such as butylated hydroxy toluene (BHT), can evaporate from the sample. The relationship between results using ambient shelf storage, oven storage, and the AOM test for oils varies with oil type and oil treatment. Protection factors usually vary with the initial stability of the oil.

Oxidative Stability Index

The OSI methods are often referred to as automated AOM tests because they measure the stability of fats and oils at accelerated temperature but without the continuous monitoring needed to run the AOM test. In the OSI procedure, purified air is passed through the oil held at temperatures ranging from 100 to 140°C. deMan and deMan (1984) described a home-built, automated AOM test that measures volatile organic acid as the end-point. AOCS official method Cd 12b-92 outlines the extensive procedures needed to run this test with either the Rancimat or the OSI (AOCS, 1994). The endpoint of the OSI test is determined by monitoring the conductivity of the effluent water to detect the levels of volatile organic acids formed during oxidation (deMan et al., 1987). Hasenhuettl and Wan (1992) used the Rancimat to show relative stabilities of six commonly used edible vege-table oils (Fig. 14.6). A collaborative study for AOCS showed an overall average coenefficient of variation (CV) of 11.3% for 12 samples tested at 110°C by 15 laboratories (Jebe et al., 1993). A CV of 10% was calculated between the results of analyses by eleven laboratories using the Rancimat for 16 samples of rapeseed and palm oils (Woestenburg and Zaalberg (1986). Laubli and Bruttel (1986) calculated a correlation coefficient of 0.99 be-tween results of the AOM and Rancimat analyses for peanut, sunflower, and olive oils, lard, butter, and margarine. The OSI cannot be used at lower temperatures because of the lack of volatile organic acid formation. The OSI is a continuous measurement that does not need periodic determina-tions for endpoint as in the AOM test. Six samples can be run at a time by the Rancimat and up to 24 by the Oxidative Stability Instrument. The OSI test was adopted in 1994 as an official method (Cd 12b-92) by the American Oil Chemists' Society (1994). The OSI has some of the limitations of the AOM test, in that it is conducted at elevated temperatures and the results may not be relevant to normal storage conditions. Results are also susceptible to error if glassware is not scrupulously clean. Finally, fat-containing foods cannot be tested by these methods unless the fat is extracted.

Light Exposure

Some oils and fat-containing foods, including snack foods and milk, are easily photoxidized. For example, soybean oil, which is susceptible to pho-toxidation, was originally packaged in amber bottles to protect it from light exposure. Light-sensitive foods may require methodology to measure the

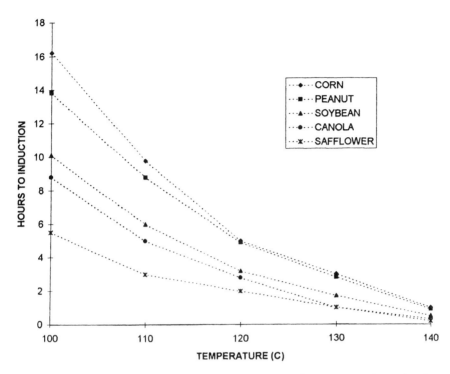

FIG. 14.6   Effect of temperature in oil stability index (OSI) analyses by the Rancimat method. (*From Hasenhuettl and Wan, 1992.*)

stability of these products to light. Early light stability tests included placing oil in clear glass contains in a north-facing window to expose the oil to sunlight to increase the development of off-flavors characteristic of photox-idation. Later, more controlled techniques were developed in which oils were exposed to fluorescent light at specific light intensities, such as 4000–8000 lux (Moser et al., 1965; Warner, 1984). AOCS does not have an official method for light exposure testing; however, a light exposure procedure has been published by Warner et al. (1984, 1987), which was used in an AOCS collaborative study (Waltking, 1981). In the method, oil was placed in a 250-mL, narrow-mouthed, clear glass bottle (2/3 full) with air in the headspace, then the sample was exposed to fluorescent light at 7535 lux (700 ftc) at 30°C. Endpoint determinations have been made by sensory analysis, perox-ide value, or volatile compound measurement. Sensory analysis can detect characteristic flavors produced from photoxidation; for example, a charac-teristic flavor in light-exposed soybean oil is referred to as light-struck and is usually described as green grassy, buttery, and metallic. Light exposure produces increased amounts of 2-heptenal in soybean oil, which can be measured by gas chromatographic volatile analysis (Warner, 1985). Peroxide analysis shows only minor changes in peroxide levels between light-exposed and control oil samples and is not recommended as an index to light stability.

Oxygen Uptake

This accelerated method measures effects of oxidation during the initial stages by measuring the levels of oxygen reacted with the oils. Headspace oxygen is most commonly measured by gas chromatography. Factors influencing oxidative stability tests are temperature, sample size, and surface area. Hahm and Min (1995) have outlined the procedures for headspace oxygen analysis. The depletion headspace oxygen is expressed as the amount of oxygen remaining in the headspace as a concentration percentage (%) or as the remaining or reacted headspace content as $\mu mol/ml$. The most common use for oxygen uptake is in biological systems, although oxidation of meat can be analyzed by this method (Melton, 1983). Two recent studies included oxygen uptake as one of several methods to determine oxidation in fish oil (Davis et al., 1993) and in sunflower, triolein, and corn oil (Roozen et al., 1994).

PROTOCOL FOR OXIDATION AND STABILITY MEASUREMENTS

The degree of oxidation should be determined at suitable time intervals, by more than one method, and by measuring different types of products, including initial and decomposition products of lipid oxidation. Initial products of oxidation, such as hydroperoxides, can be estimated by determining the peroxide value or level of conjugated dienes. Decomposition products of oxidation can be measured by analysis of carbonyl compounds or volatiles by gas chromatography. Initial products provide information on precursors of flavor compounds, and decomposition products are directly related to the flavor compounds affecting quality. If claims are being made about the flavor quality or flavor stability, then sensory evaluation should be incorporated as part of an oil or fat-containing food analysis program that also includes other methods that monitor primary and secondary oxidation products. We have found that sensory evaluation, gas chromatographic volatiles, and peroxide values provide the most information about the quality and stability of salad oils (Warner, 1985). Before gas chromatographic volatile analysis was perfected, Going (1968) reported that flavor and peroxide values effectively measured the deterioration of partially processed soybean oil. No test should stand alone as a measure of quality or stability.

According to Frankel (1993), accelerated conditions must be kept as close as practical to the conditions under which protection against autoxidation is required. A rapid test does not mean that it is a true representation of flavor quality. Frankel (1993) reviewed tests to measure oxidation and concluded that stability tests conducted at high temperatures (100°C and above) may not be indicative of shelf-life stability at lower temperatures. Valid comparisons of oxidative stabilities of edible oils and of the activity of antioxidants in lipids require testing at different storage temperatures, preferably 40–60°C, depending on the rate of oxidation. Each test should be calibrated for each fat or food formulation.

REFERENCES

AOCS. 1994. *Official and Tentative Methods.* American Oil Chemists' Society, Champaign, IL

ASTM. 1990. *Annual Book of ASTM Standards*, pp. 66–68. American Society for Testing and Materials, Philadelphia, PA.

Boki, K., Wada, T., and Ohno, S. 1991. Effects of filtration through activated carbons on peroxide, thiobarbituric acid and carbonyl values of autoxidized soybean oil. *J. Am. Oil Chem. Soc.* 68: 561–565.

Cowan, J. C. 1965. Advances in research on the flavor stability of edible soybean oil—a review. *Food. Technol.* 19: 107–110.

deMan, J. M. and deMan, L. 1984. Automated AOM test for fat stability. *J. Am. Oil Chem. Soc.* 61: 534–536.

deMan, J. M., Tie, F., and DeMan, L. 1987. Formation of short chain volatile organic acids in the automated AOM method. *J. Am. Oil Chem. Soc.* 64: 993–996.

Dugan, L. 1955. Stability and rancidity. *J. Am. Oil Chem. Soc.* 32: 605.

Dupuy, H. P., Fore, S. P., and Goldblatt, L. A. 1971. *J. Am. Oil Chem. Soc.* 48: 876.

Erickson, D. R. and Bowers, R. H. 1976. In *Objective Methods for Food Evaluation*, pp. 133–144. National Academy of Sciences, Washington, DC.

Evans, C. D. 1967. Hydrocarbons derived from autoxidized vegetable oils through thermal splitting. Presented at AOCS Annual Meeting, October 15–18.

Evans, C. D., List, G. R., Dolev, A., McConnell, and Hoffman, R. L. 1967. Pentane from thermal decomposition of lipoxidase-derived products. *Lipids* 2: 432–434.

Evans, C. D., List, G. R., Hoffman, R. L., and Moser, H. 1969. Edible oil quality as measured by thermal release of pentane. *J. Am. Oil Chem. Soc.* 46: 501–504.

Ewbank, F. C. and Gould, I. A. 1942. The oven and aeration methods as means of accelerating fat oxidation. *Oil Soap* 19: 205.

Frankel, E. N. 1980. Lipid oxidation. *Prog. Lipid Res.* 19: 1–22.

Frankel, E. N. 1982. Volatile lipid oxidation products. *Prog. Lipid Res.* 22: 1–33.

Frankel, E. N. 1984a. *Prog. Lipid Res.* 23: 127–145.

Frankel, E. N. 1984b. Chemistry of free radical and singlet oxidation of lipids. *Prog. Lipid Res.* 23: 197–222.

Frankel, E. N. 1993. In search of better methods to evaluate natural antioxidants and oxidative stability in food lipids. *Trends Food Sci. Technol.* 4: 220.

Frankel, E. N. and Huang, S-W. 1994. Improving the oxidative stability of polyunsaturated vegetable oils by blending with high-oleic sunflower oil. *J. Am. Oil Chem. Soc.* 71: 255–259.

Gearhart, W. M., Stuckey, B. N., and Austin, J. J. 1957. Comparison of methods for testing the stability of fats and oils, and of foods containing them. *J. Am. Oil Chem. Soc.* 34: 427.

Going, L. H. 1968. Oxidative deterioration of partially processed soybean oil. *J. Am. Oil Chem. Soc.* 34: 427.

Gray, J. I. 1978. Measurement of lipid oxidation: A review. *J. Am. Oil Chem. Soc.* 45: 632–634.

Gray, J. I. 1985. Simple chemical and physical methods for measuring quality of fats and oils. In *Flavor Chemistry of Fats and Oils*, D. B. Min and T. H. Smouse (Ed.), p. 237. American Oil Chemist's Society, Champaign, IL.

Gray, J. I. and Monahan, F. J. 1992. Measurement of lipid oxidation in meat and meat products. *Trends Food Sci. Technol.* 31: 315.

Gutteridge, J. M. C. 1990. The measurement and mechanism of lipid peroxidation in biological systems. *TIBS* 15: 129.

Hartman, L., Antunes, A. J., Garruti, R. S., and Chaib, M. A. 1975. The effect of free fatty acids on the taste, induction periods, and smoke points of edible oils and fats. *Lebensm. Wiss. Technol.* 8: 114–118.

Hasenhuettl, G. L. and Wan, P. J. 1992. Temperature effects on the determination of oxidative stability with the Metrohm Rancimat. *J. Am. Oil Chem. Soc.* 69: 525–527.

Henick, A. S., Benca, M. F., and Mitchell, J. H. 1954. Estimating carbonyl compounds in rancid fats and foods. *J. Am. Oil Chem. Soc.* 31: 88–91.

Holm, U., Ekbom, K., and Wobe, G. 1957. *J. Am. Oil Chem. Soc.* 34: 606.

IUPAC. 1987. *Standard Methods for the Analysis of Oils, Fats, and Derivatives*, 7th ed. Method Number 2.504. Determination of the p-anisidine value (p-A./V.), Blackwell Scientific Publications, Oxford, UK.

Jebe, T. A., Matlock, M. G., and Sleeter, R. T. 1993. Collaborative study of the oil stability index analysis. *J. Am. Oil Chem. Soc.* 70: 1055–1060.

Joyner, N. T. and McIntyre, J. E. 1938. The Oven test as an index of keeping quality. *Oil Soap* 15: 184–187.

King, A. E., Roschen, H. L., and Irwin, W. H. 1933. *Oil Soap* 10: 105–108.

Laubli, M. W. and Bruttel, P. A. 1986. Determination of the oxidative stability of fats and oils: Comparison between the active oxygen method (AOCS Cd 12-57) and the Rancimat method. *J. Am. Oil Chem. Soc.* 63: 792–795.

Lea, C. H. 1931. *Proc. Royal Soc. London 108B:* 175–177.

Lea, C. H. 1962. The oxidative deterioration of food lipids. In *Lipids and Their Oxidation*, H. W. Schulz (Ed.), pp. 3–28. Avi Publishing Co., Inc., New York.

Liu, H-R. and White, P. J. 1992. Oxidative stability of soybean oils with altered fatty acid compositions. *J. Am. Oil Chem. Soc.* 69: 528–532.

List, G. R., Evans, C. D., Kwolek, W. F., Warner, K., Boundy, B. K., and Cowan, J. C. 1974. Oxidation and quality of soybean oil: A preliminary study of the anisidine test. *J. Am. Oil Chem. Soc.* 51: 17–21.

Malcolmson, L. J. 1995. Organization of a sensory evaluation program. In *Methods to Assess Quality and Stability of Oils and Fat-Containing Foods*, K. Warner and N. A. M. Eskin (Ed.), pp. 37–48. American Oil Chemists' Society, Champaign, IL.

Melton, S. L. 1983. Methodology for following lipid oxidation in muscle foods. *Food Technol.* July: 105.

Morrison, W. H., Lyon, B. G., and Robertson, J. A. 1981. Correlation of gas liquid chromatographic volatiles with flavor intensity scores of stored sunflower oils. *J. Am. Oil Chem. Soc.* 58: 23–27.

Moser, H. A., Evans, C. D., Cowan, J. C., and Kwolek, W. K. 1965. A light test to measure stability of edible oil. *J. Am. Oil Chem. Soc.* 42: 30–33.

Moser, H. A., Jaeger, C. M., Cowan, J. C., and Dutton, H. J. 1947. The flavor problem of soybean oil. *J. Am. Oil Chem. Soc.* 24: 291–296.

Paquette, G., Kupranycz, D. B., and van de Voort, F. R. 1985a. The mechanisms of lipid autoxidation I. Primary oxidation products. 18: 112–118.

Paquette, G., Kupranycz, D. B., and van de Voort, F. R. 1985b. The mechanisms of lipid autoxidation I. Nonvolatile secondary oxidation products. 18: 197–206.

Pongracz, G. 1986. Determination of rancidity of edible oils by headspace gas chromatographic detection of pentane. *Fette Seifen Anstrichmittel* 88: 383–386.

Przybylski, R. and Eskin, N. A. M. 1995. Methods to measure volatile compounds and the flavor significance of volatile compounds. In *Methods to Assess Quality and Stability of Oils and Fat-Containing Foods*, K. Warner and N. A. M. Eskin (Ed.), pp. 107–133. American Oil Chemists' Society, Champaign, IL.

Raghavan, S. K., Reeder, S. K., and Khayat, A. 1989. Rapid analysis of vegetable oil flavor quality by dynamic capillary gas chromatography. *J. Am. Oil Chem. Soc.* 66: 942–947.

Ragnarsson, J. O. and Labuza, T. P. 1977. Accelerated shelf-life testing for oxidative rancidity in foods—a review. *Food Chem.* 2: 291–306.

Scholz, R. G. and Ptak, L. R. 1966. *J. Am. Oil Chem. Soc.* 43: 596–599.

Selke, E. and Frankel, E. N. 1988. Dynamic headspace capillary gas chromatographic analysis of soybean oil volatiles. *J. Am. Oil Chem. Soc.* 64: 749–753.

Sherwin, E. R. 1968. Methods for stability and antioxidant measurement. *J. Am. Oil Chem. Soc.* 45: 632A.

Snyder, J. 1995. Historical and future development of volatile compounds. In *Methods to Assess Quality and Stability of Oils and Fat-Containing Foods*, K. Warner and N. A. M. Eskin (Ed.), pp. 134–145. American Oil Chemists' Society, Champaign, IL.

Snyder, J. M., Frankel, E. N., Selke, E., and Warner, K. 1988. Comparison of gas chromatographic methods for volatile lipid oxidation compounds in soybean oil. *J. Am. Oil Chem. Soc.* 65: 1617–1621.

Tautorus, C. L. and McCurdy, A. R. 1990. Effect of randomization on oxidative stability of vegetable oils at two different temperatures. *J. Am. Oil Chem. Soc.* 67: 525–530.

Warner, K. 1995. Sensory evaluation of oils and fat-containing foods. In *Methods to Assess Quality and Stability of Oils and Fat-Containing Foods*, K. Warner and N. A. M. Eskin (Ed.), pp. 49–75. American Oil Chemists' Society, Champaign, IL.

Warner, K., Evans, C. D., List, G. R., Boundy, K., and Kwolek, W. F. 1974. Pentane formation and rancidity in potato chips. *J. Food Sci.* 39: 761–765.

Warner, K., Frankel, E. N., and Mounts, T. L. 1989. Flavor and oxidative stability of soybean, sunflower and low erucic acid rapeseed oils. *J. Am. Oil Chem. Soc.* 66: 558–564.

Weiss, T. J. 1970. *Food Oils and Their Uses*, p. 21. Avi Publishing Co., New York.

Wheeler, D. H. 1932. *Oil and Soap* 9: 89–92.

White, P. J. 1995. Analyses for conjugated diene, anisidine and carbonyl values. In *Methods to Assess Quality and Stability of Oils and Fat-Containing Foods*, K. Warner and N. A. M. Eskin (Ed.), pp. 159–178. American Oil Chemists' Society, Champaign, IL.

White, P. J. and Miller, L. A. 1988. Oxidative stabilities for low-linolenate, high-stearate and common soybean oils. *J. Am. Oil Chem. Soc.* 65: 1334–1338.

Williams, J. L. and Applewhite, T. H. 1977. Correlation of the flavor scores of vegetable oils with volatile profile data. *J. Am. Oil Chem. Soc.* 54: 461–463.

Woestenburg, W. J. and Zaalberg, J. 1986. Determination of the oxidative stability of edible oils—interlaboratory test with the automated Rancimat method. *Fette Seifen Anstrichmittel* 88: 53–56.

15
Applications of Plant Biotechnology to Edible Oils

Toni Voelker

Calgene Inc.
Davis, California

INTRODUCTION

Vegetable oils are of major economic importance, representing the source for practically all plant-derived fats in our diet. Plants deposit fatty acids in triglycerides for high-density carbon and energy storage. The triglycerides accumulate predominantly in seeds, where the oil can make up a large component of the total weight of the tissue (from several to about 50%). In seeds the oil can be deposited in the resting embryo itself, predominantly in the cotyledons (soybean, rapeseed, sunflower), or in an accessory tissue, called endosperm (coconut, castor bean), or both. The oil is then metabolized by the seedling during germination. In some plants the oil is deposited outside the seed in fruit coats, for example, in the olive. Also, palm oil is extracted from the pericarp (fruit coat) of the oil palm (see Padley et al., 1986, for compositions).

The fatty acid triglyceride composition of a given oil determines its physical, chemical, and nutritional value. For example, acyl chain length and desaturation determine melting characteristics and other functional properties, such as nutritional values (Hegenbart, 1992; see Willett, 1994, for reviews). To date, the fatty acid compositions of commercial oil seeds fall into only a handful of categories. Temperate crops produce highly unsaturated C18 oils, with different degrees of unsaturation (70–94%). Palmitate (16:0) represents most of the saturated fatty acid component in these oils. All are liquid at room temperature and must be hydrogenated in order to be useful for solid fat applications.

Current medium-chain fatty acid (C8–C14) oils are exclusively of tropical origin, with coconut and palm kernel being the predominant sources. Lauric acid (12:0, 40–50%) is the major fatty acid in these oils (Padley et al., 1986). In the United States these oils are mostly used in nonfood applications, but they are found in confectionery and nondairy creamers (Weiss, 1982). Oils with rather unique compositions include palm oil (40% palmitate, 40% oleate, 18:1) and cocoa butter [high stearate (18:0), palmitate], which are used in shortenings, for frying applications, and in confectionery. This rather limited set of fatty acid compositions in commercially important vegetable oils contrasts with the extreme variability found in seed oils of different plant species, where fatty acids may vary with respect to chain length, degree of saturation, and presence of fatty acid–modifying groups (Battey et al., 1989).

Because in many cases the fatty acid composition of a natural oil is nonoptimal for certain applications, there is a history of "upgrading" the raw materials by chemical alteration after harvest or improving the oil resource itself by genetically altering the oil crops. In the past, classical breeding and mutagenesis programs succeeded in the reduction or elimination of certain unwanted fatty acids or the elevation of preferred ones. For example, erucic acid (22:1) was eliminated from rapeseed oil (Stefansson et al., 1961), leading to the highly unsaturated edible oil canola. High-oleic sunflower (Fick, 1989), high-palmitate, or high-stearate soybean varieties have been achieved via this route (Bubeck et al., 1989). In summary, the successes of classical breeding have demonstrated the plasticity of seed oil composition in that significantly large alterations in fatty acid compositions can be made with no apparent detrimental effect on the crop agronomics. Also, the wide variety of plant seed oil compositions found in nature demonstrates that plant cells can produce and accumulate a near limitless variation in storage oils (Hilditch and Williams, 1964).

BIOSYNTHESIS OF PLANT OILS

More recently, as a novel means to alter fatty acid composition, attempts have been made to apply genetic engineering to oil crops. In contrast to classical breeding, which is empirical in nature and mainly restricted to elimination of gene functions or the introduction of genes from close relatives, genetic engineering made possible a rational redesign of a given seed oil using genes from any organism. Transferring these genes to the target species allows the introduction of a novel enzyme, leading (if compatible with the new host) to a new trait, for example, deposition of a fatty acid previously not present in this plant.

In contrast to classical breeding, detailed knowledge of the biosynthetic pathway of plant lipids is necessary in order to define target genes crucial for the engineering of the desired traits. Fortunately, in the past two decades the general framework of plant lipid biosynthesis has been elucidated, and many genes have been cloned (reviewed by Somerville and Browse, 1991; Gibson et al., 1994). A brief outline of this pathway follows—as much as is necessary for the understanding of the engineering of oil composition (the particulars of membrane lipid biosynthesis are excluded).

Like all other plant carbon compounds, fatty acids are ultimately derived from photo assimilate. The de novo fatty acid biosynthesis is located in a special compartment of plant cells, the plastids (chloroplasts are a form of plastids). There, a set of enzymes assembles the carbon chains (Fig. 15.1). In

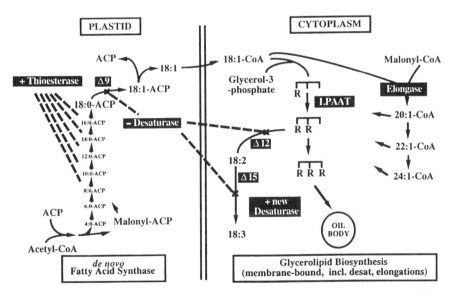

FIG. 15.1 Overview of the plant seed oil biosynthesis: the central double line represents the double membrane separating the de novo fatty acid synthase located in the plastid from the glycerolipid biosynthesis located at the ER of the cytoplasm. Shown are the metabolites important for the discussion. ACP = acyl carrier protein; R = acyl chain. Enzyme targets for engineering are highlighted by a black background; see text for more details. Broken lines point to the position of the respective enzymes in the pathway.

a first step, a 2-carbon primer is attached to a protein, the acyl-carrier protein (ACP). Subsequently, the primer is extended by repeated condensation of C2 components to its chain, i.e., the acyl-ACP grows with each step by 2 carbons. In most plants some of the chain elongation is terminated at the C16 stage, but the majority continues to 18:0-ACP, and subsequently a $\Delta 9$ desaturase ($\Delta 9$: double bond between carbon 9 and 10, when counting from the carboxyl group) forms 18:1-ACP. The fatty acid synthase reactions are terminated by specialized thioesterases, which release the acyl chains from their proteinaceous primer, the ACP, thereby producing free fatty acids. For subsequent modification and assembly into triglycerides, the free fatty acids exit the plastid, become reesterified to CoA, and enter the cytoplasmic glycerolipid biosynthesis pathway. There, a set of membrane-bound enzymes attach the three acyl chains to the glycerol backbone in sequence (see Fig. 15.1). In the same compartment, each acyl group can be desaturated further, leading to polyunsaturated fatty acids. Usually, double bonds are first introduced by specific desaturases at $\Delta 12$ and subsequently at $\Delta 15$. All of the three desaturases mentioned introduce exclusively *cis* isomers. In certain plants, for example, rapeseed, specialized elongases can further increase chain length. Finally, the completed triglycerides are deposited as oil in storage compartments, the oil bodies.

ENGINEERING PLANT OIL COMPOSITION

To engineer vegetable oil composition requires detailed knowledge of the biochemical pathways and the enzymes responsible for the determining steps. It is necessary to have the target enzyme genes available (in most cases as cDNAs) and have the means to introduce them into the genome of the crop species, together with a promoter, which confers seed specific expression. In most of the cases reported to date, promoters of seed storage protein genes have been shown to be most useful, since in many oilseeds lipid and seed storage protein synthesis takes place in the same cells and at the same developmental stage (Kridl et al., 1991; Höglund et al., 1992).

After splicing the reading frame of the target enzyme gene to the appropriate promoter, the chimeric gene must be transferred to the host genome. This can be achieved by direct DNA transformation using accelerated microparticles (biolistics), but most commonly used for plant transformation is the so-called cocultivation of the target tissue with *Agrobacterium tumefaciens*. This bacterium is able to transfer any target gene (placed in a special shuttle plasmid vector) into the plant nucleus, where it subsequently becomes stably integrated into the genome (Klee et al., 1987). After transformation, the bacteria are removed and complete plants are regenerated from the cultured tissue. To facilitate the selection of transformed tissues after cocultivation, usually a selective marker (for example, a resistance gene against a certain antibiotic) is cotransformed with the target gene (Klee et al., 1987). In principle there are two approaches for manipulating lipid biosynthesis through genetic engineering. One can either genetically repress or overexpress the gene for a certain enzyme already active in the crop plant, or one can introduce a new enzyme with a novel specificity.

SUPPRESSION OF DESATURASE REACTIONS

The following section illustrates the repression of 18:0-ACP desaturation, as demonstrated first by Knutzon et al. (1992) in rapeseed. Normally, the de novo fatty acid biosynthesis in rapeseed extends up to 18:0-ACP, and most of the output is immediately desaturated to become 18:1-ACP (Fig. 15.1). About 1–3% of the total remains saturated and accumulates as 18:0. In Figure 15.2A this is shown schematically, where enzymes are symbolized by arrows and the concentration of metabolite (containers) is shown as fill levels. The concentration of the intermediate (18:0-ACP) is one determinant for the turnover rate for both competing enzymes, desaturase (major), and cleavage by the (minor) 18:0-ACP thioesterase activity. The other determinants for the actual flow rates are the enzymatic properties (K_m, V_{max}) of the two 18:0-ACP–utilizing enzymes.

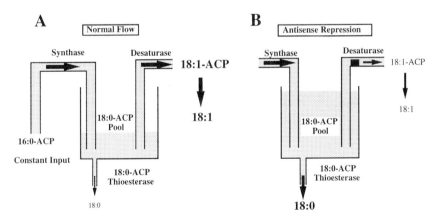

FIG. 15.2   Redirection of metabolic flux through enzyme repression: the drawing shows a detail of fatty acid biosynthesis in the plastid. Enzymes involved are symbolized by arrows; thickness of arrows indicates relative flux strength. Fill levels of the metabolite pool represent concentration of the respective metabolites. (A) Normal state; (B) repression of the Δ9 desaturase.

After efficient repression of the predominant enzyme by genetic engineering, the 18:0-ACP pool concentration should increase, facilitating increased flux through the 18:0 thioesterase and thereby diverting the flow of metabolites. Such repression was achieved by expressing the reading frame of the canola Δ9 desaturase in antisense orientation, driven by a seed storage protein gene promoter (Knutzon et al., 1992). It should be noted that the mechanism by which the production of antisense transcript in the cell can lead to a drastic (up to 95%) reduction of the (sense) mRNA of the endogenous gene of the same or very similar sequence is not understood. This reduction in mRNA then leads to reduced translation of the target mRNA and less enzyme in the cell. The in vivo results obtained with such a metabolic engineering project are shown in Figure 15.3. The highly unsaturated canola oil is transformed to a high stearate oil. Further analysis showed that stearate is not only made in dramatically increased amounts, but enters the lipid biosynthesis pathway in the cytoplasm and is deposited in the triglycerides.

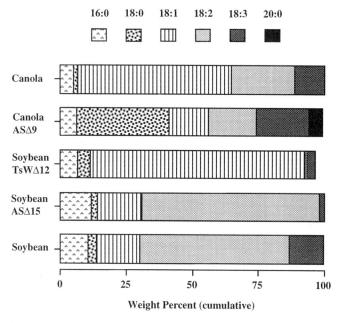

FIG. 15.3 Engineering saturation status of vegetable oils: each horizontal bar represents the fatty acid composition of a given vegetable oil (source to the left). Minor fatty acids are not included. (*Canola ASΔ9 from Knutzon et al., 1992; soybean data from Hitz et al., 1995, and T. Kinney, unpublished.*)

To date such enzyme-repression strategies have been executed with all of the three major desaturases in several oil crops, which demonstrates that the manipulation of polyunsaturation is also possible with this approach. Activities of the $\Delta12$ and $\Delta15$ desaturases (Fig. 15.1) were genetically suppressed leading to low-linolenic or high-oleic varieties (Fig. 15.3). The most dramatic reduction of polyunsaturates is demonstrated with the high-oleic soybean [to generate this phenotype, the $\Delta12$ desaturase reduction was engineering by so-called co-suppression (Matzke and Matzke, 1993; T. Kinney, personal communication)]. To date, all of these novel traits have been tested in multigeneration field trials, and the varieties are in an advanced state of product development. In summary, it is possible to redirect the bulk flux of metabolites in the plant lipid biosynthetic pathway by changing the status of a single crucial enzyme.

MANIPULATION OF CHAIN LENGTH

The enzyme repression results described in the last paragraph resulted in phenotypes that can be achieved through conventional plant breeding and mutagenesis. The recent introduction of high-oleic sunflower oil is one example. With the introduction of novel enzymes in crop plants, plant genetic engineering further transcends the limits of conventional breeding. This is discussed, using examples, in the following paragraphs.

Oils having 8:0, 10:0, 12:0, or 14:0 fatty acids are commonly referred to as medium-chain oils, with the commercially dominant sources being coconut and palm kernel (with similar, laurate-dominated, composition). Considerable interest in the possibility of the production of these fatty acids in temperate crops has emerged in the past. The current strategy used for this metabolic engineering involves thioesterases for premature chain termination. As the acyl chain is elongated in the de novo fatty acid synthase (see Fig. 15.1), pools of even chain length acyl-ACP intermediates are formed. These pools of intermediates should be accessible for chain-length engineering, as illustrated for laurate production in Figure 15.4. The model proposes the introduction of a 12:0-ACP–hydrolyzing thioesterase, which would then compete with the elongation reaction. Free laurate would be produced, ready for plastid export and triglyceride synthesis. The proportion of laurate in the overall composition should reflect the efficiency of competition with the elongation reaction at the 12:0-ACP stage.

The first successful engineering of medium-chain fatty acid production was reported in rapeseed (Voelker et al., 1992). To achieve this goal, a thioesterase specific for 12:0-ACP and to a lesser degree for 14:0-ACP was isolated from the developing seeds of the California bay tree (laurate repre-

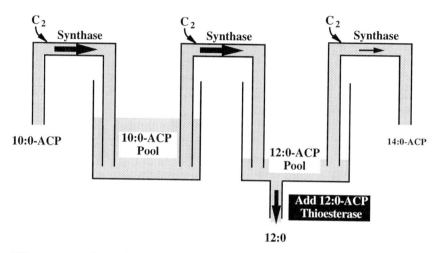

FIG. 15.4   Redirecting metabolic flux by introduction of a novel pathway: see Fig. 15.2 for explanations. A section of the de novo fatty acid biosynthesis of the plastid (Fig. 15.1) is shown.

sents 60% of its seed oil). Subsequently its cDNA was cloned and then expressed in canola under a seed storage protein promoter. The foreign gene was expressed properly during the phase of fatty acid biosynthesis, and plants with a varying degree of medium chains in their seed oil were regenerated. Figure 15.5 shows the impact of this engineering on canola oil. Medium-chain fatty acids, practically absent from canola, can accumulate to up to 60% of the total. These fatty acids accumulate in triglycerides, which demonstrates that all steps of lipid biosynthesis subsequent to the interception are flexible enough to accommodate the shorter substrates (with limitations—see below). High-laurate canola has been extensively field tested. It is the first crop variety with genetically engineered oil composition which has been recently approved by USDA and FDA. The first commercial crop was harvested in early summer 1995 in Georgia.

The thioesterase technology for premature termination of fatty acid synthesis has been shown not to be restricted to lauric acid production. To date, many thioesterases from different plants have been isolated, with specificities ranging from 8:0-ACP to 16:0-ACP. Figure 15.5 illustrates the versatility of this approach. Expressing a 16:0-ACP thioesterase from a Mexican shrub (*Cuphea hookeriana*) allowed the production of a high-palmitate canola oil (Jones et al., 1995), and a thioesterase specific for 8:0-ACP and 10:0-ACP isolated from the same species generated the canola oil composi-

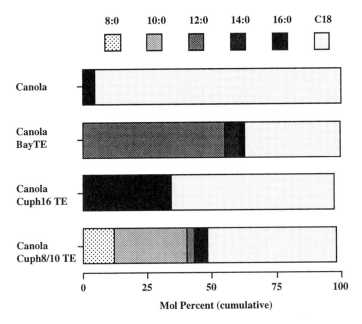

FIG. 15.5 Engineering fatty acid chain length: each horizontal bar represents the fatty acid composition of a given vegetable oil (source to the left). Minor fatty acids are not included. (*Canola Bay T.E. from Voelker, unpublished; Canola Cuph16 from T. E. Jones et al., 1995; Canola Cuph8/10 from T. E. Dehesh et al., unpublished.*)

tion displayed in the bottom bar (Dehesh et al., unpublished). In summary, the design of a canola variety with a desired composition of chain lengths has become a reality.

STRUCTURED TRIGLYCERIDES

The physical and nutritional properties of a given oil are not only defined by the nature of its fatty acids, but are also determined by the position the respective fatty acids that reside in the glycerol backbone (Hegenbart, 1992). Due to the biochemistry of plant lipid biosynthesis, triglyceride positions are usually not randomly filled. For example, in palm oil, palmitate occupies only sn1 and sn3 positions, in cocoa butter palmitate and stearate are excluded from position sn2 (Padley et al., 1986). This exclusion of saturated fatty acids from sn2 of the glycerol backbone is generally the rule for most plant species investigated (Browse and Somerville, 1991), but there are exceptions. For example, the tropical lauric oils have up to 95% saturated fatty acids; obviously these plants must have acyl transferases with modified acyl preferences. If plants not currently used commercially for oil production are included in the survey, then one can find species that accumulate almost exclusively one type of triglyceride, for example *Actinodaphne hookeri*, where 96% of all triglycerides are trilaurin (Mangold, 1994). In summary, not only have plants developed the ability to synthesize a wide range of fatty acids, but they are also able to precisely determine the triglyceride position of a given fatty acid.

It is known that temperate oil crops exclude saturated fatty acids from the middle position in their triglycerides (Browse and Somerville, 1991). This specificity is conferred by an enzyme-labeled lysophosphatidic acid acyl transferase (LPAAT) (see Fig. 15.1 for its position in the lipid biosynthesis pathway). Indeed, when high-lauric canola oil was analyzed, the medium chains were found to be excluded from the middle position of the triglycerides. Since all saturated fatty acids together account for about 60 mol% of the total oil composition, a structured triglyceride similar to cocoa butter or palm oil was created with shorter saturated fatty acids, predominantly C12. In Figure 15.6 the triglyceride compositions of coconut oil and high-laurate canola are compared to show the drastically different nature of these high-lauric oils. More recently, coconut LPAAT has been purified and its cDNA isolated. In vitro characterization showed that this LPAAT, in contrast to conventional plant LPAAT enzymes, prefers to add medium

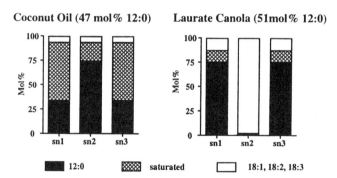

FIG. 15.6   Triglyceride composition of high-lauric oils: the graphs represent the respective average distribution of fatty acids in triglycerides in two oils. Positions 1 and 3 are assumed as equal, as calculated from sn2 data (obtained with lipase digestion). (*From Davies et al., 1995, and M. Davies, unpublished.*)

chains to position sn2 of the glycerol backbone (Davies et al., 1995; M. Davies, personal communication).

REGULATORY ASPECTS

The generation of novel crops via plant biotechnology is currently tightly supervised by the respective regulatory agencies: EPA, USDA, and FDA. There are several areas of concern, namely, the growth of the novel engineered crop itself and the properties of the new, potentially changed products derived from this plant (Redenbaugh et al., 1992, summarizes these aspects with the Flavr Savr Tomato). Two agencies are involved with the generation of crops with modified vegetable oils. USDA regulates the outdoor release and cultivation of novel crops. A major concern here is the introduction of genes into a crop plant, which might cause environmental problems (e.g., weediness, outcrossing potential of the crop plants, potential of the new genes to cause harm in the environment after transfer to another organism). FDA regulates the release of genetically engineered plant products for food. In the case of oilseed crops, FDA is concerned about changes in the meal, which is used in animal formulations, and the actual oil composition. The meal will usually contain the new genes and enzymes introduced, and it is important to assess their potential for increased toxicity, allergenicity, etc. Another concern about specific oils is the total impact on the average diet, for example, whether the use of a new oil will significantly increase the total intake of saturated fatty acids. (FDA general guidelines on plant biotechnology products can be found in Kessler, 1992.)

SUMMARY AND OUTLOOK

With the first products of single-gene manipulations nearing the marketplace, plant biotechnology is at the threshold of making its impact on the market of vegetable oil feed stocks. It has been shown that through directed genetic manipulations, near-total control over the saturation status of a given oil can be achieved. Also, acyl chain-length distributions of a given oil can be manipulated to a large extent by the introduction of a novel thioesterase. The near future will show whether these novel oils can live up to their promise and carve a niche in the current oil marketplace. Of utmost importance are not only the generation of the desired oil compositions but also the ability to produce these new feed stocks at reasonable prices. Agronomic performance of engineered crops might be influenced in some unforeseeable way. It is possible that these changes make plants more susceptible to pests, drought, or cold. There is evidence with experimental plants that genetic changes in fatty acid unsaturation can lead to growth impairment at low temperatures (Miquel and Browse, 1994). With the rapid increase in knowledge about every aspect of plant fatty acid biosynthesis and the refinement of the involved technologies, it is likely that in the next several decades nearly complete control over triglyceride fatty acid structure and composition can be achieved. This will allow the production of vegetable oils that carry traits advantageous for specific applications. Future novel triglycerides will carry new and often unexpected properties. This will influence the application spectra of these new vegetable oils in unforeseeable ways.

REFERENCES

Battey, J. F., Schmidt, K. M., and Ohlrogge, J. B. 1989. Genetic engineering for plant oils: Potential and limitations. *Trends Biotechnol.* 7: 122–126.

Browse, J. and Somerville, C. 1991. Glycerolipid synthesis: Biochemistry and regulation. *Annu. Rev. Plant Physiol. Plant Mol. Biol.* 42: 467–506.

Bubeck, D. M., Fehr, W. R., and Hammond, E. G. 1989. Inheritance of palmitic and stearic acid mutants of soybean. *Crop Sci.* 29: 652–656.

Davies, H. M., Eriqat, C. A., and Hayes, T. R. 1995. Utilization of laurate by the Kennedy pathway in developing seeds of *Brassica napus* expressing a 12:0 ACP thioesterase gene. In *Plant Lipid Metabolism*, J.-C. Kader and P. Mazliak (Ed.), pp. 503–505. Kluwer Academic Publishers.

Fick, G. N. 1989. Sunflower. In *Oil Crops of the World*, R. K. Downey et al. (Ed.), pp. 301–308. McGraw-Hill, New York.

Gibson, S., Falcone, D. L., Browse, J., and Somerville, C. 1994. Use of transgenic plants and mutants to study the regulation and function of lipid composition. *Plant, Cell Environ.* 17: 627–637.

Hegenbart, S. 1992. Taming the tempest: Health development in fats and oils. *Food Prod. Des.* (Nov.): 17–43.

Hilditch, T. P. and Williams, P. N. 1964. *The Chemical Constitution of Natural Fats.* Chapman and Hall, London.

Höglund, A.-S., Rödin, Larsson, E., and Rask, L. 1992. Distribution of napin and cruciferin in developing rape seed embryos. *Plant Physiol.* 98: 509–515.

Jones, A., Davies, H. M., and Voelker, T. A. 1995. Palmitoyl-acyl carrier protein (ACP) thioesterase and the evolutionary origin of plant acyl-ACP thioesterases. *Plant Cell* 7: 359–371.

Kessler, D. A. 1992. Statement of policy: Foods derived from new plant varieties. *Fed. Reg.* 57(104): 22984–23005.

Klee, H., Horsch, R., and Rogers, S. 1987. *Agrobacterium*-mediated plant transformation and its further applications to plant biology. *Annu. Rev. Plant Physiology* 38:467–486.

Knutzon, D. S., Thompson, G. A., Radke, S. E., Johnson, W. B., Knauf, V. C., and Kridl, J. C. 1992. Modification of *Brassica* seed oil by antisense expression of stearoyl-acyl carrier protein desaturase gene. *Proc. Natl. Acad. Sci.* 89: 2624–2628.

Kridl, J. C., McCarter, D. W., Rose, R. E., Scherer, D. E., Knutzon, D. S., Radke, S. E., and Knauf, V. C. 1991. Isolation and characterization of an expressed napin gene from *Brassica rapa. Seed Sci. Res.* 1: 209–219.

Mangold, H. K. 1994. "Einfache Triacylglycerine" in Fetten and Ölen aus den Samen von Wildpflanzen: Wertvolle Rohstoffe für die chemische Industrie. *Fat Sci. Technol.* 1: 23–27.

Matzke, M. and Matzke, A. J. M. 1993. Genomic imprinting in plants: Parental effects and *trans*-inactivation phenomena. *Annu. Rev. Plant Physiol. Plant Mol. Biol.* 44: 53–76.

Miquel, M. F. and Browse, J. A. 1994. High-oleate oilseeds fail to develop at low temperature. *Plant Physiol.* 106: 421–427.

Padley, F. B., Gunstone, F. D., and Harwood, J. L. 1986. Occurrence and characteristics of oil and fats. In *The Lipid Handbook*, F. D. Gunstone, J. L. Harwood, and F. B. Padley (Ed.), pp. 49–170. Chapman and Hall, London.

Redenbaugh, K., Hiatt, W., Martineau, B., and Emlay, D. 1994. Regulatory assessment of the FLAVR SAVR tomato. *Trends Food Sci. Technol.* 5: 105–110.

Somerville, C. and Browse, J. 1991. Plant lipids: Metabolism, mutants, and membranes. *Science* 41: 218–219.

Stefansson, B. R., Hougen, F. W., and Downey, R. K. 1961. Note on the isolation of rape plants with seed oil free from erucic acid. *Canadian J. Plant Sci.* 41: 218–219.

Voelker, T. A., Worrell, A. C., et al. 1992. Fatty acid biosynthesis redirected to medium, chains in transgenic oilseed plants. *Science* 257: 72–74.

Weiss, T. J. 1982. *Food Oils and Their Uses.* AVI Publishing, Westport, CT.

Willett, W. C. 1994. Diet and health: What should we eat? *Science* 264: 532–537.

16
Current Developments in Fat Replacers

William E. Artz

University of Illinois, Urbana, Illinois

Steven L. Hansen

Bunge Foods, Bradley, Illinois

INTRODUCTION

The most important factor in consumer food selection is taste (90%), followed by nutrition (75%), product safety (72%), and cost (71%) (Anonymous, 1992a). Fat is closely associated with the desirable taste, texture, and palatability of many foods. People are particularly desirous of fat substitutes that produce a taste comparable to traditional products (Shukla, 1992). While consumers believe that products prepared with fat substitutes would be more healthful than traditional products, they also feel that "natural" fat substitutes (e.g., Simplesse) would be more healthful than "synthetic" fat substitutes (e.g., olestra).

In an effort to develop food products with the desired taste, texture, and palatability, several companies are developing fat-based, heat-stable fat substitutes (Artz and Hansen, 1994). If approved, there could be a substantial financial reward for the successful firms. The combined U.S., European, and Japanese market for fat substitutes is estimated at nearly $7 billion, with a U.S. share of >50% (Bruhn et al., 1992).

Fat serves several important functions in a food product (Cheftel and Dumay, 1993), including having favorable effects upon the texture, acting as a carrier for fat-soluble vitamins and a source of essential fatty acids, imparting taste and flavor, including a feeling of satiety, and providing ease of processing. Product texture can be altered by (1) the lubricating effect of oil, (2) creaminess provided by emulsions, (3) a smooth plastic texture provided by semisolid fats, and (4) the desirable effects provided by the addition of fats and oils to baked goods. It can also help in achieving a desirable texture at an intermediate stage of processing, e.g., batter viscosity during the production of baked goods. Although fats and oils are generally bland in flavor, they can contribute important flavor compounds to the food product, which is particularly critical with fried foods. Fat substitutes must fulfill one or more of these functions if they are to be of any utility. Fat substitutes can be divided into three general categories: carbohydrate-based, protein-based, and fat-based. The fat-based substitutes are the only ones with the potential to provide all of above-listed functions, except for being, of course, a source of essential fatty acids.

One characteristic that could be affected by the addition of fat substitutes is flavor stability. Fats and oils that contain unsaturated fatty acids are susceptible to oxidation and the undesirable flavor changes that can occur as a result of oxidation. Addition of protein- or carbohydrate-based fat substitutes could reduce the amount of oxidative off-flavor development in a food product. Replacement of fat with a fat-based substitute that contains substantially less unsaturated fatty acids could also improve the flavor stability of a product. Although the use of aqueous protein- and carbohydrate-based fat-substitution systems could improve oxidative flavor stability, it could also result in a significant reduction in microbial stability, reducing the storage stability of the product or, worse, increasing the risk of food poisoning. This factor is an important consideration during reformulation.

Many carbohydrate- and protein-based fat substitutes either have received or will probably receive GRAS (general recognized as safe) status from the Food and Drug Administration (FDA). However, one should be aware that GRAS status for a compound approved for use as a food additive at low concentrations would not necessarily mean approval for its use as a macronutrient substitute.

All of the fat-based macronutrient substitutes are likely to require extensive safety testing prior to FDA approval. Since the carbohydrate- and protein-based fat substitutes developed to date cannot be used for frying, this discussion will include the heat-stable, low-to-noncaloric, fat-based fat substitutes in anticipation that one or more will eventually receive FDA approval. Fat-based substitutes are unique in that they contribute little to the caloric content of the food, yet they retain the important functional attributes associated with "regular" fat. Early developments in this area have been discussed elsewhere (Haumann, 1986; LaBarge, 1988; Harrigan and Breene, 1989).

The widespread use of fat-based substitutes could result in a substantial reduction in the amount of fat calories in the U.S. diet, which would have important positive implications in terms of heart disease and other cardio-vascular problems. According to the U.S. Surgeon General (1988), a substantial reduction in fat consumption would be the single most important positive change in the American diet. A significant reduction in the percentage of fat in the diet should have a positive effect on cardiovascular disease, arteriosclerosis, obesity, and numerous related health problems. Another potential positive effect of the presence of a nondigestive oil substitute in the digestive tract might be a decrease in absorption of dietary cholesterol, which would reduce the serum cholesterol concentration (Mattson et al., 1979). In contrast, fat-soluble vitamin (Hassel, 1993) and drug absorption could be depressed and laxative effects could be induced. Some studies have indicated that the caloric intake is increased to compensate for a reduction in fat intake (Beaton et al., 1992; Caputo and Mattes, 1992; Rolls et al., 1992; Birch et al., 1993).

There are important questions about fat-based fat and oil substitutes that must be answered (Munro, 1990; Borzelleca, 1992; Vanderveen, 1994) prior to approval. Until the last few years, regulatory agencies had little experience in the evaluation of macronutrient substitutes, which has compelled them to take a very cautious approach with respect to approval. There are many more limitations to the safety testing of macronutrient substitutes than of food additives used in small concentrations, because the normal level of safety guarantees cannot be attained. Luckily, many potential fat substitutes are closely related structurally to emulsifiers that have been used for decades, so it may be possible to make inferences about the effect of long-term exposure. A comprehensive and informative text titled *Low-Calorie Foods Handbook* (Altschul, 1993) included a chapter on the regulatory aspects of low-calorie foods by John E. Vanderveen of the FDA, who also presented guidelines at the 1994 IFT annual meeting that would be of particular interest to companies who intend to request regulatory approval for a macronutrient substitute (Vanderveen, 1994). These can be summarized as follows:

1. The exact chemical structure of the substitute must be known and documented. If it is composed of more than one compound, the structure of each component must be completely elucidated.

2. The stability should be well documented, especially during food production, storage, and final preparation. If partial degradation

occurs, the by-products should be identified. If any harmful impurities are present, limits should be established as to the concentration of these components.

3. Detailed exposure assessment for each population type should be included, which would include toxicological data demonstrating that the use of the macronutrient substitute, as well as any of the degradative by-products, would not cause harm to at least the levels of exposure for the intended use.

4. Additional tests may be required to provide pharmacokinetic, metabolic, and/or nutritional data not normally required for other additives.

5. It will be necessary to determine whether the macronutrient substitute is absorbed or not. If it is poorly absorbed, one needs to determine whether large concentrations of the material in the gut affect the morphology, physiology, biochemistry, or normal flora of the gastrointestinal tract.

6. Since some of the normal testing procedures used for the evaluation of micronutrients are either inappropriate or provide insufficient data, an innovative or novel approach may be required. The selection of animal models, experimental protocols, and measurement techniques must be carefully planned to provide data, which can be used to accurately assess the safety of the substitute. In addition, consideration of the appropriate controls and control experiments would be advised.

7. Sufficient data must be provided to demonstrate that the substitute or its metabolites do not interfere with absorption or metabolism of essential nutrients. If interference does occur, one must determine whether it can be safely offset with nutrient fortification. If the compound is adsorbed at a measurable rate, there must be data indicating the impact, if any, on the nutrient status of the animal. In general, traditional assessments of nutritional status should be sufficient for nutrient status assessment.

8. Another area of special concern is the effect of macronutrient substitutes on selected, particularly sensitive, population segments, such as the very young, senior citizens, or those afflicted with certain health problems. One example is aspartame due to its effect on individuals susceptible to phenylketonuria.

9. The effect of the macronutrient on drug absorption and/or activity should be assessed. Some of the oil substitutes can have a slight laxative or anal leakage effect, at least during the initial stages of

consumption until the digestive system has adapted to the product. Since this effect is often greater among children than adults, it may require additional evaluation. In addition, some consumers may not be aware of the relationship between substitute consumption and the laxative effects, as with prunes, for example. Special labeling may be needed to address the problem.

10. Postmarket surveillance will be needed in most cases. One long-term potential problem of particular concern could result from the simultaneous consumption of several macronutrient substitutes, since it is likely that more than one may be approved in the future. There may be a synergistic or interactive effect on some of the factors just discussed. This concern is also likely to limit the number of fat-based fat substitutes eventually approved.

FAT MIMETICS

The food industry has employed several methods to reduce the fat content of food: leaner cuts of meat, adding fillers such as soy protein, and formulation changes, e.g., substituting milk for cream. Carbohydrate-based ingredients previously used primarily as stabilizers or thickeners are now often used as fat substitutes. Some novel techniques used to improve food characteristics include protein concentration in fluid milk using membrane processing (Cheryan, 1991) or the controlled, partial hydrolysis of casein with rennet. In both cases, one can achieve in modified low-fat milk with ≤0.1% fat the textural and visual characteristics characteristic of milk containing 1–3.5% fat. The thin, rather translucent appearance of skim milk is replaced with the slightly thicker, more opaque, appearance typical of whole milk. Another technique discussed during the 1995 IFT annual meeting in Los Angeles was the use of hydrocolloids to reduce oil absorption during deep-fat frying (Gerrish, 1995; Kresl and Higgins, 1995).

Protein-Based Fat Mimetics

Although numerous products are discussed in detail, this chapter is not a listing of all available products—only selected products are covered. Simplesse, derived from milk or egg protein, is the best known of the protein-based fat substitutes (Anonymous, 1989, 1990a,b, 1991a; Smith 1993). The protein is particulated during a combined pasteurization and homogenization process that produces microparticles of uniform size and spherical shape approximately 1 μm in diameter (Singer and Moser, 1993). The nutritive quality of the protein is essentially unaltered during the preparative processing. Most of the protein-based fat substitutes have a similar basis, i.e., the protein is particulated into spherical particles with some combination of heat and shear, with or without added components such as gums, stabilizers, or emulsifiers. The simulated fat produced from an aqueous suspension of microparticulated protein particles of the appropriate size and characteristics has shear thinning characteristics and a smoothness and creaminess similar to fat. Particles with significantly smaller or larger dimensions than 0.5–2 μm do not seem to have the desired sensory characteristics, unless the particles are very soft, hydrated, and compressible, which can extend the size range considerably. While the protein in the fat substitutes contains 4 kcal/g, an aqueous microparticulate protein suspension contains fewer than 4 kcal/g, generally 1–2 kcal. The protein-based substitutes can be used to formulate a variety of products, including cheesecake, puddings, sauces, pie fillings, sour cream, ice cream, cream cheese, mayonnaise, dips, and spreads. Simplesse has been affirmed as GRAS by FDA for use in several products. The main limitation, which is true for all currently approved fat substitutes and mimetics, is that it cannot be used for many heated-product applications, particularly frying.

There is more than one form of Simplesse available (Frye and Setser, 1993). One of the newest versions is Simplesse 100, which is a thixotrophic fluid derived from whey protein concentrate. It can be used in a wide variety of dairy and bakery products. It is also available as a readily hydratable powder. Simplesse 300 is a mixture of egg white and milk proteins that can be used in food products that require heating. Of course, it cannot be used as a frying medium.

Other protein-based products include Trailblazer (milk/egg white protein) from Kraft General Foods, Finesse (milk/egg white protein) from Reach Associates, LITA from Opta Food Ingredients (corn protein), and Miprodan from MD Foods (milk protein) (Frye and Setser, 1993; Tamime et al., 1994). Miprodan can be used in yogurt, butter spreads, frozen yogurt, and ice cream. NutriFat, a carbohydrate/protein mixture from Reach Associates, can be used in ice cream–type products.

Once investigators realized that microparticulation could be used to produce a homogenous suspension of small protein particles with fatlike properties, other protein-based fat replacers, microparticulation processes, and systems were examined. Recent efforts in this area were reviewed by Cheftel and Dumay (1993). Membrane processing (ultrafiltration followed by diafiltration) has been used to concentrate casein micelles to four- to ninefold to produce a product that can be used to partially or completely replace fat in ice cream, chocolate mousse, dairy product–based spreads, and sauces (Habib and Podolski, 1989). The micelles are reported to function as microparticles with an approximate diameter of 0.1–0.4 μm.

Protein precipitation under carefully controlled conditions can produce a microparticulated product that can also be used as a fat substitute (Mai et al., 1990). A dilute solution of water-soluble protein (1–5%) is precipitated with heat and/or a change in pH to the isoelectric point of the protein. Starches, gums, emulsifying agents, etc., can be used to enhance product characteristics and prevent extensive aggregation.

A solution of alcohol-soluble (70–80% ethanol) proteins (prolamines from corn, wheat, rice, etc.) can be precipitated by dilution with water to produce a microparticulated spherical protein precipitate (Stark and Gross, 1990). Gums should be used to prevent extensive aggregation. To produce a concentrated protein suspension, ultrafiltration followed by diafiltration can be used. Freeze-drying can be used to produce a powdered precipitate.

One of the first thermomechanical coagulation processes for the microparticulation of protein was described by Singer et al. (1988). A whey protein concentrate is dispersed in water, acidified to approximately pH 4, and then heated (90–120°C) under high-shear conditions (500,000 s^{-1}). The resultant dispersion contains small spherical particles (0.1–2.5 μm) and has a creamy and smooth texture. Protein sources other than whey protein can also be used (Cheftel and Dumay, 1993).

In addition to the dual heating/high-shear particulation processes used to make Simplesse-type products, extrusion can be used to prepare a microparticulated protein-based fat substitute (Cheftel and Dumay, 1993). The extrusion conditions are very mild compared to typical extrusion conditions. For example, a whey protein concentrate (20%) within a pH range 3.5–3.9 (extruder conditions: barrel temperature of 85–100°C and screw speed of 100–200 rpm) can be extruded to produce a semisolid spread with a smooth and creamy texture. No die is used, so there is no pressure buildup and subsequent expansion. The particles are rather large (12 μm) on average. If the extrusion is done at a higher pH (4.5–6.8), the protein solubility is reduced and the percentage of large particles (>20 μm) is much greater and the resultant texture is coarse and grainy. The nitrogen solubility index of the protein remains relatively high, 43–47% for the acid product and 69–70% for the neutral product. The addition of 0.5% xanthan gum improved the creamy texture and reduces the particle size.

Carbohydrate-Based Fat Mimetics

There are several starch-derived fat replacers or mimetics available (Anonymous, 1990a; Glicksman, 1991; Anonymous, 1992b; Cheftel and Dumay, 1993; Frye and Setser, 1993; Mela, 1992; Yackel and Cox, 1992; Schmidt et al., 1993; Smith, 1993; Tamime et al., 1994), which are essentially maltodextrins. They are produced upon partial enzymatic or acid-catalyzed hydrolysis of starch and are fully digestible. Low–dextrose equivalent (DE) maltodextrins have fat-binding functional properties, unlike high-DE products. Starches and sugars contain 4 kcal/g, but since they are generally used at concentrations of much less than 100%, the actual caloric content is typically 0.5–2 kcal/g. They include Lycadex-100 and Lycadex-200 from Roquette Freres; Crestar SF from Euro Centre Food; N-Lite, Instant N-Oil, and N-Oil II from National Starch Co.; Maltrin M040 from Grain Processing Corp.; Paselli SA-2 from Avebe America, Inc.; Tapiocaline from Tripak; Star Dri, Stellar, and Sta-Slim from A. E. Staley; Amalean I from American Maize Products; and Rice-trin from Zumbro. Typically, a smooth viscous solution or a soft gel is formed when hydrated.

Lycadex is an enzymatically hydrolyzed cornstarch-based maltodextrin. The typical concentration used is 20%, and it is nongelling. Typical applications include sauces and salad dressings.

Maltrin M040 is a maltodextrin (DE = 5) made from cornstarch (Frye and Setser, 1993; Tamime et al., 1994), which is hot water soluble. A solution containing 30–50% solids produces a thermoreversible gel with a bland flavor, smooth mouthfeel, and texture similar to hydrogenated oils for butterfat. According to the manufacturer, it can be used for dairy products, frozen foods, sauces, salad dressings, confectionery products, and dry mixes.

Paselli SA2 is a maltodextrin derived from potato starch (Anonymous, 1989; Frye and Setser, 1993). It forms a shiny, white, thermoreversible gel with a smooth, fatlike texture and neutral taste that is also suited for acid formulations. The gel is stable with fat- and oil-containing products. A gel is formed at concentrations above 20%, and the gel strength increases with an increase in concentration.

N-Oil is a tapioca-based maltodextrin (Anonymous, 1989; Frye and Setser, 1993). An instantized version, N-Oil II, can be used with foods that require either no heat processing or very modest thermal processing, such as high-temperature, short-time thermal processing. N-Oil is heat stable, and it can withstand high temperatures, high shear, and acidic conditions. Upon cooling, a solution of hot water–soluble N-Oil will develop a texture similar to hydrogenated shortening.

Amalean I is a modified high-amylose cornstarch used at relatively low concentration (8%) compared to the maltodextrins. A gel for fat replacement can be prepared upon heating a paste or slurry to 88–90°C for 3 minutes. An Amalean II product is available for enhancing batter aeration.

StaSlim is a modified starch designed to provide a creamy texture for a wide range of food products, but it is particularly well suited for salad dressings. In contrast to other products, it is usually processed as a warm liquid in formulation. It is prepared as a slurry at a concentration of 3–20% and heated with agitation to 65–71°C to completely solubilize the starch. It is recommended for use in salad dressings, cheese products, and soups.

Stellar is a microparticulated cornstarch gel used in pastries, snack foods, frostings and fillings, cheese products, margarines, meat products, salad dressings, and other products (Anonymous, 1991b; Frye and Setser, 1993). The water is bound sufficiently such that water migration from the cake to the filling is slowed and staling is retarded. The small, intact starch granules duplicates the mouthfeel sensation of fat. The particle aggregates are 3–5 μm in diameter, slightly larger than the protein-based fat replacer products but approximately the same size as the fat crystals they are designed to replace. The microparticulate character is required to maintain the smooth creamy texture. If it is heated sufficiently to completely gelatinize and disperse the starch (105°C), much of the fat substitute or mimetic functionality is permanently lost. Applications include low-fat margarines, salad dressings, soups, confectionery products, baked goods, frostings, fillings, and certain dairy and meat products.

Scientists at American Maize were able to use an unmodified, pregelatinized waxy starch (waxy starches contain nearly 100% amylopectin) at a concentration of 2% to produce a blueberry muffin with only 3% fat, yet with textural characteristics comparable to a muffin containing 15% fat (Hippleheuser et al., 1995). The waxy starch assists in providing a uniform cell size, the appropriate crumb structure, and a strong tendency to retain moisture, which extends the shelf life and produces a desirable moist mouthfeel. Since the addition of starch allows an increased moisture content, the potential problem of rapid mold storage should be addressed (0.1% potassium sorbate).

Polydextrose is a low-calorie polymer that can be used to replace some of the fat in a food product. It is formed by the random polymerization of glucose, sorbitol, and citric acid. Sorbitol provides an upper molecular weight limit and reduces the formation of water-insoluble material. Most of the linkages are glycosidic, and the 1–6 bond, in particular, predominates. Litesse, which is a polydextrose-type product, and Veri-Lo, which consists of fat-coated carbohydrate-based gel particles, are both from Pfizer.

The fiber-based products include gums, celluloses, hemicelluloses, pectins, β-glucans, and lignins. These are isolated from a wide variety of sources, including cereals, fruits, legumes, nuts, and vegetables. Gums are typically not used as fat substitutes directly, rather they are used at low concentrations (0.1–0.5%) to form gels that increase product viscosity. Agar, alginate, gum arabic, carrageenan, konjac, guar gum, high- and low-methoxy pectin, xanthan gum, and cellulose derivatives can all potentially be used.

Fiber-based products available include Nutrio-P-fibre from the Danish Sugar Factory; Nutricol derived from Konjac flour; P-150 C and P-285 F derived from pea fiber from Grindsted Products; and Avicel, a micro-crystalline cellulose and carrageenan, both from FMC. Slendid is a pectin that form gels with fatlike meltability from Hercules. Quaker oatrim is a product of Rhône-Poulenc Food Ingredients derived from oats.

Cellulose derivatives used include α-cellulose, carboxymethyl cellulose, hydroxypropyl cellulose, microcrystalline cellulose, and methyl cellulose (Frye and Setser, 1993). The gel produced from the cellulose derivatives display several desirable fatlike functional properties, including creaminess, fatlike mouthfeel, stability, texture modification, increased viscosity, and the glossy appearance of high-fat emulsions. FMC, for example, has cellulose-based gels (Penichter and McGinley, 1991) as well as gums, which increase emulsion viscosity and, hence, product stability. This allows one to reduce the oil content because the gel mimics some of the rheological properties associated with high-fat emulsions.

Oatrim is a cold water–dispersible amylodextrin rich in β-glucans (Anon-ymous, 1990b), produced upon partial enzymatic hydrolysis of the starch. It is derived from whole oat or debranned whole oat flour. An oatrim-based gel (25% solids) can function as a fat replacer. In addition, the β-glucan compo-nents in the oatrim have a demonstrated hypocholesterolemic effect (In-glett and Grisamore, 1991).

There is evidence that the replacement of fat with either protein- or carbohydrate-based fat substitutes in a normal diet can induce increased caloric intake to compensate for the reduction in calories (Harris and Jones, 1991). However, if animals are initially on a high-fat diet rather than a normal diet, which is then altered with the addition of a fat substitute, they do not necessarily increase their caloric intake.

Reduced-Calorie, Fat-Based Fat Replacers

The objective for these products is similar to that for the protein- and carbohydrate-based fat substitutes—a substantial reduction in calories, rather than a complete elimination of fat. For example, N-Flate (National Starch and Chemical Corp.) is a blend of mono- and diglycerides, modified food starch, and guar gum in a nonfat milk base (ADA, 1991). It can be used to replace some or all of the shortening in baked goods. It contains 5.1 kcal/ g and is used in smaller amounts than the fat it replaces.

Durkee Foods has developed a fat replacer composed of mono- and diglycerides. It still contains 9 kcal/g, but, like the N-Flate, it is used in smaller amounts than the shortening it is designed to replace in cakes, cookies, and other baked goods.

Caprenin is a reduced-calorie triglyceride (Procter & Gamble Co., Cincinnati, OH) formed by the esterification of three naturally occurring fatty acids: caprylic, capric, and behenic (ADA, 1991). Since the behenic acid is only partially absorbed, the caprenin contains 5 rather than the normal 9 kcal/g. Caprenin has functional properties similar to cocoa butter and is intended to replace some of the cocoa butter in selected confectionery products. It is digested, absorbed, and metabolized by the same pathways as other triacylglycerols.

Another fabricated triacylglycerol, similar to caprenin, is Salatrim, which is comprised of a mixture of long-chain (primarily stearic acid) and short-chain (acetic, propionic and butyric) fatty acids randomly esterified to glycerol (Smith et al., 1994). It contains approximately 5 kcal/g, rather than the 9 kcal/g contained in regular fats and oils. It is a product of the Nabisco Foods Group. Twenty-one papers from a symposium on Salatrim were published in the February 1994 issue of the *Journal of Agriculture and Food Chemistry*. The research reported included structural characterization(s) of the oil, an analysis of the oil in food products, and an extensive series of papers on the metabolism and toxicology of the oil in various animal and human model systems. It has the same utility that caprenin does as a fat replacer in reduced-fat systems and could be used as a cocoa butter substitute in confectionery products and in baked products and filled dairy products. Caprenin and Salatrim may be of limited use for retail and home deep-fat frying applications, e.g., the smaller molecular weight fatty acids may cause undesirable flavor effects upon hydrolysis.

A third reduced-calorie, short-chain triglyceride is Captrin from Stepan Food Ingredients (Anonymous, 1994). It is a randomized triglyceride made from linear saturated fatty acids primarily C8 to C10 in length. Some of the proposed uses include baked goods, confections, dairy product analogs, snack foods, and soft candy.

Fat-Based Fat Mimetics

Eventually, some of the fat-based substitutes are likely to achieve FDA approval for limited uses. There are several reviews discussing the status, structure, and utility of many of the fat-based fat substitutes under development in the United States and Europe (Mieth, 1992). Carbohydrate fatty acid esters have undergone extensive development and evaluation as potential fat substitutes. Much of that work was recently reviewed in a text by Akoh and Swanson (Akoh and Swanson, 1994) titled *Carbohydrate Polyesters as Fat Substitutes*. The most well-known carbohydrate fatty acid ester is the sucrose fatty acid ester called olestra (Anonymous, 1990a; LaBarge, 1988), which is composed of hexa-, hepta-, and octa-fatty acid esters of sucrose (Procter &

Gamble) with long-chain fatty acids (predominantly C18) (Jandacek, 1991a). Olestra contains at least 70% octaester and 1% or less of the hexaester and <0.5% of the penta- and lower esters combined (Bergholz, 1992; Jandacek, 1991a). Tests indicate that olestra is not a toxin, carcinogen, mutagen, or reproductive toxin. Numerous studies have been completed, including more than 100 studies with five animal species and 25 clinical studies with more than 2500 men, women, and children. Although one study indicated some liver changes in one group of test animals, the changes were not significant and the consensus is that the product is safe (ADA, 1991). Other tests have examined its effect on intestinal cell morphology, gastric emptying, motility, pancreatic response, bile acid physiology, and colonic microflora. Olestra is not susceptible to lipase action. It does not enter the mixed micellar phase in the intestine, so absorption does not occur (Jandacek, 1991b; Bergholz, 1992). It can reduce fat-soluble vitamin (Jandacek, 1991a; Bergholz, 1992) and fat-soluble drug absorption (Benmoussa et al., 1992), although not in all cases (Jandacek, 1991b). Reduced absorption of fat-soluble vitamins can be readily compensated with fat-soluble vitamin supplementation. Microbial gut flora appear unable to metabolize olestra (Nuck et al., 1994). Sucrose fatty acid polyesters can be synthesized from a variety of fat sources, including partially hydrogenated soybean oil, olive oil, canola oil, corn oil, milkfat, etc. (Volpenhein, 1985; Chase et al., 1994; Drake et al., 1994a,b,c; Marquez-Ruiz et al., 1994; Rios et al., 1994).

In 1987 a petition was submitted to FDA for approval of olestra as a fat replacer (≤35%) in home use oils and shortenings and as a fat replacer in restaurant and commercial deep-fat frying operations (up to 75%). In 1990, the petition was limited to a request to approve olestra for use in replacing 100% of the fat used in the preparation of "savory snacks." Approval was recently granted.

Some of the physical properties of olestra are similar to those of triacylglycerols, such as the interfacial tension with water and stability under frying conditions (Jandacek, 1991b). It is completely miscible with other food oils. It can be used in place of food oils for frying, cooking, and baking applications. It can be used to replace fat in cheese, margarine, salad dressings, and ice cream.

Reports on the synthesis and analysis of carbohydrate fatty acid esters have been published by several groups (Akoh and Swanson, 1989, 1994; Rios et al., 1994; Drake et al., 1994d). Swanson's research group at Washington State University has published much on carbohydrate fatty acid esters synthesized from a variety of carbohydrate sources under a variety of catalytic conditions (Akoh and Swanson, 1990; Akoh, 1994a). They reported an optimized synthesis with yields of 99.8% utilizing a solvent-free, one-stage process for the synthesis of sucrose octaoleate. The synthesis of several carbohydrate-fatty acid–derived fat substitutes, including glucose fatty acid esters, sucrose fatty acid esters, raffinose fatty acid esters, and even larger polysaccharide oligomers, such as stachyose and verbascose fatty acid esters, were reported. Enzymatic methods for the synthesis of carbohydrate fatty acid esters are discussed in detail by Riva (1994). One of the most promising enzymes tested, particularly for fatty acid esterification of the alkylated glycosides, was a lipase from the yeast *Candida antarctica*,which had been immobilized on macroporous resin beads. Since only a limited number of successful enzymatic syntheses have been reported, much more research is needed.

Mono- and oligomeric carbohydrate esters have also been prepared from sugars or other carbohydrates and saturated fatty acids and/or ester-forming fatty acid derivatives (Hoechst AG, Frankfurt, FRG) (Mieth et al., 1982; Deger et al., 1988) that contain branched or unbranched carboxylic acids of various chain lengths. For example, glucose laurate was examined for its acceptability as a fat substitute in chocolate.

Alkyl glycoside fatty acid esters could be used to replace fat (5–95%) in such items as frying oils and white or Italian salad dressings (Curtice-Burns, Inc., Rochester, NY) (Meyer et al., 1989). Alkyl glycosides can be formed by reacting a reducing saccharide with a monohydric alcohol. Soybean, safflower, corn, peanut, and cottonseed oils are preferred since they contain C_{16}–C_{18} fatty acids that do not volatilize at the temperatures used for interesterification. The preferred alkyl glucosides are the reaction products between glucose, galactose, lactose, maltose, and ethanol and propanol. Blending of unsaturates and saturates (>25% C_{12} or larger) produces a heterogeneous alkyl glycoside fatty acid polyester, which does not induce undesirable anal leakage. Anal leakage may be prevented if the alkyl glycoside fatty acid polyesters have a melting point greater than or equal to 37°C.

A patent was awarded for the incorporation of the alkyl glycoside fatty acid polyester into food products (Curtice-Burns, Inc., Rochester, NY) (Winter et al., 1990). The fat substitute could replace "visible fats" in such products as shortening, margarine, butter, salad and cooking oils, mayonnaise, salad dressing, and confectionery coatings or "invisible fats" in such foods as oilseeds, nuts, dairy, and animal products. "Visible fats" are defined as the fats and oils that have been isolated from animal tissues, oilseeds, or vegetable sources. "Invisible fats" are fats and oils that are not isolated from animal or vegetable sources and are consumed along with the protein and carbohydrate components of the sources as they naturally occur. Substitution at 10–100% is possible; however, less than 100% is preferred, preferably in the range 33–75%. The addition of an anti–anal leakage (AAL) agent is not necessary, especially if the diet has "invisible fats" containing fatty acids with melting points about 37°C.

Glucosides containing from 1 to 50 alkoxy groups can be used as fat substitutes at substitution ranges of 10–100% in low-calorie salad oils, plastic shortenings, cake mixes, icing mixes, mayonnaise, salad dressings, and margarines (Procter & Gamble) (Ennis et al., 1991). The alkoxylated alkyl glucoside (i.e., propoxylated or ethoxylated methyl glucoside) is esterified with four to seven C_2–C_{24} fatty acids. For example, ethoxylated glucoside tetraoleate was prepared by reacting oleyl chloride with Glucam E-20 (ethoxylated methyl glucoside obtained from reacting methyl glucoside with ethylene oxide).

The ARCO Chemical Technology Limited Partnership (Wilmington, DE) has patented a fatty acid esterified polysaccharide (PEP) that is partially esterified with fatty acids. The PEP can be used as a fat substitute in salad oils, cooking oils, margarine, butter blends, mayonnaise, and shortening at a substitution range of 10–100% (White, 1990). It is nonabsorbable, indigestible, and nontoxic. Suitable oligo/polysaccharide materials include xanthan gum, guar gum, gum arabic, alginates, cellulose hydrolysis products, hydroxypropyl cellulose, starch hydrolysis products ($n < 50$), karaya gum, and pectin. The degree of esterification is controlled by the length of the acyl ester chain and the total number of hydroxyl groups available for esterification. The preferred level of esterification involves one or more hydroxyl groups per saccharide unit with one or more C_8–C_{24} fatty acids. The preferred fatty acid sources are soybean, olive, cottonseed, corn oil, tallow, and lard. Preparation may involve direct esterification or transesterification, with the metal-catalyzed (sodium methoxide, potassium hydroxide, titanium isopropoxide, or tetraalkoxide) transesterification preferred due to the charring of saccharides that can occur during direct esterification.

Milkfat sucrose fatty acid esters can be used as a fat substitute for the production of cheese (Drake et al., 1994c). Sensory analysis indicated that cheese samples prepared with sucrose polyesters were significantly different from the control samples, which was attributed to the preparation of the fat-based substitute oil, since it was not steam-deodorized. Mixtures of glucose and sucrose fatty acid esters have been examined for their utility for emulsion stabilization. Several physical parameters were examined after preparation of oil-in-water and water-in-oil emulsions, e.g., surface tension, interfacial tension, and emulsion stability. It was suggested that blends of the sugar esters would be useful for the preparation of low-fat salad dressings (Akoh, 1992; Akoh and Nwosu, 1992).

Fatty acid esterified propoxylated glycerols (EPGs) (ARCO Chemical Company, Newtown Square, PA) were developed for use as fat substitutes. Glycerol is propoxylated with propylene oxide to form a polyether polyol, which is then esterified with fatty acids (Gillis, 1988; White and Pollard,

1988, 1989a,b,c; Dziezak, 1989; Anonymous, 1990a; Cooper, 1990; Arci-szewski, 1991; Duxbury and Meinhold, 1991; Hassel, 1993). The preferred fatty acids are in the C_{14}–C_{18} range. The resulting triacylglycerol is similar to natural fats in structure and functionality. Fatty acid EPG is a low-calorie or noncaloric oil, heat-stable and only very slightly digestible. The in vivo threshold for nondigestibility occurs when the number of added propylene oxide groups equals four. It can be used in table spreads, ice cream, frozen desserts, salad dressings, bakery products, salad and cooking oils, mayon-naise, and shortenings. Feeding experiments with rats (White and Pollard, 1989b) and mice (White and Pollard, 1989c) indicated no toxicity. Prepara-tion of propoxylated glycerides for use as fat substitutes involved trans-esterifying propoxylated glycerol with esters of C_{10}–C_{24} fatty acids in a solvent-free, nonsaponifying system (ARCO Chemical Technology Limited Partnership, Wilmington, DE) (Cooper, 1990) to avoid reagents unaccept-able in food systems.

Dialkyl dihexadecylmalonate (DDM) (Frito-Lay, Inc., Dallas, TX) is a fatty alcohol ester of malonic and alkylmalonic acids, which could be used in high-temperature applications (Fulcher, 1986; Gillis, 1988; Dziezak, 1989). The fatty acids most preferred are myristic, palmitic, stearic, oleic, and linoleic. Suitable acids include malonic acid and monoalkyl and dialkyl malonic acids. A blend of DDM and soybean oil resulted in potato and tortilla chips that were less oily and as crisp as those fried in soybean oil (White and Pollard, 1989c). The aforementioned blend resulted in a 33% reduction in calories and a 60% reduction in fat intake. DDM was also evaluated as a fat substitute in mayonnaise and margarine-type products. The lower molecular weight DDM could be used in mayonnaise and marga-rine, while the higher molecular weight DDM could be used as a frying oil (Fulcher, 1986; Gillis, 1988; Dziezak, 1989).

Nabisco Brands Inc. (East Hanover, NJ) has developed a partially digest-ible, carboxylate ester–based fat substitute synthesized with fatty acids or fatty alcohols (Huhn et al., 1989; Anonymous, 1991c). Suitable fatty alcohols include n-hexadecyl alcohol, oleyl alcohol, and n-octadecyl alcohol. Al-though citric acid is not recommended for some applications due to its thermal instability, the three carboxyl groups and a hydroxyl group make it particularly useful. The functionality of the fat-based substitute can be controlled by the choice of the fatty alcohol. Possible applications include margarine, mayonnaise, and baked goods.

Esters of fatty alcohols and/or fatty acids with other hydroxycarboxylic acids have also been developed for use as fat replacers (Nabisco Brands, Inc., East Hanover, NJ) (Klemann and Finley, 1989a,b). Dioleyl 1-myristoyl-oxy-1,2-ethanedicarboxylate was prepared and evaluated using animal studies. Only 4% of the potentially available calories were digestible. Possible applications include butter, ice cream, vanilla wafers, coconut oil mimetic, and crackers.

Glycerol esters of α-branched carboxylic acids could be used as partial (10%) or complete (100%) fat substitutes in such products as cakes, bread, mayonnaise, dairy products, salad oils, cooking oils, and margarine (Procter & Gamble) (Whyte, 1971). Preparation involves esterifying glycerol to an α-branched carboxylic acid. The α-branched carboxylate structure prevents the ester from being hydrolyzed by pancreatic lipase in the intestine.

Acylated glycerides could be used to replace normal triacylglycerols in fat-containing foods (Procter & Gamble) (Volpenhein, 1986). As the number of acylated groups is increased, the acylated glyceride is less digestible with pancreatic enzymes. The α-acylated glyceride may provide partial to total replacement (10–100%) of fat in a food system. Possible applications include salad or cooking oils, plastic shortening, prepared cake and icing mixes, mayonnaise, salad dressings, and margarine.

Dialkyl glycerol ethers have been developed for use as a fat substitute (Swift and Co., USA) (Trost, 1981). A mixture of didodecyl glycerol ether (20%), *cis*-9-octadecenyl octadecyl ether (35%), *cis*-9-octadecenyl tallow alcohol glycerol ether (35%), and dioctadecyl glycerol ether (10%) may be used as a shortening substitute in bakery products or in margarines.

Tris(hydroxymethyl) alkane esters are different from most engineered fats in that the esters are partially hydrolyzed in vivo and may contribute 0.5–6 kcal/g, as compared to 9 kcal/g for conventional fats (Nabisco Brands) (Klemann et al., 1990a,b). Mixtures of fatty acids obtained from non-hydrogenated or hydrogenated soybean, safflower, sunflower, sesame, peanut, corn, olive, rice bran, canola, babassu nut, coconut, cottonseed, and/or palm oils can be used. Fatty acid derivatives can be used, such as halogenated or dicarboxylate-extended (malonic, succinic, glutaric, or adipic acids) fatty acid residues. The monomeric and dimeric tris(hydroxymethyl) alkane esters can be used in combination in partial or full replacement of fat in such products as frozen desserts, puddings, pie fillings, margarine substitutes, pastries, mayonnaise, filled dairy products, flavored dips, frying fats and oils, meat substitutes, whipped toppings, compound coatings, frostings, cocoa butter replacements, fatty candies, and chewing gum.

Phenyldimethylpolysiloxane (PDMS) (Dow Corning Corp., Midland, MI) has been examined as a noncaloric frying media (Morehouse and Zabik, 1989) and as a fat replacer (Hamm, 1984). Morehouse and Zabik (1989) examined samples of PDMS with four different viscosities for frying fish patties, French fries, and doughnut holes. PDMS is thought to be a suitable frying medium due to its thermal and oxidative stability, minimal change in viscosity over a wide temperature range, water repellent ability, and biological inertness. The heat transfer characteristics of PDMS depend upon the food composition and temperature. Frying in low-viscosity PDMS resulted in a lighter, less red product with a softer and more consistent texture than products fried in corn oil. The fat content of the PDMS fried foods was one-fourth or less that of corn oil–fried foods.

Phenylmethylpolysiloxane (PS) (Dow Corning 550 Fluid, Contour Chemical CO., North Reading, MA) has also been examined as a possible fat substitute (Bracco et al., 1987). PS is chemically inert, nonabsorbable, and nontoxic. The viscosity is dependent upon the molecular weight of the polymers. Obese female Zucker rats lost weight while on a PS (22% w/w) low-fat diet, as compared to a low-fat diet only. The PS-fed rats did not compensate for their caloric reduction by increasing food intake (Labell, 1991). According to Dow Corning Corp. (Midland, MI) (Ryan, 1990), research has established the safety and lack of toxicity of PDMS and related organosilicones. Applications include baked goods, mayonnaise, peanut butter, cereals, icings, and frying oils (Frye, 1986), although at very small concentrations, silicone-based antifoams can be deleterious to cake texture, potato chip, and doughnut quality. Other possible applications include dairy products and shortening substitutes (Ryan, 1989). Rats fed a diet containing 6.5% (by weight) PDMS exhibited an undesirable anal leakage. Anti–anal leakage (AAL) agents should be used and consist of fatty acids with a melting point of $\geq 37°C$. Other AAL agents include particulate silica with a surface area greater than 10 m^2/g, preferably 300–400 m^2/g. The third type of AAL agent is edible, nondegradable, water-insoluble plant fiber.

Linear polyglycerol esters have been reported as a potential cooking oil substitute (Dobson et al., 1993). The compounds resist hydrolysis by digestive enzymes and are poorly absorbed. However, if small amounts are absorbed, hydrolysis should eventually occur. Except for slightly greater viscosities, the oil has properties similar to natural triacylglycerols in color, odor, taste, and other physical characteristics. Linear polyglycerol esters (LPGs) are prepared via the alkaline polymerization of glycidol, followed by the addition of oleyl chloride to form the octaglyceroldecaoleate oil. LPGs are enzyme resistant and poorly absorbed as reported from animal feeding studies. The LPG esters have a color, odor, taste, and other physical properties similar to normal triglycerides.

Colestra (Food Ingredients and Innovations) and Prolestra (Reach Associates) (Anonymous, 1990a) are olestra-type fat-based fat substitutes. Prolestra is a mixture of sugar fatty acid esters and protein, while Colestra is a sugar fatty acid ester.

Hamm (1984) compared five separate potential low-caloric oil substitutes: trialkoxytricarballyate, trialkoxycitrate, trialkoxyglyceryl ether, jojoba oil, and sucrose fatty acid polyester. The oils were synthesized or refined, depending upon the required procedures. An extensive series of compositional analyses, physical property analyses, and functional property analyses were completed. He concluded that the physical properties of all five substitutes were similar to liquid edible triacylglycerols, such as corn oil. Generally, the functional properties of the fat substitutes could be changed by altering the source of the fatty acid side chains. However, the trialkoxycitrate did not appear to have the thermal stability needed for frying and the jojoba oil solidified well above room temperature, limiting its use in liquid salad dressings, margarines, and possibly mayonnaise. The trialkoxytricarballyate and the sucrose fatty acid polyester appeared to have the most potential as fat substitutes. The difficulty in synthesizing trialkoxyglyceryl ether will probably limit its utility.

SELECTED APPLICATIONS

Numerous factors must be considered when selecting a fat substitute, in addition to the obvious and critical sensory quality questions. Is any thermal processing applied to the product? How severe is the thermal processing (pasteurization vs. sterilization)? How pH sensitive is the fat substitute? How long will the product be stored, i.e., are there undesirable textural or flavor changes that occur during long-term storage or during some excessively turbulent shipping? Will it be refrigerated? Must it be refrigerated? What are the home preparation steps involved? Is the product microbiologically stable? Are there "opportunities" for abuse in the home, i.e., if opened and left on the counter overnight, is food poisoning a possibility? The technical sales and support personnel of companies that sell fat substitutes should be knowledgeable about the use of their fat substitute in products similar to your product. If not, find a company that is knowledgeable. They should be able to demonstrate, with a concrete example, the utility of their fat substitute in your specific product. All of these companies should welcome an opportunity to show that their product works in your product.

A comparison of yogurts produced with one of seven selected fat substitutes was made with a control yogurt sample containing milkfat. The overall acceptability and organoleptic quality was comparable to the control for five of the seven fat substitutes: Litesse, N-Oil II, Lycadex-100, Lycadex-200, and Paselli SA2. Interestingly, the overall acceptability, including the flavor and aroma, generally improved after 20 days of storage (Barrantes et al., 1994a,b), in contrast to the control. Yogurt made with Simplesse was very similar to the control yogurt made with anhydrous milk fat (Barrantes et al., 1994c), except that the Simplesse-containing product had less sour flavor intensity and more serum separation than the control.

Ice milk samples made with fat mimetics (Simplesse or N-Lite D) and 2.1% milk fat were compared to control ice milk samples containing 4.8% milk fat (Schmidt et al., 1993). Overall, the protein- or Simplesse-containing product was more similar to the control sample than the sample containing the carbohydrate-based fat mimetic. The Simplesse-based ice milk samples had rheological properties that were generally the same as the control. However, the maximum overrun was over 40% greater for the Simplesse-containing sample than for the control. The maximum overrun for the carbohydrate-based fat mimetic was approximately 60% that of the control.

Milkfat content can be substantially reduced in frozen dairy dessert products with the addition of gums or maltodextrin gels (Frye and Setser, 1993; White, 1993). Low-DE maltodextrins, such as Paselli SA2, can be used with frozen dairy desserts if they are thermostable, cold water soluble and able to form stable mixtures with other components. Other thermostable, cold water–soluble carbohydrate-based fat substitutes include selected gums, e.g., carrageenan, guar gum, and carboxymethylcellulose.

Mono- and diglyceride emulsifiers can be used to replace as much as 50% of the fat in baked goods, since they can be used as a 50/50 emulsifier/water mixture (Frye and Setser, 1993; Vetter, 1993). Additional emulsifiers used similarly include sodium stearoyl lactylate, sorbitan monostearate, and poly-sorbate 60 at high hydration levels. A hydrated blend of emulsifiers developed specifically for fat replacement include stearyl monoglyceridyl citrate, glycol monostearate, and lactylated monoglycerides. Some of the products that can be used to make acceptable frozen dessert products include oatrim, Maltrin 40, and N-Oil. Simplesse, protein hydrolysates, Sta-Slim 143, and sucrose fatty acid esters have been used as fat substitutes in yogurt, sour cream, cream cheese, cheese spread, and frozen dairy desserts. Additional applications are discussed by Frye and Setser (1993).

Olestra can be used as a partial fat substitute in shortening, margarines and frying oils (Hollenback and Howard, 1983; Robbins and Rodriguez, 1984; Roberts, 1984). Simplesse and selected maltodextrins can be used in soft margarine applications for reduced-calorie spreads. The product has the mouthfeel, flavor, and spreading properties of a soft margarine (Frye and Setser, 1993).

Gums are used extensively in salad dressings to provide the viscosity associated with high-fat products (Quesada and Clark, 1993). Low pH stability by each gum is also required. Maltodextrins can be used, providing better product characteristics than gums (Frye and Setser, 1993). A 25% maltodextrin solution can replace 30–50% of the fat in salad dressings. Simplesse, as well as the fat-based substitutes, can be used in salad dressings and mayonnaise.

Meat applications for fat substitutes include breakfast sausages, hamburger, hot dogs, gravies, and soups. Some of the products used include Paselli SA2, N-Oil, carrageenan, hydrolyzed vegetable protein, cellulose gum, alginate, and maltodextrins (Frye and Setser, 1993). Carrageenan was used to produce a ground beef patty similar in product characteristics to the high-fat product (Egbert et al., 1991). Spices and a mixture of hydrolyzed vegetable protein and salt (1:2) were added (0.375%) to enhance beef flavor intensity, and 0.5% carrageenan and 10% water were added to enhance other product organoleptic attributes. (That formulation was adapted by McDonalds as their "McLean Deluxe.") Others have reported that hydrolyzed soy protein (McMindes, 1991) and oat bran (Pszczola, 1991) can both be effective as the major component in a fat-reduction system for ground meat.

One rather creative idea for using fat substitutes was the suggestion that sucrose fatty acid esters could be used to inhibit lipoxygenase and thereby improve food quality (Nishiyama et al., 1993). An increase in binding strength of the sucrose fatty acid monoester and soybean lipoxygenase-1 (L-1) occurred as the fatty acid carbon chain length was increased from 8 to 12. Thermodynamic analysis of the binding constants indicated that the binding was hydrophobic in character. Sucrose fatty acid esters also suppress lipase activity and have an antibacterial effect in some cases.

EFFECTS OF HEATING

During heating and deep-fat frying, numerous oxidative and thermally induced changes occur in triacylglycerols (TAGs). The TAG decomposition rate, as well as nonvolatile and volatile decomposition products that occur, are dependent upon the composition of the fatty acids that are present. If the fat-based fat substitutes contain the same fatty acids as found in native fats and oils, they are likely to have similar stabilities and produce most, if not all, of the same compounds that occur in heated, native TAGs. Some new compounds may be produced as well. These new compounds may or may not affect product flavor, oil stability, and product safety, depending upon the compounds produced and the amount formed.

Extensive reports of heating studies have been published on only one fat substitute. The first report on olestra, referred to prior to that time as sucrose polyester, was in 1990 (Gardner and Sanders, 1990). Two samples were heated and compared: the first was a sample of heated olestra, while the second was a heated mixture of olestra and partially hydrogenated soybean oil. The 100% olestra sample was heated at 190°C for 6 12-hour days in a 15-lb capacity fryer, while the mixture was heated at 185°C for 7 12-hour days in a 15-lb fryer. Raw, French-style cut potatoes were heated in the mixture through the 7 days of heating (49 batches/day at 380 g/batch). As expected, the relative percentage of polyunsaturated fatty acids decreased after heating, while the relative percentages of saturated fatty acids increased after heating for both samples.

The dimers in the heated olestra were fractionated with preparative thin-layer chromatography (TLC), while the dimers contained in the heated mixture of olestra and soybean oil were fractionated with preparative size exclusion chromatography (SEC). Fractions containing suspected dimers were transesterified. The methyl ester fatty acid dimers were separated with capillary gas chromatography (GC) and tentatively identified based on their retention times relative to methylated dimer fatty acid standards (Emery Chemical Co., Henkel-Emery Group, Cincinnati, OH) (Gardner and Sanders, 1990). In addition, mass spectral analysis, after gas chromatographic separation, was completed on the methyl ester fatty acid dimers. Polymer linkages identified were very similar to those occurring in thermal oxidized vegetable oils containing the same fatty acids.

Nuclear magnetic resonance (NMR) and infrared (IR) spectra were obtained for the intact olestra monomer and dimer isolates. Plasma desorption mass spectrometry (PDMS) of intact olestra dimers (Gardner and Sanders, 1990), as well as the olestra monomer (Sanders et al., 1992), were completed. During heating there was an increase in the high molecular weight components, as indicated by high-performance SEC analysis. The PDMS characterization of the high molecular weight olestra fraction isolated with HPSEC indicated that the fraction was an olestra dimer. In addition, PDMS analysis indicated the presence of an olestra-triglyceride component in the heated olestra-triglyceride mixture. The IR, carbon-13 NMR, and proton NMR spectra of the olestra monomer were virtually identical to those of the olestra dimer, indicating that changes in the sucrose backbone structure did not occur and that the high molecular weight components are olestra dimers. GC-MS analysis indicated the presence of dehydro dimers of methyl linoleate in the methylated dimer fatty acid fraction isolated from dimerized olestra and the HPSEC isolated olestra-triglyceride fraction, which indicates that the linkages are the same for the olestra dimers and the olestra-triglyceride component. In total, the results strongly suggest that the changes were occurring in the polyunsaturated fatty acids, rather than the sucrose backbone.

In 1992, two articles (Gardner et al., 1992; Henry et al., 1992) were published on the analysis of heated olestra. In the first report, Gardner et al. (1992) described in detail an analytical scheme developed for detailed qualitative comparisons of heated fats and oils. The oils (soybean oil and olestra) were transesterified, and the fatty acid methyl esters (FAMEs) were isolated. The FAMEs were separated on the basis of their polarity by adsorption chromatography and solid-phase extraction. Mass spectrometry and infrared spectroscopy were used to identify specific structural components in the compounds separated with capillary GC. The FAMEs (and other components soluble in the hexane phase) were first fractionated with silica gel column chromatography into four fractions: I and II, unaltered FAMEs; III, altered FAMEs; and IV, polar materials. Fraction III was further separated with solid phase extraction (C18) into A, oxidized FAMEs, and B, FAME dimers. GC separation of fraction IIIA resulted in the detection of FAMEs of various chain lengths with aldehydic, hydroxy, epoxy, and keto functional groups. GC separation of fraction IIIB resulted in the detection of three plant sterols and some dimer FAMEs. HPLC separation of fraction IV produced components consisting of oxidized di- and triglycerides, monoglycerides, and two very polar FAMEs, one of which was tentatively identified as 9-hydroxyperoxy-10,12-octadecadienoate.

The second report (Henry et al., 1992) used the fractionation methods presented in the first paper (Gardner et al., 1992) to provide a detailed qualitative comparison of the transesterified fatty acids from the heated olestra and heated soybean oil. The olestra was produced from partially hydrogenated soybean oil. Olestra and soybean were separately used to fry potatoes. The heated oils were transesterified and fractionated into four fractions based on polarity with the fractionation scheme presented in Gardner et al. Analysis indicated that the fatty acid components of both oils undergo similar chemical reactions and changes upon frying, and that the altered FAMEs found were similar to those found in heated fats and oils by other investigators (Henry et al., 1992).

The oxidative stability index (OSI) is commonly used in the food industry to measure oil quality, particularly concerning the expected life of an oil upon heating. Akoh (1994b) compared eight different oils, including some fat substitutes, with an Omnion OSI instrument. The four vegetable oils examined were crude soybean oil, crude peanut oil, refined, bleached, and deodorized (RBD) soybean oil, and RBD peanut oil. The four oil substitutes analyzed included a soybean oil–derived sucrose polyester, a high oleate/stearate sucrose polyester, a butterfat-derived sucrose polyester, and a methyl glucoside polyester of soybean oil. As determined by the OSI, the crude oils were the most stable, RBD oils were second, and the least stable were the oil substitutes.

SUMMARY AND CONCLUSIONS

Fat can impart some very desirable flavor and textural characteristics to food. However, fat has some very undesirable characteristics, which include a high caloric content and a strong association with cardiovascular disease and obesity. As a result, substantial commercial effort has been expended to develop reduced-fat/reduced-calorie food products and fat substitutes. The fat substitutes include the protein-based and carbohydrate-based fat mimetics, reduced-calorie fat replacers, and the fat-based fat substitutes. The protein-based and carbohydrate-based fat mimetics are used extensively in food products and are available from a variety of commercial sources. The reduced-calorie fat replacers are limited in number and commercial use, but could see substantial increase in use over the next few years. None of the fat-based fat substitutes has been approved, but since they could provide the desirable flavor and textural characteristics without little, if any, caloric impact, their use could be substantial soon after FDA approval.

The protein-based fat mimetics generally consist of an aqueous suspension of microparticulated protein. The concentration and particle size of the small protein spheres produces a product that has some of the textural characteristics of fats and oils. The carbohydrate-based fat mimetics are designed to increase the viscosity of the water/carbohydrate solution or suspension such that oil or fat textural characteristics are imparted to the product. In addition, carbohydrate-based materials are used to increase emulsion stability in food products.

The reduced-calorie, fat-based products are designed to either be used at reduced concentrations relative to regular fat and/or have a reduced caloric content due to reduction in the absorption of the product, e.g., Salatrim. The fat-based fat substitutes generally use food-grade materials as a starting point to produce a product that is not susceptible to lipase activity due to a change in the components on each side of the ester bond from the normal glycerol and fatty acid. These changes include substituting glucose for glycerol, switching a fatty alcohol and organic acid for the fatty acid and glycerol, or adding a small extension to the glycerol so that the fatty acid is no longer adjacent to the glycerol, thereby reducing the susceptibility of the ester bond to lipase.

Numerous applications have been examined and are commercially available for the protein-based and carbohydrate-based products, including low-fat dairy products, low-fat baked goods, and low-fat meat products. The fat-based fat substitutes could be used just as easily in the same products.

During heating, fats and oils undergo thermolytic and oxidative changes, changes that can impart very desirable flavor characteristics to fried foods during deep-fat frying. The fat-based fat substitutes have the potential to produce the same effect, but carefully designed investigations on their heat stability and flavor profiles during heating must be undertaken to confirm this assumption. It appears that the American public is willing, perhaps even anxious, to include low-fat foods in their diet, particularly if product taste and textural characteristics are similar to those found in high-fat products.

REFERENCES

Akoh, C. C. 1992. Emulsification properties of polyesters and sucrose ester blends I: Carbohydrate fatty acid polyesters. *J. Am. Oil Chem. Soc.* 69: 9–13.

Akoh, C. C. 1994a. Synthesis of carbohydrate fatty acid polyesters. In *Carbohydrate Polyesters as Fat Substitutes*, pp. 9–35. Marcel Dekker, Inc., New York.

Akoh, C. C. 1994b. Oxidative stability of fat substitutes and vegetable oils by the oxidative stability index method. *J. Am. Oil Chem. Soc.* 71: 211–216.

Akoh, C. C. and Swanson, B. G. 1989. Synthesis and properties of alkyl glycoside and stacyose fatty acid polyesters. *J. Am. Oil Chem. Soc.* 66: 1295–1301.

Akoh, C. C. and Swanson, B. G. 1990. Optimized synthesis of sucrose polyesters: Comparison of physical properties of sucrose polyesters, raffinose polyesters and salad oils. *J. Food Sci.* 55: 236–243.

Akoh, C. C. and Swanson, B. G. 1994. A background and history of carbohydrate polyesters. In *Carbohydrate Polyesters as Fat Substitutes*, pp. 1–8. Marcel Dekker, Inc., New York.

Akoh, C. C. and Nwosu, C. V. 1992. Emulsification properties of polyesters and sucrose ester blends II: Alkyl glycoside polyesters. *J. Am. Oil Chem. Soc.* 69: 14–19.

Altschul, A. M. 1993. *Low-Caloric Foods Handbook*. Marcel Dekker, Inc., New York.

American Dietetic Association (ADA). 1991. Position of the American Dietetic Association: Fat replacements. *J. Am. Diet. Assoc.* 90(11): 1285–1288.

Anonymous. 1989. Fats, oils and fat substitutes. *Food Technol.* 43(7): 72–73.

Anonymous. 1990a. Fat substitute update. *Food Technol.* 44(3): 92–97.

Anonymous. 1990b. USDA's oatrim replaces fat in many food products. *Food Technol.* 44(10): 100.

Anonymous. 1991a. Fat substitute for dairy and oil-based products. *Food Technol.* 42(4): 96–97.

Anonymous. 1991b. Carbohydrate-based ingredient performs like fat for use in a variety of food applications. *Food Technol.* 45(8): 262–265.

Anonymous. 1991c. Quest for fat substitutes taking many routes. *INFORM* 2(2): 115–119.

Anonymous. 1992a. Six fat mimetics developed for specific food applications. *Food Technol.* 46(4): 110–111.

Anonymous. 1992b. Consumers receiving conflicting messages. *INFORM* 3: 676–677.

Anonymous. 1994. Stepan seeks GRAS status for Caprin. *INFORM* 5: 1167.

Arciszewski, H. 1991. Fat functionality, reduction in baked foods. *INFORM* 2(4): 392–399.

Artz, W. E. and Hansen, S. L. 1994. Other fat substitutes. In *Carbohydrate Polyesters as Fat Substitutes*, C. C. Akoh and B. G. Swanson (Ed.), pp. 197–236. Marcel Dekker, Inc., New York.

Barrantes, E., Tamime, A. Y., Davies, G., and Barclay, M. N. I. 1994a. Production of low-calorie yogurt using skim milk powder and fat-substitute. 2. Compositional quality. *Milchwissenschaft* 49: 135–139.

Barrantes, E., Tamime, A. Y., and Sword, A. M. 1994b. Production of low-calorie yogurt using skim milk powder and fat-substitute. 3. Microbiological and organoleptic qualities. *Milchwissenschaft* 49: 85–88.

Barrantes, E., Tamime, A. Y., Muir, D. D., Sword, A. M. 1994c. The effect of substitution of fat by microparticulate whey protein on the quality of set-type, natural yogurt. *J. Soc. Dairy Technol.* 47(2): 61–68.

Beaton, G. H., Tarasuk, V., and Anderson, G. H. 1992. Estimation of possible impact of non-caloric fat and carbohydrate substitutes on macronutrient intake in the human. *Appetite* 19: 87–103.

Benmoussa, K., Sabouraud, A., Scherrmann, J.-M., Brossard, D., and Bourre, J.-M. 1992. Effect of fat substitutes, sucrose polyester and tricarballyate triester, on digitoxin absorption in the rat. *J. Pharm. Pharmacol.* 45: 692–696.

Bergholz, C. M. 1992. Safety evaluation of olestra, a nonabsorbed fatlike fat replacement. *Crit. Rev. Food Sci. Nutr.* 32: 141–146.

Birch, L. L., Johnson, S. L., Jones, M. B., and Peters, J. C. 1993. Effects of a nonenergy fat substitute on children's energy and macronutrient intake. *Am. J. Clin. Nutr.* 58: 326–333.

Borzelleca, J. F. 1992. Macronutrient substitutes: Safety evaluation. *Regul. Toxicol. Pharmacol.* 16: 253–264.

Bracco, E. F., Baba, N., and Hashim, S. A. 1987. Polysiloxane: Potential noncaloric fat substitutes; effects on body composition of obese Zucker rats. *Am. J. Clin. Nutr.* 46: 784–789.

Bruhn, C. M., Cotter, A., Diaz-Knauf, K., Sutherlin, J., West, E., Wightman, N., Williamson, E., and Yakkee, M. 1992. Consumer attitudes and market potential for foods using fat substitutes. *Food Technol.* 46(4): 81–86.

Caputo, F. A., and Mattes, R. D. 1992. Human dietary responses to covert manipulations of energy, fat and carbohydrate in a mid-day meal. *Am. J. Clin. Nutr.* 56:36–43.

Chase, Jr., G. W., Akoh, C. C., and Eitenmiller, R. R. 1994. Evaporative light scattering mass detection for high-performance liquid chromatographic analysis of sucrose polyester blends in cooking oils. *J. Am. Oil Chem. Soc.* 71: 1273–1276.

Cheftel, J. C. and Dumay, E. 1993. Microcoagulation of proteins for development of creaminess. *Food Rev. Int.* 9: 473–502.

Cheryan, M. 1991. Membranes in food processing. In *Effective Industrial Membrane Processes—Benefits and Opportunities*, M. Cheryan (Ed.), pp. 157–180. Elsevier Science Publishers Ltd., England.

Cooper, C. F. 1990. Preparation of propoxylated glycerides as dietary fat substitutes. Eur. Patent 353,928.

Deger, H. M., Fritsche-Lang, W., Reng, A., Schlingman, M., and Lawson, C. J. 1988. Verfahren zur Herstellung von Gemischen aus mono-und oligomeren Kohlenhydratestern, die so erhaeltlichen Kohlenhydratestergemische und ihre Verwerdung. GFR Patent 3,639,878.

Dobson, K. S., Williams, K. D., and Boriack, C. J. 1993. The preparation of polyglycerol esters suitable as low-caloric fat substitutes. *J. Am. Oil Chem. Soc.* 70: 1089–1092.

Drake, M. A., Ma, L., Swanson, B. G., and Canovas, G. V. B. 1994a. Rheological characteristics of milkfat and milkfat-blend sucrose polyesters. *Food Res. Int.* 27: 477–481.

Drake, M. A., Boutte, T. T., Younce, F. L., Cleary, D. A., and Swanson, B. G. 1994b. Melting characteristics and hardness of milkfat blend sucrose polyesters. *J. Food Sci.* 59: 652–654.

Drake, M. A., Boutte, T. T., Luedecke, L. O., and Swanson, B. G. 1994c. Milkfat sucrose polyesters as fat substitutes in cheddar-type cheeses. *J. Food Sci.* 59: 652–654.

Drake, M. A., Nagel, C. W., and Swanson, B. G. 1994d. Sucrose polyester content in foods by a colorimetric method. *J. Food Sci.* 59: 655–656.

Duxbury, D. D. and Meinhold, N. M. 1991. Dietary fats and oils. *Food Process.* 52(3): 58–61.

Dziezak, J. D. 1989. Fats, oils, and fat substitutes. *Food Technol.* 43(7): 66–74.

Egbert, W. R., Huffman, D. L., Chen, C., and Dylewski, D. P. 1991. Development of low-fat ground beef. *Food Technol.* 45(6): 69–73.

Ennis, J. L., Kopf, P. W., Rudolf, S. E., and van Buren, M. F. 1991. Esterified alkoxylated alkyl glycosides useful in low calorie fat-containing food compositions. Eur. Patent 415,636.

Frye, C. L. 1986. Fat and oil replacements as human food ingredients. Eur. Patent 205,273.

Frye, A. M. and Setser, C. S. 1993. Bulking agents and fat substitutes. In *Low-Calorie Foods Handbook*, A. M. Altschul (Ed.), pp. 211–251. Marcel Dekker, Inc., New York.

Fulcher, J. 1986. Synthetic cooking oils containing dicarboxylic acid esters. U.S. Patent 4,582,927.

Gardner, D. R. and Sanders, R. A. 1990. Isolation and characterization of polymers in heated Olestra and an Olestra/triglyceride blend. *J. Am. Oil Chem. Soc.* 67: 788–796.

Gardner, D. R., Sanders, R. A., Henry, D. E., Tallmadge, D. H., and Wharton, H. W. 1992. Characterization of used frying oils. Part I: Isolation and identification of compound classes. *J. Am. Oil Chem. Soc.* 69: 499–508.

Gerrish, T. C. 1995. The use of pectin as an oil barrier for deep fat fried potatoes. Abstract No. 61-4. 1995 IFT Annual Meeting *Abstract Book*, Los Angeles, CA.

Gillis, A. 1988. Fat substitutes create new issues. *J. Am. Oil Chem. Soc.* 65: 1708–1711.

Glicksman, M. 1991. Hydrocolloids and the search for the oily grail. *Food Technol.* 45(10): 94–103.

Habib, M. and Podolski, J. S. 1989. Concentrated, substantially non-aggregated casein micelles as a fat/cream substitute. Eur. Patent Application 0,334,226. NutraSweet Co.

Hamm, D. J. 1984. Preparation and evaluation of trialkoxytricarballyate, trialkoxycitrate, trialkoxyglycerylether, jojoba oil, and sucrose polyester as low calories replacements of edible fats and oils. *J. Food Sci.* 49: 419–428.

Harrigan, K. A. and Breene, W. M. 1989. Fat substitutes: Sucrose esters and simplesse. *Cereal Foods World* 34: 261–267.

Harris, R. B. S. and Jones, W. K. 1991. Physiological response of mature rats to replacement of dietary fat with a fat substitute. *J. Nutr.*: 1109–1116.

Hassel, C. A. 1993. Nutritional implications of fat substitutes. *Cereal Foods World* 38: 142–144.

Haumann, B. F. 1986. Getting the fat out. *J. Am. Oil Chem. Soc.* 63: 278–288.

Henry, D. E., Tallmadge, D. H., Sanders, R. A., and Gardner, D. R. 1992. Characterization of used frying oils. Part 2: Comparison of Olestra and triglyceride. *J. Am. Oil Chem. Soc.* 69: 508–519.

Hippleheuser, A. L., Landberg, L. A., and Turnak, F. L. 1995. A system approach to formulating a low-fat muffin. *Food Technol.* 49(3): 92–95.

Hollenbach, E. J. and Howard, N. B. 1983. Emulsion concentrate for palatable polyester beverage. U.S. Patent 4,368,213.

Huhn, S. D., Given, P. S. Jr., and Klemann, L. P. 1989. Ether bridged polyesters and food compositions containing ether bridged polyesters. U.S. Patent 4,888,195.

Inglett, G. E. and Grisamore, S. B. 1991. Maltodextrin fat substitute lowers cholesterol. *Food Technol.* 45(6): 104.

Jandacek, R. J. 1991a. The development of Olestra, a noncaloric substitute for dietary fat. *J. Chem. Educ.* 68: 476–479.

Jandacek, R. J. 1991b. Developing a fat substitute. *Chemtech* 21: 398–402.

Klemann, L. P. and Finley, J. W. 1989a. Low calorie fat mimetics comprising carboxy/carboxylate esters. Eur Patent 303,523.

Klemann, L. P. and Finley, J. W. 1989b. Low calorie fat mimetics comprising carboxy/carboxylate esters. International Patent 89/01293.

Klemann, L. P., Finley, J. W., and Simone, A. 1990a. Tris-hydroxymethyl alkane esters as low calorie fat mimetics. U.S. Patent 4,927,658.

Kelmann, L. P., Finley, J. W., and Simone, A. 1990b. Tris-hydroxymethyl lower alkane esters as fat mimetics. U.S. Patent 4,927,659.

Kresl, K. E. and Higgins, C. A. 1995. Oil reduction in batter and breaded food items using calcium reactive pectin chemistry. Abstract No. 61-5. 1995 IFT Annual Meeting *Abstract Book*, Los Angeles, CA.

LaBarge, R. G. 1988. The search for a low-caloric oil. *Food Technol.* 42(1): 84–90.

Labell, F. 1991. MCT oil metabolizes like carbohydrate. *Food Process.* 52(2): 60–64.

Mai, J., Breitbar, D., and Fischer, C. D. 1990. Proteinaceous material. Eur. Patent Application 0,400,714. Unilever, NV.

Marquez-Ruiz, G., Perez-Camino, M. C., Rios, J. J., and Dobarganes, M. C. 1994. Characterization of sucrose polyesters-triacylglycerol mixtures. *J. Am. Oil Chem. Soc.* 71: 1017–1020.

Mattson, F. H., Glueck, C. J., and Jandacek, R. J. 1979. The lowering of plasma cholesterol by sucrose polyester in subjects consuming diets with 800, 300 or less than 50 mg cholesterol per day. *Am. J. Clin. Nutr.* 32: 1636–1644.

McMindes, M. K. 1991. Applications of isolated soy protein in low-fat meat products. *Food Technol.* 45(12): 61–64.

Mela, D. J. 1992. Nutritional implications of fat substitutes. *J. Am. Diet. Assoc.* 92: 472–476.

Meyer, R. S., Root, J. M., Campbell, M. L., and Winter, D. B. 1989. Low calorie alkyl glycoside fatty acid polyester fat substitutes. U.S. Patent 4,840,815.

Mieth, V. G. 1992. Akalorische Lipide—Enwicklungstrends und Probleme ihrer Applikation als Fettaustauschstoffe. *Fat Sci. Technol.* 94: 496–505.

Mieth, G., Weiss, A., Behrens, H., Pohl, J., and Brueckner, J. 1982. Verfahren zur Herstellung von Kohlenhydrat-fettsäureestern. GDR Patent 3,156,283.

Morehouse, S. E. and Zabik, M. E. 1989. Evaluation of polydimethylsiloxane fluids as non-caloric frying media. *J. Food Sci.* 54: 1062–1065.

Munro, I. C. 1990. Issues to be considered in the safety evaluation of fat substitutes. *Food Chem. Tox.* 28: 751–753.

Nishiyama, J., Shizu, Y., and Kuninori, T. 1993. Inhibition of soybean lipoxygenase-1 by sucrose esters of fatty acids. *BioSci. Biotech. Biochem.* 57: 557–560.

Nuck, B. A., Schlagheck, T. G., and Federle, T. W. 1994. Inability of the human fecal microflora to metabolize the nonabsorbable fat substitute, Olestra. *J. Indust. Micro.* 13: 328–334.

Penichter, K. A. and McGinley, E. J. 1991. Cellulose gel for fat-free food applications. *Food Technol.* 45(6): 105.

Pszczola, D. E. 1991. Oat-bran-based ingredient blend replaces fat in ground beef and pork sausage. *Food Technol.* 45(11): 60–66.

Quesada, L. A. and Clark, W. L. 1993. Low-calorie foods: General category. In *Low-Calorie Foods Handbook*, A. M. Altschul (Ed.), pp. 293–321. Marcel Dekker, Inc., New York.

Rios, J. J., Perez-Camino, M. C., Marquez-Ruiz, G., and Dobarganes, M. C. 1994. Isolation and characterization of sucrose polyesters. *J. Am. Oil Chem. Soc.* 71: 385–390.

Riva, S. 1994. Enzymatic synthesis of carbohydrate esters. In *Carbohydrate Polyesters as Far Substitutes*, pp. 37–64. Marcel Dekker, Inc., New York.

Roberts, B. A. 1984. Oleaginous compositions. U.S. Patent 4,446,165.

Robbins, M. B. and Rodriguez, S. S. 1984. Low calorie baked products. U.S. Patent 4,461,782.

Rolls, B. J., Pirraglia, P. A., Jones, M. B., and Peters, J. C. 1992. Effects of Olestra, a noncaloric fat substitute, on daily energy fan fat intakes in lean men. *Am. J. Clin. Nutr.* 56: 84–92.

Ryan, J. W. 1989. Prevention of anal leakage of polyorganosiloxane fluids used as fat substitutes in foods. Eur. Patent 368,534.

Ryan, J. W. 1990. Food composition containing a siloxane polymer and a particulate silica. U.S. Patent 4,925,692.

Sanders, R. A., Gardner, D. R., Lacey, M. P., and Keough, T. 1992. Desorption mass spectrometry of Olestra. *J. Am. Oil Chem. Soc.* 69: 760–771.

Schmidt, K., Lundy, A., Reynolds, J., and Lee, L. N. 1993. Carbohydrate or protein based fat mimicker effects on ice milk properties. *J. Food Sci.* 58: 761–763.

Shukla, T. P. 1992. Low-fat foods and fat substitutes. *Cereal Foods World* 37: 452–453.

Singer, N. S., Yamamoto, S., and Latella, J. 1988. Protein product base. U.S. Patent 4,734,287 and European Patent Application 0,250,623. John Labatt, Ltd.

Singer, N. S. and Moser, R. H. 1993. Microparticulated proteins as fat substitutes. In *Low-Calorie Foods Handbook*, A. M. Altschul (Ed.), pp. 171–179. Marcel Dekker, Inc., New York.

Smith, R. E. 1993. Food demands of the emerging consumer: The role of modern food technology in meeting that challenge. *Am. J. Clin. Nutr.* 58(suppl): 307S–312S.

Smith, R. E., Finley, J. W., and Leveille, G. A. 1994. Overview of SALATRIM, a family of low-calorie fats. *J. Agric. Food Chem.* 42: 432–434.

Stark, L. E. and Gross, A. T. 1990. Hydrophobic protein microparticles and preparation thereof. World Patent Application WO 90/03123. Enzytech, Inc.

Tamimie, A. Y., Barclay, M. N. I., Davies, G., and Barrantes, E. 1994. Production of low-calorie yogurt using skim milk powder and fat-substitute. 1. A review. *Milchwissenschaft* 49: 85–88.

Trost, V. W. 1981. Low calorie fat substitutes. Canada Patent 1,106,681.

U.S. Surgeon General. 1988. *The Surgeon General's Report on Nutrition and Health.* U.S. Department of Health and Human Services, DHHS (PHS) Publication No. 88-50210.

Vanderveen, J. E. 1994. Regulatory status of macronutrient substitutes: what FDA needs to assure safety. Paper No. 15-1. 1994 IFT Annual Meeting *Abstract Book*, Atlanta, GA.

Vetter, J. L. 1993. Low-calorie bakery foods. In *Low-Calorie Foods Handbook*, A. M. Altschul (Ed.), pp. 273–291. Marcel Dekker, Inc., New York.

Volpenhein, R. 1985. Synthesis of higher polyol fatty acid polyesters using carbonate catalysts. U.S. Patent 4,517,360.

Volpenhein, R. A. 1986. Acylated glycerides useful in low calorie fat-containing food compositions. U.S. Patent 4,582,715.

White, C. H. 1993. Low-fat dairy products. In *Low-Calorie Foods Handbook*, A. M. Altschul (Ed.), pp. 253–271. Marcel Dekker, Inc., New York.

White, J. F. 1990. Partially esterified polysaccharides (PEP) fat substitutes. U.S. Patent 4,959,466.

White, J. F. and Pollard, M. R. 1988. Esterified epoxide-extended polyols as nondigestiable fat substitutes of low-caloric value. Eur. Patent 254,547.

White, J. F. and Pollard, M. R. 1989a. Non-digestible fat substitutes of low-calorie value. U.S. Patent 4,861,613.

White, J. F. and Pollard, M. R. 1989b. Non-digestible fat substitutes of low-calorie value. Eur. Patent 325,010.

White, J. F. and Pollard, M. R. 1989c. Low-calorific and non-digestive substitute of fat/oil. China Patent 1,034,572.

Whyte, D. D. 1971. Triglyceride esters of α-branched carboxylic acids. U.S. Patent 3,579,548.

Winter, D. B., Meyer, R. S., Root, J. M., and Campbell, M. L. 1990. Process for producing low calorie foods from alkyl glycoside fatty acid polyesters. U.S. Patent 4,942,054.

Yackel, W. C. and Cox, C. 1992. Application of starch-based fat replacers. *Food Technol.* 46(6): 146–148.

17
The Role of Lipids in Medical and Designer Foods

Mary K. Schmidl

Humanetics Corporation
St. Louis Park, Minnesota

INTRODUCTION

Medical foods are unique formulas that are used widely in the nutritional support of patients with disease or clinical conditions. Often these formulas are administered via enteric feeding tubes to hospitalized, nursing home, or at-home patients. They may provide complete nutritional support or be used in conjunction with total parenteral nutrition (TPN) or as a supplement (partial feeding). Lately they are being designed to meet the needs of various age groups ranging from older adults to pediatric patients.

The term designer foods may have evolved from the National Academy of Sciences–National Research Council's report "Designing Foods," which discusses future trends and developments in the creation of nutritionally based products for the U.S. population (NRC, 1988). Specific items of interest are the breeding of animals with less fat and more desirable types of fat (e.g., unsaturated), the development of genetically engineered dairy starter cultures that digest the cholesterol in butterfat during fermentation of cheese, resulting in a no-cholesterol product, and the use of microorganisms to remove offending amino acids from protein for those with inborn errors of metabolism. Research is also recommended to determine the extent of genetic variation in the cholesterol content of animals, the reduction of oxidative rancidity of animal products through feeding or management, and the development of more cost-effective methods of efficiently producing low-fat animal products by integrated production management systems.

More recently, other novel terms for designation of special diets have infiltrated the marketing and scientific literature. These include nutraceuticals, functional foods, and pharmafoods (Schmidl and Labuza, 1994). Whatever term is used, the end goal is to provide a product that will improve the health or disease condition of the individual or patient, maintain optimum health, or promote longevity.

Medical food is the only term from this group that has a legal definition. In 1988, Congress amended the Orphan Drug Act to include the first legal definition of medical foods [21 U.S. Code 360ee (b)]. The definition was later codified in 21 CFR 101.9(8):

> A medical food is a food which is formulated to be consumed or administered enterally under the supervision of a physician and which is intended for the specific dietary management of a disease or condition for which distinctive nutritional requirements, based on recognized scientific principles, are established by medical evaluation. A food is subject to this exemption only if:
>
> (i) It is a specially formulated and processed product (as opposed to a naturally occurring foodstuff used in its natural state) for the partial or exclusive feeding of a patient by means of oral intake or enteral feeding by tube;
>
> (ii) It is intended for the dietary management of a patient who, because of therapeutic or chronic medical needs, has limited or impaired capacity to ingest, digest, absorb or metabolize ordinary food stuffs or certain nutrients, or who has other special medically determined nutrient requirements, the dietary management of which cannot be achieved by the modification of the normal diet alone;
>
> (iii) It provides nutritional support specifically modified for the management of the unique nutrient needs that result from the specific disease or condition, as determined by medical evaluation;
>
> (iv) It is intended to be used under medical supervision; and
>
> (v) It is intended only for a patient receiving active and ongoing medical supervision wherever the patient requires medical care on a recurring basis for, among other things, instructions on the use of the medical food.

BACKGROUND

The use of medical foods in the clinical setting is a relatively recent phenomenon and in some ways has developed due to the limitations put on parenteral nutrition (PN) technology (Schmidl et al., 1988). In the 1990s, health care reform has driven many health care professionals to carefully scrutinize their practices, review and conduct scientific clinical trials, and carefully monitor the needs of the patient. This has created a renewed interest in enteral nutrition when compared to PN.

Enteral nutrition products that are fed by tube are commonly used basically to meet the needs of patients who will not or cannot normally ingest what they require. Compared to TPN, enteral nutrition is the preferred route for the following reasons:

1. Enteral nutrition is more cost-effective in terms of materials, equipment and professional supervision.

2. Mechanical metabolic and septic complications of intravenous feeding can be significant or are not required for enteral foods. Catheter infections are of major concern to the clinician.

3. The apparent physiological benefits of providing nutrients directly to the gastrointestinal (GI) tract and preserving GI integrity along with providing preferred gut fuels (e.g., glutamine) continues to be essential in prevention of bacterial translocation and associated metabolic complications.

4. The effectiveness of enteral nutrition has been validated in numerous clinical studies over the past two decades (Randall, 1990).

PRODUCT CLASSIFICATION

Medical foods are indicated for patients who cannot ingest adequate amounts of food but have enough GI function to allow digestion and absorption of feeding solutions delivered into the GI tract. Examples of specific clinical indications include:

Severe dysphagia from obstruction or dysfunction

Disease or disorders requiring administration of specific solutions

Fistulas of the distal small bowel or colon

Severe malabsorption

Long-term anorexia

Coma

Recurrent aspiration (avoid feeding into the stomach)

Examples of disease or clinical conditions include cancer, general surgery, inflammatory bowel disease, renal disorder, neurological disorder, pulmonary disease, diabetes, HIV/AIDS, and hypermetabolism.

There are numerous medical food products and classification systems (Heimburger and Weinsier, 1985; Hatton and MacKey, 1989; IFT Status Summary, 1992; Shike, 1994). FDA's Compliance Program Guidance (FDA, 1989) identifies four major categories of products: (1) nutritionally complete products, (2) nutritionally incomplete (modular) products, (3) products for metabolic disorders, and (4) rehydration products.

Nutritionally Complete Products

The majority of medical foods currently in use are nutritionally complete enteral formulations. These formulations supply all the required protein, fat, carbohydrates, vitamins, and minerals in sufficient quantities to maintain the nutritional status of individuals receiving no other source of nourishment and are used for nutritional sustenance of patients with a wide variety of clinical conditions. The products within this class can be further subdivided on the basis of compositional profile (i.e., amount of fiber, caloric density, milk-based, lactose-free, etc.) and range from those composed of whole protein, carbohydrates, and fats to those consisting of simple sugars, amino acids, and medium-chain triglycerides (MCTs). The latter are indicated for individuals with impaired ability to digest or absorb intact nutrients. The raw materials used in the manufacture of nutritionally complete enteral formulations are supplied in such forms as calcium and sodium caseinate, soy protein isolate, crystalline amino acids, hydrolyzed cornstarch, and corn, canola, soy, and safflower oils.

Nutritionally Incomplete Products

These enteral formulations supply a single nutrient or combinations of nutrients in quantities insufficient to maintain the nutritional status of normal, healthy individuals. Known as modular components, these products can be used as supplemental sources of nutrients and calories in otherwise normal diets (e.g., whey protein as a nitrogen source), or they can be combined with other modular components to produce a nutritionally complete formula.

The number of modular components in the marketplace has steadily increased. They permit flexibility because they can be tailored to meet special individual requirements. However, the disadvantages of modular products may outweigh their advantages and limit their widespread use. Disadvantages include (1) lack of sufficient labor in most institutions to properly mix the formulations, (2) need for considerable expertise in mixing and calculating the amounts of modular components required to fulfill the dietary needs of the patients, (3) expense of these individually tailored formulations, (4) increased potential for environmental and/or microbial contamination during preparation, in the hospital or at home, by individuals untrained in dietetics or clinical nutrition, and (5) potential for induction of metabolic disorders or deficiency states resulting from the lack of or excess of specific nutrients in the blended formula.

Formulas for Metabolic (Genetic) Disorders

These formulations are manufactured specifically for individuals with in-born errors of metabolism, e.g., phenylketonuria (PKU), maple syrup urine disease (MSUD), urea cycle disorder, glycogen storage disease, propionic acidemia, or methylmalonic acidemia. Although not nutritionally complete in the traditional sense (e.g., PKU products have a reduced level of aromatic amino acids to which the minimum amount of phenylalanine needed to meet the growth requirement of the infant is added), these formulas are designated to provide the nutrient composition necessary for the growth and development of persons afflicted with a specific metabolic disorder. The National Organization for Rare Disease has been formed to help promote research into the dietary restrictions and requirements for these diseases, as well as to enable third-party insurance payments for special medical foods. In these metabolic disorders and others treated with special individual formulations, histopathology may change with age, affecting nutrient requirements and eliciting the need to modify the medical food in unknown dimensions.

Oral Rehydration Solutions

These medical foods consist of products indicated for replacement of water and electrolytes that have been lost through mild to severe diarrhea. Standard components of these formulations include sodium, chloride, potassium, citrate, dextrose, and water. Recent scientific literature also suggests the use of rice syrup solids and other carbohydrate-related compounds (i.e., fibers) in these supplements (Molina et al., 1995; Lebenthal et al., 1995).

LIPIDS AND ENTERAL NUTRITION

From the 1970s to the early 1990s, when the majority of enteral formulas were being developed, the focus was on designing formulas based on a typical American diet using the knowledge base of fatty acid metabolism and nutritional requirements. For example, it was known that the normal American diet constituted 40–45% of calories mainly in the form of long-chain triglycerides, the major source of fat coming from butterfat, corn oil, soybean oil, and safflower oil. The role of fat was to provide a concentrated source of calories (9 kcal/g) and the essential fatty acid linoleic acid (Burr and Burr, 1930). It was determined then that linoleic acid (18:2 omega-6) should be supplied in amounts of 2–4% of the total calories. Small quantities of α-linolenic acid, an omega-3 fatty acid found to be essential for growth and development in children and adults (Holman et al., 1982; Bjerve et al., 1987), were also recommended. Table 17.1 illustrates the high level of linoleic acid found in selected vegetable oils commonly used at that time for medical foods. Additionally, these oils were chosen based on (1) availability, (2) flavor, (3) cost, (4) ease of processing (ability to incorporate into emulsions), (5) stability, and (6) FDA approval status. They were often used in amounts ranging from 30 to 50% of the total calories.

It should also be remembered that, in this time period, physicians and patients were bombarded with information concerning dietary fats and health (Kris-Etherton et al., 1988). This campaign focused primarily on lowering serum cholesterol levels in the population to reduce the nation's high level of coronary artery disease, primarily through serum cholesterol screening and convincing those in the upper percentile (>200 mg/dL) to take corrective action. In addition to a reduction in dietary cholesterol, one of the most popular dietary changes to lower serum cholesterol was to reduce dietary saturated fat and partially replace it with polyunsaturated fats. The National Cholesterol Education Program augmented by industry-sponsored advertising and the Nutrition Labeling and Education Act (NLEA) of 1990, followed by the regulations in 1994, continue to promote foods that do not contain cholesterol as well as those that are higher in polyunsaturated fats.

TABLE 17.1 Typical Linoleic Acid (18:2 omega-6) Content in Vegetable Oils

Oil source	% Linoleic acid
Safflower oil	78
Sunflower oil	66
Corn oil	58
Soybean oil	54

All of these efforts at reducing the coronary risk of the American population through dietary changes are laudable but in general have little or no significance in the choice of fatty acids for many medical foods. Medical and designer foods are often designed for specific well-defined metabolic conditions, and therefore to mimic the typical American diet or to add high levels of polyunsaturated fatty acids (PUFAs) to lower serum cholesterol may be inherently incorrect. Many disease conditions may not require reduction of cholesterol, in fact some disease conditions may suggest the need to have cholesterol added to the diet. In addition, excess polyunsaturated fatty acids (especially omega-6) may be detrimental to specific patient groups. These will be discussed below.

NOMENCLATURE OF FATTY ACIDS

Fatty acids are characterized according to carbon chain length, presence and number of double bonds, and position of these double bonds. Physical and chemical properties are in part related to the carbon chain length of a given fatty acid, with the length being categorized as short chain (2–4 carbons), medium chain (6–12 carbons), and long chain (14–24 carbons). PUFAs have two or more double bonds per fatty acid. Fatty acids with one double bond are called monounsaturated, and those with no double bonds are referred to as saturated. PUFAs may be divided into four families according to the location of the double bond closest to the terminal methyl end of the carbon chain: omega-3, omega-6, omega-7, and omega-9. The structure of a given fatty acid can be briefly described by noting its overall carbon chain length, the number of double bonds, and the position of the first double bond. For example, the PUFA linoleic acid (LA) has 18 carbon atoms in its carbon chain with two double bonds, the first being at the sixth carbon from the methyl terminal end, and is denoted 18:2 omega-6. Table 17.2 lists names and formulas for many of the clinically or nutritionally important fatty acids.

LONG-CHAIN FATTY ACIDS

Dietary lipids in medical foods are commonly composed of long-chain triglycerides (LCTs). These lipids supply a source of noncarbohydrate calories. The respiratory quotient (RQ), which is the ratio of carbon dioxide production to oxygen consumption, is lower for fat than for carbohydrate fuels. This may be a benefit for patients with pulmonary compromise having difficulty expiring CO_2 (Askanazi et al., 1981). The incidence of malnutrition in patients with chronic obstructive pulmonary disease is very high, and

TABLE 17.2   Common Dietary Fatty Acids

Symbol	Systematic name	Common name
Saturated fatty acids		
8:0	Octanoic	Caprylic
10:0	Decanoic	Capric
12:0	Dodecanoic	Lauric
14:0	Tetradecanoic	Myristic
16:0	Hexadecanoic	Palmitic
18:0	Octadecanoic	Stearic
Unsaturated fatty acids		
18:1 omega-9	9-Octadecenoic	Oleic
18:2 omega-6	6,9,12-Octadecadienoic	Linoleic
18:3 omega-3	9,12,15-Octadecatrienoic	Linolenic
20:4 omega-6	5,8,11,14-Eicosatetraenoic	Arachidonic
20:5 omega-3	5,8,11,14,17-Eicosaoentaenoic	EPA, timnodinic
22:6 omega-3	4,7,10,13,16,19-Docosahexaenoic	DHA, cervonic

nutrition support with high-fat diets may be considered for successful weaning of ventilator-dependent patients (Deitel et al., 1983; Noller and Mobarban, 1986).

Goldstein et al. (1988) studied the effect of nutrition support on the nitrogen and energy balance of malnourished patients with and without emphysema. In a randomized, crossover study, these investigators compared the effects of nutrition support that was either carbohydrate based (53% of calories from carbohydrates) or fat based (55% of energy from fat). Both regimens were equally effective in increasing weight, lean body mass, maximal inspiratory pressure, and skeletal muscle strength and endurance and in improving nitrogen balance. The respiratory quotient and the ventilator demand was higher in both groups when the subjects were switched from the fat-based to the carbohydrate-based regimen. As both dietary regimens were equally effective in improving nutritional status, effects on RQ may well be the deciding factor in choosing a therapeutic approach for these patients.

Substituting lipid calories for a portion of glucose calories can also be advantageous in diabetes (Reader et al., 1994). Several recent studies have evaluated the efficacy of diets rich in monounsaturated fatty acids in comparison to diets high in carbohydrate in patients with diabetes mellitus. Rasmussen et al. (1993) compared the influence of a diet rich in monounsaturated fatty acids (50% of energy as fat, 30% as monounsaturated fatty acids, and 30% as carbohydrate) versus an isocaloric high-carbohydrate diet (50% of energy as carbohydrate, 30% as fat, 10% as monounsaturated fatty acids) on blood pressure, glucose, and lipid levels in 15 persons with non–insulin-dependent diabetes mellitus (NIDDM) for 3 weeks. The monounsaturated fatty acid–rich diet significantly reduced systolic and diastolic blood pressure. Further, it improved glycemic control (reflected by lower fasting blood glucose levels, reduced postprandial blood glucose levels, and lowered average blood glucose levels) without adversely affecting lipid profiles.

In another study, Parillo et al. (1992) compared the effects of a high–monounsaturated fatty acid diet and a high-carbohydrate diet on peripheral insulin sensitivity and metabolic control in 10 patients with NIDDM. Patients were randomly assigned to 15 days of either a high–monounsaturated fatty acid diet (40% carbohydrate, 40% fat, 20% protein, 24 g fiber) or a high-carbohydrate diet (60% carbohydrate, 20% fat, 20% protein, 24 g fiber). Postprandial glucose levels decreased more for patients on the high–monounsaturated fatty acid diet than among patients on the high-carbohydrate diet (8.76 vs. 10.08 mM/liter). Furthermore, fasting plasma triglyceride levels were significantly lower in individuals receiving the high–monounsaturated fatty acid diet compared with those administered the high-carbohydrate diet (1.16 vs. 1.37 mM/liter). Insulin sensitivity was significantly increased with the high–carbohydrate diet (1.16 vs. 1.37 mM/liter). Insulin sensitivity was significantly increased with the high–monounsaturated fatty acid diet, as evaluated by insulin-mediated glucose disposal. The authors concluded that partially replacing carbohydrate-rich foods with monounsaturated fatty acid–rich foods also improved the cardiovascular risk profile and peripheral insulin sensitivity.

The clinical significance of these studies is that monounsaturated fats can be used instead of carbohydrates to replace saturated fatty acids in the diets of patients with NIDDM. High–monounsaturated fat diets may not only improve glycemic control but may also favorably affect the plasma lipoprotein profile, lessening the risk of coronary heart disease.

LCTs are generally recognized as useful nutrient substrates. However, there are several concerns regarding their clinical application. The digestion, absorption, and processing of LCTs requires a normally functioning GI tract, which may be compromised in patients with malabsorption, maldigestion, and critical illness. These fats are slowly cleared from the systemic circulation and may not be readily oxidized. Tumor necrosis factor and interleukin-1, which are cytokines that increase as part of the stress response to injury, are known to inhibit the activity of lipoprotein lipase, thereby impairing fat clearance (Kinsella et al., 1990). There has been some concern that excessive linoleic acid may result in an outpouring of eicosanoids, which may adversely affect immune competence and vascular integrity during the stress response to acute injury. In a study of severely burned patients being given enteral products with a variety of lipid-based formulas, the intravenous solution highest in linoleic acid content was associated with increased length of hospital stay and the highest mortality rate (Gottschlich et al., 1990). This research was confirmed by Daly et al. (1991) in a study using postsurgical patients in which two diets—one high in linoleic acid and the other with only 2% of the total calories from linoleic acid—were compared. The diet, Impact® (Sandoz Nutrition, Minneapolis, MN), which contains low levels of linoleic acid, resulted in decreased infections and decreased length of stay as compared to the other enteral formula. More recently, a multicenter study has also demonstrated a decreased length of stay and decreased infection rate using diets with a low level of linoleic acid and added fish oil (Bower et al., 1995).

MEDIUM-CHAIN TRIGLYCERIDES

Medium-chain triglycerides (MCTs) offer an alternative fat source to LCTs (Bach and Babayan, 1982). MCTs are commonly derived from coconut oil, which naturally contains approximately 65% medium-chain fatty acids. MCTs may also be prepared from palm kernel oil. Their low melting points, small molecular size, and ionization at neutral pH account for their easy absorption, transport, and metabolism compared to LCTs. MCTs are hydrolyzed by pancreatic lipase more rapidly and completely than are LCTs. They may be directly absorbed by the intestinal mucosa with minimum pancreatic or biliary function. They are transported to the liver predominately via the portal venous system (Fig. 17.1). There they can cross the mitochondrial membrane and be oxidized independent of carnitine to produce acetyl-CoA and ketone bodies.

MCTs may offer several advantages over LCTs, however, they do not provide essential fatty acids for the production of arachidonic acid. MCTs are well tolerated by the enteral route and are frequently used in patients with maldigestion or malabsorption. In many medical foods, an MCT/LCT mixture is used to provide both rapidly metabolized and slowly metabolized fuel as well as essential fatty acids. MCTs have utility in disorders of pancreatic and/or biliary insufficiency as well as a variety of diseases that comprise fat digestion or absorption including: cystic fibrosis, blind loop syndrome, massive small bowel resection, celiac disease, Whipple's disease, Crohn's disease, enteritis, gluten enteropathy, sprue, and neonatal malabsorption. MCTs are increasingly utilized in the feeding of critically ill or septic pa-

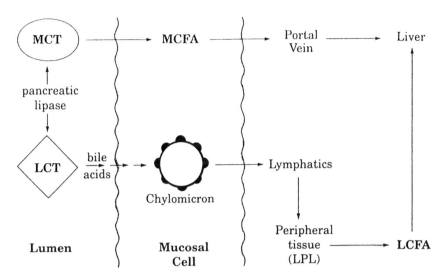

FIG. 17.1   Simplified diagrammatic representation of digestion, absorption, and transport of medium- and long-chain triglycerides.

tients, who presumably gain benefits in the setting of associated intestinal dysfunction. The minimal contribution of MCT to lymph production and flow may be utilized to advantage in disorder of lymphatic engorgement or leakage.

Further investigation should clarify potential roles for MCT in patients with lipid disorders associated with lipoprotein lipase deficiency and carnitine or carnitine palmityl transference deficiency. The thermogenesis and weight loss that may be seen with MCT use suggest possible application in weight reduction for obese patients (Mascioli et al., 1991).

STRUCTURED TRIGLYCERIDES

Structured triglycerides (STs) have been developed to fully optimize the benefit of fat substrate mixtures. They are created by hydrolysis of the fatty acid moieties from a mixture of triglycerides followed by random reesterification back onto the glycerol backbone (Babayan, 1987). Typically, a variety of fatty acids are used in this process, including different classes of saturated, monounsaturated, polyunsaturated, and MCTs, depending on the desired metabolic effect. Thus, a mixture of fatty acids is incorporated onto

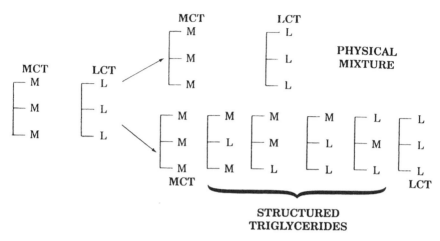

FIG. 17.2   Triglyceride: structured vs. physical mix.

the same glycerol molecule. STs differ from physical mixtures (PMs), in which a collection of triglycerides is simply mixed together (Fig. 17.2).

Early studies showed that STs synthesized from a mixture of MCTs and LCTs conferred several unique advantages over PMs of the same fatty acid mix, including an ability to improve nitrogen retention while preserving reticuloendothelial function (Sobrado et al., 1985). The reason for this benefit is not entirely clear but may relate to the more rapid oxidation and clearance of the long-chain fatty acid part of the ST.

Short-term infusions of four lipid emulsions (STs, PMs, LCTs, and MCTs) in thermally injured animals showed that animals receiving STs maintained overall body weight, lean body mass, and visceral protein stores better than those receiving the other emulsions (Mok et al., 1984). In a similar study, two ST emulsions were fed enterally to burned rats who were hyper-metabolic. The diets were shown to reduce postburn catabolism, improve nitrogen utilization, and increase protein synthesis rates for skeletal muscle and the liver (DeMichele et al., 1988). Enhanced absorption of linoleic acid (18:2 omega-6) was observed in cystic fibrosis patients fed structured tri-glycerides containing long- and medium-chain fatty acids (McKenna et al., 1985; Hubbard and McKenna, 1987). In vitro lipase digestions and isolated intestinal loop absorption studies revealed rapid hydrolyses and absorption of a structured triglyceride containing 18:2 omega-6 in the 2 position and medium-chain fatty acids in the 1 and 3 positions (Jandacek et al., 1987).

An ST with a high percentage of PUFAs provided as fish oil has been shown to inhibit tumor growth while improving body weight and nitrogen retention in sarcoma-bearing rats (Ling et al., 1991). These studies compared STs composed of MCTs and fish oil (with only enough LA to meet EFA requirements) with similar physical mixtures and lipid emulsions with excessive amounts of LA. A similar study, which provided an enteral formula with MCT/fish oil ST to thermally injured animals, found all of the previously noted benefits regarding nitrogen metabolism and also noted a diminution in energy expenditure, which was attributed to the unique ability of omega-3 PUFAs to modulate the injury response (Teo et al., 1989).

The metabolic advantages of STs over PMs are likely due to the position, or stereospecificity, of certain fatty acids on the glycerol backbone. One theory is the STs with medium-chain fatty acids in the 2 position of the glycerol molecule are more slowly removed from circulation than if they are given as standard MCT. This stereospecificity is maintained by enhanced lymphatic absorption of medium-chain fatty acids in the 2 position of enterally administered STs, which has been shown in animals (Jensen and Jensen, 1992) and humans (Jensen et al., 1989). The enhanced absorption is believed to be the result of the action of pancreatic lipase, which preferentially cleaves the fatty acid moieties from the 1 and 3 positions of a triglyceride molecule. This monoglyceride can then be repackaged into a triglyceride, which is transported via the intestinal lymphatics to the systemic circulation. Further investigation is required to completely explain the nutritional effects of STs.

OMEGA-3 VERSUS OMEGA-6 FATTY ACIDS

Sources of omega-3 PUFAs include seafood and certain plants. Marine oils contain moderately high levels of eicosapentaenoic acid (EPA) and docosahexaenoic acid (DHA), while plant sources including linseed, canola, rapeseed, walnut, and soybean oils contain α-linolenic acid (Hepburn et al., 1986).

Linoleic acid, an omega-6 PUFA, is desaturated and elongated by a series of enzymes leading to the production of arachondic acid. Though the conversion of α-linolenic acid to EPA parallels that of linoleic acid to arachidonic acid (Fig. 17.3), the extent of this biochemical reaction in humans is small because α-linolenic acid competes for the same enzyme system as linoleic acid, and linolenic acid is present in much lower concentrations. Thus, most of the α-linolenic acid consumed is actually oxidized (Nettleton, 1991).

The PUFAs of the omega-3 and omega-6 series are of clinical interest because they serve as precursors for the synthesis of prostaglandins (PGs), leukotrienes (LTs), and thromboxanes (TXs), which are collectively re-

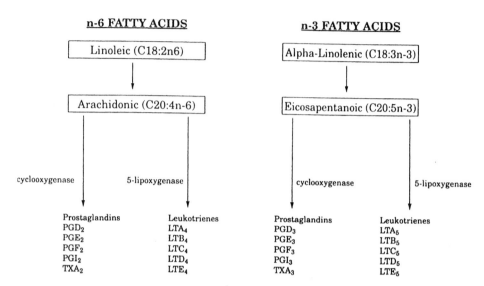

FIG. 17.3 Eicosanoids derived from omega-6 fatty acid, the precursor of arachidonic acid, and omega-3 fatty acid, the precursor of eicosapentanoic acid.

ferred to as eicosanoids. When macrophages, neutrophils, and other cells are stimulated, arachidonic acid is processed by cyclo-oxygenase and lipoxygenase to form 2 series prostaglandins and 4 series leukotrienes. These molecules are potent regulators of immune function and differentiation; high concentrations are immunosuppressive because of their many effects on lymphocytes and macrophages (Table 17.3). The leukotriene LTB_4 is an important mediator for endothelial cell adhesion and chemotaxis of neutrophils. LTC_4, LTD_4, and LTE_4, formerly referred to as the slow-reacting

TABLE 17.3 Effects of PGE_2 on Immunological Functions

Suppress macrophage- and lymphocyte-mediated reactions
Lymphocyte (B- and T-cell) proliferation and migration
Cell-mediated toxicity and cytolysis
Reduce lymphokine production
Reduce mitogen-induced proliferation of lymphocytes
Reduce macrophage proliferation
Modification of macrophage membrane receptor functions (1a antigen)

substances of anaphylaxis, are potent mediators of capillary and postcapillary venule vasodilation and permeability. The thromboxane TXA_2 causes vasoconstriction and platelet aggregation.

A diet enriched in EPA leads to the incorporation of this fatty acid into the phospholipid fraction of the cell membrane, where it is available as a substrate for eicosanoid production (Lee et al., 1985). These PUFAs have been shown to diminish the production of series-2 PG, TX, and series-4 leukotrienes in humans by competitively inhibiting their synthesis from amino acids. Because of the position and number of double bonds in EPA, the enzymes of the eicosanoid cascade produce series-3 PG and TX and series-5 leukotrienes, which are generally less metabolically active than the amino acid metabolites (Fig. 17.3). It is through this sequence of events that omega-3 PUFAs derive their anti-inflammatory and immunomodulatory effect.

The therapeutic benefits of omega-3 PUFAs are quite varied, involving a broad range of metabolic, cardiovascular, and immunological conditions. Epidemiological studies have attributed the low incidence of cardiovascular disease in Eskimos to their relatively high dietary intake of omega-3 and omega-6 PUFAs (Bang and Dyerberg, 1972). Fish oil supplementation has been shown to lower systemic blood pressure in patients with mild hypertension in a double-blind, controlled crossover study (Radack et al., 1991). Fish oil has also been shown to decrease serum triglyceride and cholesterol levels while increasing concentrations of HDL cholesterol (Sirtori et al., 1992). Chronic immunologically mediated diseases including atopic dermatitis, psoriasis, rheumatoid arthritis, ulcerative colitis, and lupus nephritis have been shown to improve with short-term use of fish oil supplementation (Yetive, 1988). The major risks of this therapy include bleeding, vitamin E deficiency, and vitamin A and D toxicity. The importance of generating biologically less active eicosanoids may also be extended to the critical care setting. Prefeeding guinea pigs with fish oil has been shown to improve survival when the animals are exposed to lethal doses of endotoxin (Mascioli et al., 1988). In addition, the febrile response to recombinant interleukin-1 has been shown to be blunted with the use of fish oil supplementation (Pomposelli et al., 1989). Animals fed omega-3 PUFAs from fish oil have a lesser degree of lactic acidemia following endotoxin infusion than those fed omega-6 PUFAs. This is believed to be due to improved microvascular muscle perfusion (Pomposelli et al., 1991). Pulmonary infiltrates were less pronounced in animals that received fish oil. Fish oil also appears to reduce the propensity to develop fatty infiltration in the liver and to improve glucose utilization in models of septic injury (Ling et al., 1992).

The consumption of large quantities of fish oil by healthy human volunteers resulted in diminished production of interleukin-1 and tumor necrosis factor by stimulated peripheral blood monocytes in vitro (Endres et al., 1989). This finding suggests one of several mechanisms whereby omega-3 PUFAs might reduce the severity of the injury response.

CONCLUSION

Fats are not simply sources of fuel. They play important roles in the structure and function of many metabolic and immunological systems. This brief review has examined the physiological effect of TG, medium- and long-chain and polyunsaturated fatty acids and structured triglycerides (omega-6 and omega-3) and the use of these fats in medical and designer foods. Future investigation should help to further define the metabolic advantages of these lipids, leading to a clarification of the clinical application of this unique class of substrate.

REFERENCES

Askanazi, J., Nordenstrom, J., Rosenbaum, S. H., Elwyn, D. H., Hyman, A. I., Carpentier, Y. A., and Kinney, J. M. 1981. Nutrition for the patient with respiratory failure: Glucose versus fat. *Anesthesiology* 54: 373–377.

Babayan, V. K. 1987. Medium chain triglycerides and structured lipids. *Lipids* 22: 417–420.

Bach, A. and Babayan, V. K. 1982. Medium chain triglycerides: An update. *Am. J. Clin. Nutr.* 36: 950–962.

Bang, H. O. and Dyerberg, J. 1972. Plasma lipids and lipoproteins in Greenlandic west coast Eskimos. *Acta Med. Scan.* 192: 85–94.

Bjerve, K. S., Mostad, I., and Thoresen, L. 1987. Alpha-linolenic acid deficiency in patients on long term gastric tube feeding: Estimation of linolenic acid and long-chain unsaturated n-3 fatty acid requirement in man. *Am. J. Clin. Nutr.* 15: 66–77.

Bower, R. H., Daly, J. M., Lieberman, M. D., Goldfine, J., Shou, J., Weintraub, F., Rosato, E. F., and Lavin, P. 1995. Early enteral administration of a formula (Impact®) supplemented with arginine, nucleotides, and fish oil in intensive care unit patient: Results of a multicenter prospective, randomized clinical trial. *Crit. Care Med.* 23(3): 436–449.

Burr, G. O. and Burr, M. M. 1930. On the nature and the role of fatty acids essential in nutrition. *J. Biol. Chem.* 86: 587–621.

Daly, J. M., Lieberman, M. D., Goldfine, J., Shou, J., Weintraub, F., Rosato, E. F., and Lavin, P. 1992. Enteral nutrition with supplemental arginine,

RNA, and omega-3 fatty acids in patients after operation: immunologic, metabolic and clinical outcome. *Surgery* 112: 56–76.

Deitel, M., Williams, V. P., and Rice, T. W. 1983. Nutrition and the patient requiring mechanical ventilatory support. *J. Am. Coll. Nutr.* 2: 25–32.

DeMichele, S. J., Karlstad, M. D., Babayan, V. K., Istfan, N., Blackburn, G. L., and Bistrian, B. R. 1988. Enhanced skeletal muscle and liver protein synthesis with structured lipid in enterally fed burned rats. *Metabolism* 37: 787–795.

Endres, S., Ghorbani, R., Kelly, V. E., Georgilis, K., Lonnemann, G., vander Meer, J. W., Cannon, J. G., Rogers, T. S., Klempner, M. S., Weber, P. C., Schaefer, E. J., Wolff, S. M., and Dinarello, C. A. 1989. The effect of dietary supplementation with n-3 polyunsaturated fatty acids on the synthesis of interleukin-1 and tumor necrosis factor by mononuclear cells. *N. Engl. J. Med.* 320: 265–271.

FDA. 1989. *Compliance Program Guidance Manual*, Chapter 21, Program No. 7321.002 (1989–91). Food and Drug Administration, Washington, DC.

Goldstien, S. A., Thomashow, B. M., Kuetan, V., Askanazi, J., Kinney, J. M., and Elwyn, D. H. 1988. Nitrogen and energy relationships in malnourished patients with emphysema. *Am. Rev. Respir. Dis.* 138: 636–644.

Gottschlich, M. M., Jenkins, M., Warden, G. D., Baumer, T., Havens, P., Snook, J. T., and Alexander, J. W. 1990. Differential effects of three enteral dietary regimens on selected outcome variables in burn patients. *JPEN* 14: 225–236.

Hattan, D. G. and Mackey, D. 1989. A review of medical foods: Enterally administered formulation used in the treatment of disease and disorders. *Food Drug Cosmetic Law J.* 44: 479–501.

Heimburger, D. C. and Weinsier, R. L. 1985. Guidelines for evaluating and categorizing enteral feeding formulas according to therapeutic equivalence. *J. Parenter. Enteral Nutr.* 9: 61–67.

Hepburn, F. N., Exler, J., and Weihrauch, J. L. 1986. Provisional tables on the conduct of omega-3 fatty acids and other fat components of selected foods. *J. Am. Diet. Assoc.* 86: 788–793.

Holmon, R. T., Johnson, S. B., and Hatch, T. F. 1982. A case of human linolenic acid deficiency involving neurological abnormalities. *Am. J. Clin. Nutr.* 35: 617–623.

Hubbard, V. S. and McKenna, M. C. 1987. Absorption of safflower oil and structured lipid preparations in patients with cystic fibrosis. *Lipids* 22: 424–428.

Jandacek, R. J., Whiteside, J. A., Holcombe, B. N., Volpenhein, R. A., and Tavlbee, J. D. 1987. The rapid hydrolyses and efficient absorption of triglycerides with octanoic acids in the 1 and 3 position and long-chain fatty acid in the 2 position. *Am. J. Clin. Nutr.* 45: 940–945.

Jensen, G. L. and Jensen, R. G. 1992. Specialty lipids for infant nutrition II: Concerns, new developments, and future applications. *Pediatr. Gastro. Nutr.* 15: 382–394.

Jensen, G. L., McGarvey, N., Taraszewski, R., Wixson, S. K., Seidner, D. L., Pai, T., Yeh, Y. Y., Lee, T. W., and DeMichele, S. J. 1994. Lymphatic absorption of enterally fed structured triacylyglycerol versus physical mix in a canine model. *Am. J. Clin. Nutr.* 60(4): 518–524.

Jensen, G. L., Mascioli, E. A., Meyer, L. P., Lopes, S. M., Bell, S. J., Babayan, V. K., Blackburn, G. L., and Bistrian, B. R. 1989. Dietary modification of chyle composition in chylothorax. *Gastroenterology* 97(3): 761–765.

Kinsella, J. E., Lokesh, B., Broughton, S., and Whelan, J. 1990. Dietary polyunsaturated fatty acids and eicosanoids: Potential effects on the modulation of inflammatory and immune cells: An overview. *Nutrition* 6(1): 24–44.

Kris-Etherton, P. M., Krummel, D., Russell, M. E., Dreon, D., Mackey, S., Borchers, J., and Wood, P. D. 1988. National Cholesterol Education Program: The effect of diet on plasma lipids, lipoproteins, and coronary heart disease. *J. Am. Diet. Assoc.* 88(11): 1373–1400.

Lebenthal, E., Khin-Maung, U., Rolston, D., Khin-Myat-Tun, Tin-Nu-Swe, Thein-Thein-Myint, Jirapinyo, P., Visitsuntorn, N., Firmansyah, A., Sunoto, S., et al. 1995. Thermophilic amylase-digested rice-electrolyte solution in the treatment of acute diarrhea in children. *Pediatrics* 95: 198–202.

Lee, T. H., Hoover, R. L., Williams, J. D., Sperling, R. I., Ravalese, J., 3d, Spur, B. W., Robinson, D. R., Corey, E. J., Lewis, R. A., and Austen, K. F. 1985. Effect of dietary enrichment with eicosapentaenoic and docosahexaenoic acids on in vitro neutrophil and monocyte leukotriene generation and neutrophil function. *NEJM* 312: 1217–1224.

Ling, P. R., Istfan, N. W., Lopes, S. M., Babayan, V. K., Blackburn, G. L., and Bistrian, B. R. 1991. Structured lipid made from fish oil and medium-chain triglycerides alters tumor and host metabolism in Yoshida-sarcoma-bearing rats. *Am. J. Clin. Nutr.* 53: 1177–1184.

Ling, M. K., Istran, N., and Colon, E. 1992. Effect of fish oil on glucose metabolism in the interleukin-1 alpha (IL-1) treated rate. *JPEN* 15 (suppl.): 215.

Mascioli, E. A., Randall, S., Porter, K. A., Kater, G., Lopes, S., Babayan, V. K., Blackburn, G. L., and Bistrian, B. R. 1991. Thermogenesis from intravenous medium chain triglycerides. *JPEN* 15: 27–31.

Mascioli, E., Leader, L., Flores, E., Trimbo, S., Bistrian, B., and Blackburn, G.

1988. Enhanced survival to endotoxin in guinea pigs fed IV fish oil emulsion. *Lipids* 23: 623–625.

McKenna, M. C., Hubbard, V. S., and Pieri, J. G. 1985. Linoleic acid absorption for lipid supplements in patients with cystic fibrosis with pancreatic insufficiency and in control subjects. *J. Pediatr. Gastro. Nutr.* 4: 45–51.

Mok, K. T., Maiz, A., Yamazaki, K., Sobrado, J., Babayan, V. K., Moldawer, L. L., Bistrian, B. R., and Blackburn, G. L. 1984. Structured medium-chain and long-chain triglyceride emulsions are superior to physical mixtures in sparing body protein in the burned rat. *Metabolism* 33: 910–915.

Molina, S., Vettorozzi, C., Peerson, J., Solomons, N. W., and Brown, K. H. 1995. Clinical trial of glucose-oral rehydration solution (ORS), rice dextrin-ORS, and rice flour-ORS for the management of children with acute diarrhea and mild or moderate dehydration. *Pediatrics* 95: 191–197.

National Research Council. 1988. *Designing Foods. Animal Product Options in the Marketplace.* National Academy Press, Washington, DC.

Nettleton, J. 1991. ω-3 Fatty acids: Comparison of plant and seafood sources in human nutrition. *J. Am. Diet. Assoc.* 91: 331–337.

Noller, C. and Mobarhan, S. 1986. Enteral feeding in patients with advanced chronic obstructive pulmonary disease. *Nutr. Support Serv.* 6: 37–39.

Parillo, M., Rivellese, A. A., Ciardullo, A. V., Capaldo, B., Giacco, A., Genovese, S., and Riccardi, G. 1992. A high monounsaturated fat/low carbohydrate diet improve peripheral insulin sensitivity in non-insulin diabetic patients. *Metabolism* 41: 1373–1378.

Pomposelli, J. J., Flores, E. A., Blackburn, G. L., Zeisel, S. H., and Bistrian, B. R. 1991. Diets enriched with n-3 fatty acids ameliorate lactic acidosis by improving endotoxin-induced tissue hypoperfusion in guinea pigs. *Ann. Surg.* 213: 166–176.

Pomposelli, J. J., Mascioli, E. A., Bistrian, B. R., Lopes, S. M., and Blackburn, G. L. 1989. Attenuation of the febrile response in guinea pigs by fish oil enriched diets. *JPEN* 13: 136–140.

Radack, K., Deck, C., and Huster, G. 1991. The effects of low doses of n-3 fatty acid supplementation on blood pressure in hypertensive subjects. *Arch. Intern. Med.* 151: 1173–1180.

Randall, H. T. 1990. The history of enteral nutrition. In *Enteral and Tube Feeding*, 2nd ed., J. L. Rombeau and M. D. Caldwell (Ed.), pp. 1–9. W.B. Saunders, Philadelphia.

Rasmussen, O. W., Thomsen, C., Hansen, K. W., Vesterlund, M., Winther, E., and Hermansen, K. 1993. Effects on blood pressure, glucose, and lipid levels of a high-monounsaturated fat diet compared with a high-carbohydrate diet in NIDDM subjects. *Diabetes Care* 16(12): 1565–1571.

Reader, D. M., Fish, L. H., and Franz, M. J. 1994. Response to isocaloric quantities of enteral feedings in non-insulin dependent diabetes mellitus (NIDDM). *J. Am. Diet. Assoc.* 94(9): A-39.

Schmidl, M. K., Massano, S. S., and Labuza, T. P. 1988. Parenteral and enteral food system. *Food Technol.* 42(7): 77–87.

Schmidl, M. K. and Labuza, T. P. 1994. *Medical Foods, Inc. Functional Foods*, I. Goldberg (Ed.), pp. 151–182. Chapman & Hall, New York.

Scientific Status Summary. 1992. Medical foods. A scientific status summary by the Institution of Food Technologist's Expert Panel on Food Safety and Nutrition. *Food Technol.* 46: 87–96.

Shike, M. 1994. Enteral feeding. In *Modern Nutrition in Health and Disease*, 8th ed. M. E. Shils, J. A. Olsen, and M. Shike (Ed.), Lea and Febiger, Philadelphia, PA.

Sirtori, C. R., Gatti, E., Tremoli, E., Galli, C., Gianfranceschi, G., Franceschini, G., Colli, S., Maderna, P., Marangoni, F., Perego, P., and Stragliotto, E. 1992. Olive oil, corn oil, and n-3 fatty acids differently affect lipids, lipoproteins, platelets and superoxide formation in Type II hypercholesterolemia. *Am. J. Clin. Nutr.* 56: 113–122.

Sobrado, J., Moldawer, L. L., Pomposelli, J. J., Mascioli, E. A., Babayan, V. K., Bistrian, B. R., and Blackburn, G. L. 1985. Lipid emulsions and reticuloendothelial system function in healthy and burned guinea pigs. *Am. J. Clin. Nutr.* 42: 855–863.

Teo, T. C., DeMichele, S. J., Selleck, K. M., Babayan, V. K., Blackburn, G. L., and Bistrian, B. R. 1989. Administration of structured lipid composed of MCT and fish oil reduces net protein catabolism in enterally fed burned rats. *Ann. Surg.* 210: 100–107.

Yetive, J. Z. 1988. Clinical application of fish oil. *JAMA* 260: 665–670.

18
Determinants of Dietary Fat Intake in Humans

Richard D. Mattes

Purdue University
West Lafayette, Indiana

INTRODUCTION

Moderation of fat intake has been a public health recommendation for more than 75 years (U.S. Department of Health and Human Services, 1988), yet despite widespread concern by the public about the potential adverse health effects of a high-fat diet (Calorie Control Council, 1993), consumption has declined only slightly over this time period (Stephen and Wald, 1990). This suggests the presence of powerful forces opposing such a dietary change. Identification of these influences and characterization of their relative significance in the population are required to develop strategies for dietary change. Many influences can be hypothesized, but few have compelling data to support their purported role. This overview will summarize current knowledge relating to genetic, neural, metabolic, cognitive, and sensory contributions to the preference for and intake of dietary fats. Sociodemographic determinants such as age, gender, income, education, ethnicity, race, and household size are also clearly involved (Axelson, 1986; Towler and Shepherd, 1992), but these fall outside the scope of this chapter.

Recent work indicates that these latter factors may be less strongly associated with attitudes towards consumption of high-fat foods than the sensory and cognitive influences, which will be described (Tuorila and Pangborn, 1988; Towler and Shepherd, 1992).

GENETIC INFLUENCE ON FAT PREFERENCE AND INTAKE

A recent meta-analysis of the relationship between the food preferences of children and their parents found correlations between mothers and offspring of 0.19 and between fathers and offspring of 0.14 (Borah-Giddens and Falciglia, 1993). The overall correlation between parents and children was 0.17, and while statistically significant, it is clearly weak. Knowledge of a parent's food preferences accounts for less than 3% of the variance in his or her child's preferences. These findings are surprising, because they reflect the contributions of both genetics and shared family environment. They suggest that preferences are shaped more by siblings, peers, the media, and other environmental influences. This view is bolstered by evidence that (1) associations between parents and their college-aged offspring are stronger (Pliner, 1983; Rozin et al., 1984), (2) siblings show greater similarity than children and parents (Pliner and Pelchat, 1986), (3) there are clear gender and age trends in food preferences (Logue et al., 1988) that reflect cultural norms, (4) associations of a similar order of magnitude to those observed among family members are observed between individuals who are unknown to each other but have a similar cultural background (Pliner and Pelchat, 1986), and (5) there is little difference in associations between monozygotic and dizygotic twins for taste (Green et al., 1975) or food preferences (Rozin and Millman, 1987).

More limited data are available on preferences specifically for foods contributing significant amounts of dietary fat. One family study that obtained ratings for only five foods, and therefore had limited statistical power, observed little similarity in ratings of parents and children (Weidner et al., 1985). Twin studies that reveal a heritable basis for food preferences indicate that the association is based largely on items not high in fat (Krondl et al., 1983; McKee and Harden, 1990; Falciglia and Norton, 1994). It is important to note that the association between food preferences and actual intake is not straightforward; indeed, these studies have generally not found a significant association between reported preferences and intake.

Twin studies exploring the genetic basis of total energy and macronutrient intake have yielded discrepant findings. In one investigation (Wade et al., 1981), no genetic basis for fat intake was reported, whereas a significant contribution for protein and carbohydrate was demonstrated.

Another trial noted a higher concordance among monozygotic twins than dizygotic siblings for fat intake, but this effect was eliminated when information about frequency of social interactions was entered into the analyses (i.e., the more frequent contact of monozygotic twins could account for their greater similarity in food intake) (Fabsitz et al., 1978). Similarly, a recent study noted a heritable component to fat intake, but this was attributable to the genetic contribution to total energy intake (deCastro, 1993). Comparisons of parent-offspring intake similarities typically indicate a weak association (r ≃ 0.25) for fat (Laskarzewski et al., 1980; Patterson et al., 1988; Perusse, 1988; Oliveria et al., 1992) that, again, may just reflect a relationship for total energy intake.

In summary, there is little evidence for a genetic basis for dietary fat preference or intake. Shared environment also contributes little to the variance in these measures. Cultural factors appear to play the predominant role (Rozin, 1980), although, here too, the mechanisms (e.g., health beliefs, body image ideals, flavor exposure) are unclear.

NEURAL MECHANISMS INFLUENCING FAT PREFERENCE AND INTAKE

Alterations of mood and feelings of well-being associated with food intake are a common experience. The potential for diet-induced changes in neurochemistry to underlie shifts in mood and further nutrient selection has recently attracted considerable research attention, much of it focused on endogenous opiates and the neurotransmitter serotonin. Alteration of plasma levels of tryptophan, the precursor of serotonin, has been associated with shifts in mood of humans (Young et al., 1988; Delgado et al., 1990). Endorphins may exert an anxiolytic effect through interactions with neurotransmitters (Cooper, 1983).

Several mechanisms can be constructed whereby a high-fat meal could enhance serotonin synthesis and thereby potentially influence mood. One is predicated on the assumption that increased serum levels of free tryptophan will facilitate uptake of the amino acid in the brain, where serotonin synthesis occurs. The pool of free tryptophan may rise due to the postprandial elevation of serum nonesterified fatty acids, which compete with tryptophan for binding sites on the transport protein albumin (Fernstrom, 1994). However, large variations of free tryptophan levels in the blood of rats do not lead to changes in brain tryptophan levels (Fernstrom and Fernstrom, 1993). Evidently, the displacement of tryptophan from albumin is not a rate-limiting step in brain uptake of the amino acid. Thus, this mechanism may hold little practical significance. The observation that a diet contributing 34% of energy as saturated fat leads to increased brain serotonin levels in rats (Mullen and Martin, 1992) suggests another potential mechanism. Such a diet can elevate serum insulin, which would promote uptake of branched-chain amino acids by muscle. As a result, competition for the carriers of tryptophan into the brain would be reduced. Whether this mechanism holds physiological importance is uncertain, since marked differences in saturated fat intake (5% vs. 34%) do not lead to altered macronutrient selection (Mullen and Martin, 1992), a purported effect of altered serotonin levels. The preponderance of data indicate that a high-fat meal does not result in elevated levels of tryptophan in the brain (Fernstrom and Fernstrom, 1993). Dietary fat levels could also exert an influence on enzymes involved in serotonin synthesis or neuronal function, but there are no data to support such mechanisms.

Another proposed mechanism whereby fat ingestion could enhance mood and promote further fat intake involves endogenous opiates. In rats, the opioid agonist morphine enhances food intake and, in particular, selection of fat (Marks-Kaufman, 1982; Gosnell and Krahn, 1993). The antagonist naloxone disproportionately decreases fat intake (Markus-Kaufman and Kanarek, 1981). Further, oral stimulation with oil elicits responses that are, at least in part, attributable to endogenous opiates, since they can be blocked by an opiate antagonist (Shide and Blass, 1991; Blass, 1991). The mechanism by which opiates stimulate appetite has not been determined, but likely involves a general enhancement of the rewarding properties of food intake (Reid, 1985; Gosnell et al., 1990). However, this effect attenuates over time (Triscari et al., 1989; Davidson et al., 1992; Gosnell and Krahn, 1992), raising questions about its ecological significance. In humans, ingestion of a palatable high-fat meal (48% of energy) has not elicited a rise in β-endorphin levels (Melchior et al., 1991). Whether this lack of effect is attributable to methodological issues (e.g., attenuation of a response due to customary ingestion of a high-fat diet) or fat not being an effective stimulus for opiate release is not clear. Individuals with eating disorders reportedly have elevated β-endorphin levels (Waller et al., 1986; Olson et al., 1991). They show reduced hedonic ratings for fats when treated with Naloxone (Drewnowski et al., 1992) and indulge in high-fat items when binging (Kales, 1990; Yanovski et al., 1992), yet they express aversions to high-fat foods when questioned (Drewnowski et al., 1988). Although there is suggestive evidence that opiates influence dietary fat intake in humans (Bertino et al., 1991), the preponderance of data does not support an opiate-based influence on hedonic ratings of high-fat foods (Hetherington, 1991) or macronutrient selection (Maggio et al., 1985; Atkinsen, 1987).

Overall, reported correlations between the level of fat intake and selected measures of mood and performance are extremely weak. Associations have been explored immediately after a meal, 60 minutes after a meal, over the interval between successive spontaneous meals, or averaged over a 9-day period (deCastro, 1987; Smith et al., 1994). It is possible that diets with especially high or low levels of fat could elicit some acute or chronic effect, but this appears unlikely under "normal" dietary conditions.

METABOLIC INFLUENCE ON FAT PREFERENCE AND INTAKE

Whether humans possess "nutritional wisdom" whereby they innately select foods to optimize health has not been resolved (Galef, 1991; Reed et al., 1992). Nevertheless, constancy of a behavior under conditions of varying influences suggests an underlying biological basis for the behavior. In this context, the consistently high levels of fat intake across cultures is noteworthy (Hegsted and Ausman, 1988; Prentice et al., 1988; Kromhout et al., 1989). Interestingly, under normal laboratory conditions, where separate sources of macronutrients are readily available, rats will also self-select diets with a similar fat composition to that noted in western populations (~34% of energy) (Bernardini et al., 1993). Does this high level of intake provide some unrecognized, metabolically-based health benefit?

Fats have many physiological effects, independent of their energy value (Reilly and Rombeau, 1993; Dannenberg and Reidenberg, 1994), that may reinforce or promote current intake levels. For example, short-chain fatty acids stimulate epithelial growth and enhance colonic blood flow, resulting in increased vascular fuel delivery. The n-3 fatty acids hold anti-inflammatory activity that may provide benefit to individuals with certain disorders (e.g., rheumatoid arthritis, ulcerative colitis). They also alter drug and xenobiotic metabolism through an influence on cytochrome P-450 enzymes and have a wide range of potential effects through modification of membrane properties (Clandinin et al., 1991). The possibility that high levels of fat serve to dilute adverse properties of other macronutrients is feasible as well. Such, presumably subtle, effects have not been explored.

Given that there is a requirement for linoleic and linolenic acids (Food and Nutrition Board, 1989), the preference for fat may reflect a mechanism to secure an adequate intake of these essential nutrients. The fact that the need is easily met in present-day, free-living, healthy individuals does not negate the argument, since there has been little evolutionary pressure to select against the trait, which may have developed when fat was not readily available. Nevertheless, the absence of any apparent abatement of desire for fat in individuals consuming more than 10 times the apparent level of need casts doubt on this mechanism.

Attributes of fat related to its energy content that may influence ingestion include its high energy density and weak satiety effect. Fat has the highest energy density of the macronutrients. Teleologically, the innate ability to detect such an energy source and find it palatable would have conferred an adaptive advantage throughout most of human evolution where acquisition of adequate energy was a challenge. Because the adverse health consequences of a high-fat, high-energy diet in a relatively sedentary population are not manifest until the most active reproductive period has passed, such a trait would be preserved.

Support for the view that energy density is a critical determinant of fat intake is equivocal. If true, it could be hypothesized that high-fat foods would be preferentially desired by individuals in negative energy balance. Findings from the Minnesota starvation experiment indicate that when released from a period of severe energy restriction, participant cravings were primarily directed towards high-fat items (e.g., ice cream, pastries, cheese, nuts) (Keys et al., 1950). However, actual food selection and ingestion did not reveal any macronutrient-specific orientation, and fat represented approximately 32% of total energy intake, a level well below that of the general population at the time and slightly lower than the current level of consumption (Stephen and Wald, 1990). Energy deprivation can promote an increased preference for fat suspensions in rats, but the effect is nonspecific since a similar response is observed for polycose (a carbohydrate) (Sclafani and Akeroff, 1993). Dietary responses to more moderate energy deficits created by covert reductions of the energy density of meals also fail to reveal a preferential selection of fat to compensate for the experimental manipulation (Blundell and Burley, 1991; Rolls et al., 1992; Caputo and Mattes, 1992).

Studies of flavor-nutrient conditioning provide ambiguous support for a rewarding property of fat's energy density. In this paradigm, exposure to flavors is paired with administration of different energy loads. Within limits, a preference generally develops for the flavor that has been paired with the more energy-dense load of a given macronutrient (Hayward, 1983; Capaldi et al., 1987; Elizaldi and Sclafani, 1990; Warwick and Weingarten, 1994). This has been demonstrated in young children with carbohydrates (Birch et al., 1990) and fats (Johnson et al., 1991; Kern et al., 1993). However, rat studies indicate that higher fat loads do not consistently lead to stronger flavor preferences than loads of lower fat content (Lucas and Sclafani, 1989). Further, fat is not as effective at promoting a flavor preference as carbohydrate (Sclafani, 1992), indicating that its energy density alone is not the key conditioning attribute.

Because of a long-held view that gastric distention suppresses hunger and knowledge that fat is the slowest of the macronutrients to clear from the gut, fat is commonly believed to have a high satiety value. However, more recent studies present compelling evidence that just the opposite is true. A particularly strong suppression of hunger and reduction of energy intake anticipated with consumption of fat is not observed. Intravenous infusion of lipid in excess of energy needs leads to a smaller adjustment of free-feeding energy intake than a comparable infusion of carbohydrate (Gill et al., 1991). Dietary supplementation with fat also elicits a lesser effect on reported hunger (Rolls et al., 1988; Blundell et al., 1993) or dietary compensation (Rolls et al., 1988; Caputo and Mattes, 1992; Rolls et al., 1994) relative to ratings following loads of carbohydrate or protein. In addition, fixed meals high in fat lead to lower or equal reported satiety compared meals high in the other macronutrients (Van Amelsvoort et al., 1989; deGraff et al., 1992). Further, free feeding from foods high in fat or carbohydrate results in greater total energy intake with the high-fat foods (Blundell et al., 1993). Finally, when a diet higher in fat than is customarily consumed is provided over several weeks, energy intake and body weight increase (Lissner et al., 1987), and when one lower in fat is ingested, weight is lost (Kendall et al., 1991).

The low satiety effect of fat reflects the weak metabolic response it elicits. Human studies generally reveal that increased ingestion of carbohydrate and protein promotes a shift in substrate oxidation and a compensatory change in energy expenditure. Excess fat intake does not provoke a similar response (Schutz et al., 1989; Bennett et al., 1992; Rising et al., 1992). Short-term (24-hour) manipulation of the macronutrient content of diets intended to match energy needs has also indicated that regulation of protein and carbohydrate balance is considerably stronger than that for fat (Abbott et al., 1988), although not uniformly (Hill et al., 1991).

Taken together, these findings do not indicate that fat provides a metabolically-based physiological health benefit due to its energy density, contribution of essential fatty acids, or other nonspecific effects in the body. Further, findings that free-feeding fat ingestion is not specifically adjusted when levels of the macronutrient are covertly altered in meals or diets demonstrates that fat balance is not closely regulated. Indeed, the most noteworthy aspect of fat ingestion is the lack of metabolic or dietary response it evokes. Thus, rather than providing a positive incentive for its ingestion, metabolism appears to play a permissive role in fat intake, that is, it fails to limit intake.

COGNITIVE INFLUENCE ON FAT PREFERENCE AND INTAKE

Culture defines what edible substances are food as well as how, when, where, and with whom these items should be obtained, stored, prepared, presented, consumed, and, when necessary, disposed of. These guidelines serve not only to identify safe and wholesome foods, but also to instill in them value unrelated to their nutritional properties. For example, within a culture, foods can facilitate social interactions, reflect social status, are used to cope with stress and tension, can influence the behavior of others, hold religious significance, and are an outlet for creative expression. Consequently, knowledge of an item and its components can influence its acceptability.

Because fat has highly desirable sensory properties but is the target of negative health claims, information about the fat content of foods evokes mixed feelings among individuals. This complicates predictions of how information about fat content will influence hedonic ratings for foods and dietary behavior.

Questionnaire studies indicate that beliefs about the sensory attributes and health consequences of eating high-fat foods are strong predictors of reported consumption (Shepherd and Stockley, 1987; Tuorila and Pangborn, 1988). In studies eliciting responses to specific foods or food groups (e.g., meats, dairy products, fried foods), correlation coefficients between reported health beliefs and consumption range from 0.43 to 0.59, and for sensory appeal the values range from 0.56 to 0.69. In contrast, coefficients for expense or convenience are below 0.20 (Towler and Shepherd, 1992).

Several studies have examined the independent influence of belief about the fat content of foods on hedonic ratings for the items. In one study (Eiser et al., 1984), adolescents provided information about the fat content of 21 common foods did not exhibit a pattern of hedonic responses consistent with the information. However, participants who received information about fat levels gave reduced "pleasantness" ratings for the high-fat items compared to uninformed participants. This paralleled the reported health beliefs about the products (i.e., products evoking the most concern were rated lowest). Interpretation of these data is complicated by the fact that different foods were used to represent items with varying fat levels [e.g., liver (a high-fat item) and sugar (a low-fat item)]. Thus, views about the particular items, rather than their fat levels, could account for the findings. This potential problem has been circumvented in other work, where different messages were provided about the fat content of a single food (sausage) (Solheim, 1992). When equated for palatability, false information that a sausage containing 20% fat had only 12% fat resulted in a 12% increase in reported liking. Similarly, true information that a sausage contained only 12% fat led to a 12% reduction in liking. It should be noted, however, that these significant informational effects were not sufficiently strong to overcome differences in liking for items that actually varied in sensory quality. The prepotence of sensory quality is a consistent observation (Light et al., 1992). Studies with other foods have also yielded significant effects of information about fat content on hedonic ratings, but reveal that the nature of the effect is not consistent. For example, information that an ice cream was high in fat enhanced its sensory appeal, whereas similar information about a cheese product had the opposite effect (Light et al., 1992). The rationale underlying the typical use of individual products (e.g., occasional treat, staple nutrient source) may influence the impact of nutrient information on hedonic ratings. Within the limited scope of existing data, information about fat content exerts a stronger effect on product liking than knowledge of other macronutrients or energy value (Eiser et al., 1984; Light et al., 1992).

Given recent concerns about the information contained on food labels, which is designed to aid consumers in selecting healthful diets, surprisingly little information is available on how information influences food selection in free-living individuals. We explored the issue by providing a midday meal to healthy subjects for 12-day periods along with information that the meals contained less, a similar amount, or more fat than each individual's customary midday meal (determined during a baseline period) (Caputo and Mattes, 1993). In fact, the identical meal was provided on all occasions. Daily food intake was monitored by dietary records during each period to evaluate the effects of the information on dietary behavior. When subjects were informed that a meal contained less fat than their customary midday meal, self-selected intake rose significantly so that daily energy intake was elevated by about 245 kcal. This was observed in 16 of the 17 subjects studied. Moreover, about 80% of the increased energy intake was derived from dietary fats. Less dramatic effects were noted when subjects were informed that the meal was higher in fat, although 12 of the 17 participants did reduce their self-selected energy intake and 10 subjects reduced their fat intake. The asymmetry in responses is likely due to differences in the perceived obstacles to make adjustments. Compensation for a purported high-fat meal would require the selection of items viewed as less palatable and ones that are often less convenient and more expensive. Alternatively, belief that a meal was reduced in fat permitted subjects to indulge in readily available, high-fat items regarded as superior in sensory quality. These data, collected on subjects who reportedly were not highly concerned about their level of fat intake, highlight the importance of information about fat content on dietary behavior. Further, they suggest that provision of information about fat reduction in products may not result in anticipated behavioral change. Clearly, reduced-fat products can aid in the adoption of a total diet reduced in fat. However, casual use of such products, where consumers consciously or unconsciously compensate for the perceived savings in fat, may be ineffective or even counterproductive.

It is clear that information about the fat content of foods can markedly alter their hedonic appeal and level of use. The direction and magnitude of the effect will be idiosyncratic, reflecting an individual's health beliefs, expectations of the product, and a host of culturally mediated influences (e.g., ideal body image).

SENSORY INFLUENCE ON FAT PREFERENCE AND INTAKE

Questionnaire studies document that the sensory appeal of high-fat foods is the primary influence on their consumption (Tuorila and Pangborn, 1988; Towler and Shepherd, 1992; Light et al., 1992; Anonymous, 1993; Lloyd et al., 1995). Given the importance of this factor, an understanding of the basis for fat preference becomes central for development of strategies for modifying its level of consumption.

Studies in rats suggest there is an innate liking for the sensation provided by fats (Ackroff et al., 1990; Sclafani, 1992). Twelve- to 15-day-old rat pups as well as adult rats show comparable hedonic responses to lipid emulsions and chow with added nutritive or nonnutritive fats. Moreover, responses to both are greater than that noted for water or chow alone. This initial acceptance for items providing the mouthfeel of fats is consistent with a view that they are innately appealing. However, a learning component can also be demonstrated. Weaning rats fed low- or high-fat diets for 4 weeks exhibit a preference for the diet on which they were reared (Warwick et al., 1990). Later reversal of diets does not lead rats initially exposed to the high-fat diet to switch their preference to one lower in fat. This suggests that early exposure to a high-fat diet may result in a particularly stable preference for a diet of this composition. Whether the learned preference for a high-fat diet is based upon metabolic or other influences has not been determined.

A metabolic basis is supported by evidence that preferences develop over time for nutritive fats over nonnutritive substances with similar sensory, but not metabolic, properties (e.g., mineral oil, petrolatum). Presumably, the sensory property of each fat is associated with its metabolic consequence. Those fats that provide energy acquire a heightened appeal relative to those that are ineffective at promoting energy balance. Consumption of a high-fat diet could promote the formation of a positive association by leading to enhanced efficiency of fat absorption and utilization (Reed et al., 1991). Fat preference is correlated with indices of utilization, but no causal association has been established. An effect of fat on glucose metabolism may be involved since diets containing high levels of saturated fat, which promote glucose intolerance, lead to avoidance of carbohydrate. This is not seen with diets high in unsaturated fat (Mullen and Martin, 1992; Uusitupa et al., 1994).

The observation that newborn infants suck more vigorously for high-fat milk compared to low-fat milk is the only suggestive evidence for an innate liking for fat in humans (Nysenbaum and Smart, 1982). No data are available on the effects of early exposure on long-term preferences in humans. However, there is considerable evidence that preferences can be modified through dietary experience. Studies with dietary fats (e.g., butter, margarine) and dairy products demonstrate that preferences are strongly associated with the product most commonly used (Prattala et al., 1992; Raats and Shepherd, 1993). A metabolic basis for this observation is unlikely since the products tested represent only a fraction of the fat and total energy consumed by respondents.

A direct test of the relative importance of sensory and metabolic factors in shaping the preferred fat level of foods has demonstrated the prepotence of the former in humans (Mattes, 1993). Subjects were divided into three dietary groups. One was prescribed a reduced-fat diet and was prohibited from using reduced-fat versions of high-fat foods for 12 weeks. Thus, they were restricted in fat intake and sensory exposure. The second group consumed diets comparably reduced in fat to the first group, but, through the use of fat-modified products, they maintained their normal level of sensory exposure to the mouthfeel of fat. No modification of diet was imposed on a third group. Monthly hedonic ratings of an array of commercially available, reduced- and normal-fat versions of foods revealed that after 8–12 weeks of dietary modification, subjects in the group deprived of sensory exposure to fats exhibited a heightened preference for the reduced-fat versions of test foods. No such shift was observed among the controls or subjects consuming a diet of comparable fat level that included foods providing oral stimulation that mimicked fats. Other studies exploring this issue have had less complete control over dietary exposure. Two have noted trends consistent with these findings (Pangborn and Giovanni, 1984; Pangborn et al., 1985), while one that used laboratory prepared test foods, rather than commercially available products, failed to note an association (Mela and Sacchetti, 1991).

The mechanism by which sensory exposure influences fat preference has not been determined. Tests of ability to discriminate fat levels of the foods revealed no changes over time (Mattes, 1993). A simple exposure effect may be involved. This view holds that familiarity promotes acceptability, and the concept is supported by controlled studies and observational data (Pliner, 1982; Sullivan and Birch, 1994). By reducing sensory exposure to the mouthfeel of fats, that sensation loses its desirability. However, this effect may not hold equally across foods. The shift was not apparent in all foods assessed in the investigation described above, and other studies have failed to alter hedonic ratings for selected fat-modified items (e.g., cheddar cheese and potato chips) by varying exposure level (Mela et al., 1993). The motivation to consume items may alter their susceptibility to an hedonic shift. Products consumed largely for the mouthfeel they impart (e.g., whipped cream) may be less likely to change than items consumed for other reasons (e.g., milk). Differences in the discriminability of gradations in fat levels of different products may also account for varying susceptibilities to hedonic shifts.

Overall, there is compelling evidence that the sensory properties that fats impart to foods exert a strong influence on their appeal. An innate basis for the appeal of dietary fats in humans has not been established, but there is clear evidence that the preferred level of fat in foods can be modified through dietary experience. The degree to which an induced hedonic shift towards low and reduced-fat foods will promote long-term dietary moderation of fat intake has not been determined.

SUMMARY

The factors promoting fat intake are multiple and diverse, reflecting the dietary importance of this macronutrient. The redundancy of determinants accounts, in part, for the difficulty that individuals encounter when attempting to moderate consumption. While strategies can be devised to circumvent some mechanisms for a period of time, no approach that effectively overrides all influences for a substantial period of time has been identified.

The weak association between level of fat intake and either compensatory dietary behavior or metabolic adjustments indicates that metabolism plays a permissive role in fostering fat intake rather than a regulatory or promotional influence. This review indicates that the predominant force driving a high level of fat intake is the sensory appeal of dietary fats. Cognitive influences are also clearly involved as individuals attempt to balance concerns about the health implications of dietary fats with the sensory appeal they offer. Sociodemographic trends probably reflect the role of variables such as education and income on how the balance between sensory appeal and health concerns is weighed. The immediate gratification of fat consumption contrasted with a potential adverse health impact from repeated indulgences many years in the future apparently sways the decision towards intake for all but the most highly motivated.

Given the prepotence of sensory input, there are two principal approaches for adopting a fat-modified diet. One involves reliance on the food industry to develop convenient, reasonably priced, appealing products that are reduced in fat. If this is undertaken on a wide scale, it will enable consumers to reduce intake without marked disruption of their normal dietary practices. The success of this approach will depend upon the degree to which consumers use fat-reduced products in a fat-controlled total diet or merely as a means to offset indulgences on high-fat items. Alternatively, individuals may elect to develop a heightened preference for products that are low in fat and do not provide its sensory impression. Evidence now suggests that this can be accomplished by restricting exposure to the mouth-feel of fats for at least 8–12 weeks. However, the degree to which this hedonic shift will promote long-term adherence to a reduced-fat diet has not been determined. It must be recognized that just as limited sensory exposure can lead to heightened preference for reduced-fat products, increased exposure can reverse the effect. Thus, the success of this approach will require individuals to be vigilant. These two approaches do not appear to be mutually reinforcing since use of products containing fat substitutes can block an hedonic adjustment. However, the possibility that more selective restrictions on exposure can elicit hedonic shifts for specific items warrants additional study. In particular, it would be useful to know the conditions under which shifts can be induced for items that are significant contributors of fat, but do not lend themselves to modifications involving fat substitutes (e.g., fluid milk, meats). Trends towards increased use of reduced-fat milk in populations where total fat intake has not been markedly reduced and use of fat-substituted products has increased suggest that this may be possible.

ACKNOWLEDGMENTS

Preparation of this manuscript was supported, in part, by Public Health Service Grant #5 RO1 DK45294 from the National Institute of Diabetes and Digestive and Kidney Diseases.

REFERENCES

Abbott, W. G. H., Howard, B. V., Christin, L., Freymond, D., Lillioja, S., Boyce, V. L., Anderson, T. E., Bogardus, C., and Ravussin, E. 1988. Short-term energy balance: relationship with protein, carbohydrate, and fat balances. *Am. J. Physiol.* 255: 332–337.

Ackroff, K., Vigorito, M., and Sclafani, A. 1990. Fat appetite in rats: The response of infant and adult rats to nutritive and non-nutritive oil emulsions. *Appetite* 15: 171–188.

Anonymous. 1993. Trends 93: *Consumer Attitudes and the Supermarket.* Food Marketing Institute, pp. 45–54.

Atkinson, R. L. 1987. Opioid regulation of food intake and body weight in humans. *Fed. Proc.* 46: 178–182.

Axelson, M. L. 1986. The impact of culture on food-related behavior. *Annu. Rev. Nutr.* 6: 345–363.

Bennett, C., Reed, G. W., Peters ,J. C., Abumrad, N. N., Sun, M., and Hill, J. O. 1992. Short term effects of dietary fat-ingestion on energy expenditure and nutrient balance. *Am. J. Clin. Nutr.* 55: 1071–1077.

Bernardini, J., Kamara, K., and Castonguay, T. W. 1993. Macronutrient choice following food deprivation: Effect of dietary fat dilution. *Brain Res. Bull.* 32: 543–548.

Bertino, M., Beauchamp, G. K., and Engelman, K. 1991. Naltrexone, an opioid blocker, alters taste perception and nutrient intake in humans. *Am. J. Physiol.* 261: 59–63.

Birch, L. L., McPhee, L., Steinberg, L., and Sullivan, S. 1990. Conditioned flavor preferences in young children. *Physiol. Behav.* 47: 501–505.

Blass, E. M. 1991. Suckling: Opioid and non-opioid processes in mother-infant bonding. In *Chemical Senses*. Vol. 4. *Appetite and Nutrition*, M. I. Friedman, M. G. Tordoff, and M. R. Kare (Ed.), pp. 283–302. Marcel Dekker, Inc., New York.

Blundell, J. E. and Burley, V. J. 1991. Evaluation of the satiating power of dietary fat in man. In *Progress in Obesity Research*, Y. Oomura, S. Tarui, S. Inoue, and T. Shimazu (Ed.), pp. 453–457. Libbey & Co., London.

Blundell, J. E., Burley, V. J., Cotton, J. R., and Lawton, C. L. 1993. Dietary fat and the control of energy intake: Evaluating the effects of fat on meal size and postmeal satiety. *Am. J. Clin. Nutr.* 57: 772–778.

Borah-Giddens, J. and Falciglia, G. A. A meta-analysis of the relationship in food preferences between parents and children. *J. Nutr. Educ.* 25: 102–107.

Calorie Control Council. 1993. Reduced-fat, low-calorie eating more popular than ever. *Calorie Control Commentary* (ISSN 1049-1791). Vol. 15: 1–2.

Capaldi, E. D., Campbell, D. H., Sheffer, J. D., and Bradford, J. P. 1987. Conditioned flavor preferences based on delayed caloric consequences. *J. Exp. Psych.* 13: 150–155.

Caputo, F. A. and Mattes, R. D. 1992. Human dietary responses to covert manipulations of energy, fat, and carbohydrate in a midday meal. *Am. J. Clin. Nutr.* 56: 36–43.

Caputo, F. A. and Mattes, R. D. 1993. Human dietary responses to perceived manipulation of fat content in a midday meal. *Int. J. Obes.* 17: 237–240.

Clandinin, M. T., Cheema, S., Field, C. J., Garg, M. L., Venkatraman, J., and

Clandinin, T. R. 1991. Dietary fat: Exogenous determination of membrane structure and cell function. *FASEB J.* 5: 2761–2769.

Cooper, S. J. 1983, Benzodiazepine-opiate antagonist interactions in relation to anxiety and appetite. *TIPS* 4: 456–458.

Dannenberg, A. J. and Reidenberg, M. M. 1994. Dietary fatty acids are no drugs. *Clin. Pharmacol. Ther.* 55: 5–9.

Davidson, T. L., McKenzie, B. R., Tujo, C. J., and Bish, C. K. 1992. Development of tolerance to endogenous opiates activated by 24-h food deprivation. *Appetite* 19: 1–13.

deCastro, J. M. 1993. Genetic influences on daily intake and meal patterns of humans. *Physiol. Behav.* 53: 777–782.

deCastro, J. M. 1987. Macronutrient relationships with meal patterns and mood in the spontaneous feeding behavior of humans. *Physiol. & Behav.* 39: 561–569.

deGraaf, C., Hulshof, T., Weststrate, J. A., and Jas, P. 1992. Short-term effects of different amounts of protein, fats, and carbohydrates on satiety. *Am. J. Clin. Nutr.* 55: 33–38.

Delgado, P. L., Charney, D. S., Price, L. H., Aghajanian, G. K., Landis, H., and Heninger, G. R. 1990. Serotonin function and the mechanism of antidepressant action. *Arch. Gen. Psychiatry* 47: 411–418.

Drewnowski, A., Krahn, D. D., Demitrack, M. A., Nairn, K., and Gosnell, B. A. 1992. Taste responses and preferences for sweet high-fat foods: Evidence for opioid involvement. *Physiol. Behav.* 51: 371–379.

Drewnowski, A., Pierce, B., and Halmi, K. A. 1988. Fat aversion in eating disorders. *Appetite* 10: 119–131.

Eiser, J. R., Eiser, C., Patterson, D. J., and Harding, C. M. 1984. Effects of information about specific nutrient content on ratings of "goodness" and "pleasantness" of common foods. *Appetite* 5: 349–359.

Elizalde, G. and Sclafani, A. 1990. Fat appetite in rats: Flavor preferences conditioned by nutritive and non-nutritive oil emulsions. *Appetite* 15: 189–197.

Fabsitz, R. R., Garison, R. J., Feinleib, M., and Hjortland, M. 1978. A twin analysis of dietary intake: Evidence for a need to control for possible environmental differences in MZ and DZ twins. *Behav. Genet.* 8: 15–25.

Falciglia, G. A. and Norton, P. A. 1994. Evidence for a genetic influence on preference for some foods. *J. Am. Diet. Assoc.* 94: 154–158.

Fernstrom, J. D. 1994. Dietary amino acids and brain function. *J. Am. Diet. Assoc.* 94: 71–77.

Fernstrom, M. H. and Fernstrom, J. D. 1993. Large changes in serum free tryptophan levels do not alter brain tryptophan levels: Studies in streptozotocin-diabetic rats. *Life Sci.* 52: 907–916.

Food and Nutrition Board. 1989. *Recommended Dietary Allowance*, 10th ed. National Academy Press, Washington, DC.

Galef, G. B. 1991. A contrarian view of the wisdom of the body as it relates to dietary self-selection. *Psych. Rev.* 98: 218–223.

Gill, K. M., Skeie, B., Kvetan, V., Askanazi, J., and Friedman, M. I. 1991. Parenteral nutrition and oral intake: Effect of glucose and fat infusions. *JPEN* 15: 426–432.

Gosnell, B. A. and Krahn, D. D. 1992. The effects of continuous naltrexone infusions on diet preferences are modulated by adaptation to the diets. *Physiol. Behav.* 51: 239–244.

Gosnell, B. A. and Krahn, D. D. 1993. The effects of continuous morphine infusion on diet selection and body weight. *Physiol. Behav.* 54: 853–859.

Gosnell, B. A., Krahn, D. D., and Majchrzak, M. J. 1990. The effects of morphine on diet selection are dependent upon baseline diet preferences. *Pharm. Biochem. Behav.* 37: 207–212.

Greene, L. S., Desor, J. A., and Maller, O. 1975. Heredity and experience: Their relative importance in the development of taste preference in man. *J. Comp. Physiol. Psychol.* 89: 279–284.

Hayward, L. 1983. The role of oral and postingestional cues in the conditioning of taste preferences based on differing caloric density and caloric outcome in weanling and mature rats. *Anim. Learn. Behav.* 11: 325–331.

Hegsted, D. M. and Ausman, L. M. 1988. Diet, alcohol and coronary heart disease in men. *J. Nutr.* 118: 1184–1189.

Hetherington, M. M., Vervaet, N., Blass, E., and Rolls, B. J. 1991. Failure of naltrexone to affect the pleasantness or intake of food. *Pharm. Biochem. Behav.* 40: 185–190.

Hill, J. O., Peters, J. C., Reed, G. W., Schlundt, D. G., Sharp, T., and Greene, H. L. 1991. Nutrient balance in humans: Effects of diet composition. *Am. J. Clin. Nutr.* 54: 10–17.

Johnson, S. L., McPhee, L., and Birch, L. L. 1991. Conditioned preferences: Young children prefer flavors associated with high dietary fat. *Physiol. Behav.* 50: 1245–1251.

Kales, E. F. 1990. Macronutrient analysis of binge eating in bulimia. *Physiol. Behav.* 48: 837–840.

Kendall, A., Levitsky, D. A., Strupp, B. J., and Lissner, L. 1991. Weight loss on a low fat diet: consequence of the imprecision of the control of food intake in humans. *Am. J. Clin. Nutr.* 53: 1124–1129.

Kern, D. L., McPhee, L., Fisher, J., Johnson, S., and Birch, L. L. 1993. The postingestive consequences of fat condition preferences for flavors associated with high dietary fat. *Physiol. Behav.* 54: 71–76.

Keys, A., Brozek, J., Henschel, A., Mickelsen, O., and Taylor, H. L. 1950. Behavior and complaints in experimental starvation and rehabilitation. In *The Biology of Human Starvation*, pp. 819–853. North Central Publishing Company, St. Paul, MN.

Kromhout, D., Keys, A., Aravanis, C., Buzina, R., Fidanza, F., Giampaoli, S., Jansen, A., Menotti, A., Nedeljkovic, S., Pekkarinen, M., Simic, B. S., and Toshima, H. 1989. Food consumption patterns in the 1960s in seven countries. *Am. J. Nutr.* 49: 889–894.

Krondl, M., Coleman, P., Wade, J., and Milner, J. 1983. A twin study examining the genetic influence on food selection. *Hum. Nutr. Appl. Nutr.* 37A: 189–198.

Laskarzewski, P., Morrison, J. A., Khoury, P., Kelley, K., Glatfelter, L., Larsen, R., and Glueck, C. J. 1980. Parent-child nutrient intake relationships in school children ages 6 to 19: The Princeton School District Study. *Am. J. Clin. Nutr.* 33: 2350–2355.

Light, A., Heymann, H., and Holt, D. L. 1992. Hedonic responses to dairy products: Effects of fat levels, label information, and risk perception. *Food Technol.* 46: 54–57.

Lissner, L., Levitsky, D. A., Strupp, B. J., Kalkwarf, H. J., and Roe, D. A. 1987. Dietary fat and the regulation of energy intake in human subjects. *Am. J. Clin. Nutr.* 46: 886–892.

Lloyd, H. M., Paisley, C. M., and Mela, D. J. 1995. Barriers to the adoption of reduced-fat diets in a UK population. *J. Am. Diet. Assoc.* 95(3): 316–322.

Logue, A. W., Logue, C. M., Uzzo, R. G., McCarty, M. J., and Smith, M. E. 1988. Food preferences in families. *Appetite* 10: 169–180.

Lucas, F. and Sclafani, A. 1989. Flavor preferences conditioned by intragastric fat infusions in rats. *Physiol. Behav.* 46: 403–412.

Maggio, C. A., Presta, E., Braco, E. F., Vasselli, J. R., Kissileff, H. R., Pfohl, D. N., and Hashim, S. A. 1985. Naltrexone and human eating behavior: A dose-ranging inpatient trial in moderately obese men. *Brain Res. Bull.* 14: 657–661.

Marks-Kaufman, R. 1982. Increased fat consumption by morphine administration in rats. *Pharmacol. Biochem. Behav.* 16: 949–955.

Marks-Kaufman, R. and Kanarek, R. B. 1981. Modifications in nutrient selection induced by naloxone in rats. *Psychopharmacology* 74: 321–324.

Mattes, R. D. 1993. Fat preference and the adherence to a reduced-fat diet. *Am. J. Clin. Nutr.* 57: 373–381.

McKee, L. M. and Harden, M. L. 1990. Genetic and environmental origins of food patterns. *Nutr. Today* 25: 26–31.

Mela, D. J. and Sacchetti, D. A. 1991. Sensory preferences for fats: relationships with diet and body composition. *Am. J. Clin. Nutr.* 53: 908–915.

Mela, D. J., Trunck, F., and Aaron, J. I. 1993. No effect of extended home use on liking for sensory characteristics of reduced-fat foods. *Appetite* 21: 117–129.

Melchior, J. C., Fantino, M., Colas-Linhart, N., Rigaud, D., Petiet, A., LaForest, M. D., Fumeron, F., and Apfelbaum, M. 1991. Lack of plasmatic beta-endorphin response to a gastronomic meal in healthy humans. *Physiol. Behav.* 49: 1217–1221.

Mullen, B. J. and Martin, R. J. 1992. The effect of dietary fat on diet selection may involve central serotonin. *Am. J. Physiol.* 363: 559–563.

Nysenbaum, A. N. and Smart, J. L. 1982. Sucking behaviour and milk intake of neonates in relation to milk fat content. *Early Hum. Dev.* 6: 205–213.

Oliveria, S. A., Ellison, R. C., Moore, L. L., Gillman, M. W., Garrahie, E. J., and Singer, M. R. 1992. Parent-child relationships in nutrient intake: The Framingham children's study. *Am. J. Clin. Nutr.* 56: 593–598.

Olson, G. A., Olson, R. D., and Kastin, A. J. 1991. Endogenous opiates. *Peptides* 13: 1247–1287.

Pangborn, R. M., Bos, K. E. O., and Stern, J. S. 1985. Dietary fat intake and taste responses to fat in milk by under-, normal, and overweight women. *Appetite* 6: 25–40.

Pangborn, R. M. and Giovanni, M. E. 1984. Dietary intake of sweet foods and of dairy fats and resultant gustatory responses to sugar in lemonade and to fat in milk. *Appetite* 5: 317–327.

Patterson, T. L., Rupp, J. W., Sallis, J. F., Atkins, C. J., and Nader, P. R. 1988. Aggregation of dietary calories, fats, and sodium in Mexican-American and Anglo families. *Am. J. Prev. Med.* 4: 75–82.

Perusse, L., Tremblay, A., Leblanc, C., Cloninger, C. R., Reich, T., Rice, J., and Bouchard, C. 1988. Familial resemblance in energy intake: Contribution of genetic and environmental factors. *Am. J. Clin. Nutr.* 47: 629–635.

Pliner, P. 1982. The effects of mere exposure on linking for edible substances. *Appetite* 3: 283–290.

Pliner, P. 1983. Family resemblance in food preferences. *J. Nutr. Educ.* 15: 137–140.

Pliner, P. and Pelchat, M. L. 1986. Similarities in food preferences between children and their siblings and parents. *Appetite* 7: 333–342.

Prattala, R., Pelton, G. H., Pelto, P., Ahola, M., and Rasanen, L. 1992.

Perceptions of spreading fats among women in Helsinki whose households use only butter or margarine. *Appetite* 18: 185–191.

Prentice, R. L., Kakar, F., Hursting, S., Sheppard, L., Klein, R., and Kushi, L. H. 1988. Aspects of the rationale for the women's health trial. *J. Natl. Cancer Inst.* 80: 802–814.

Raats, M. M. and Shepherd, R. 1993. The use and perceived appropriateness of milk in the diet: A cross-country evaluation. *Ecol. Food Nutr.* 30: 253–273.

Reed, D. R., Friedman, M. I., and Tordoff, M. G. 1992. Experience with a macronutrient source influences subsequent macronutrient selection. *Appetite* 18: 223–232.

Reed, D. R., Tordoff, M. G., and Friedman, M. I. 1991. Enhanced acceptance and metabolism of fats by rats fed a high-fat diet. *Am. J. Physiol.* 261: 1084–1088.

Reid, L. D. 1985. Endogenous opioid peptides and regulation of drinking and feeding. *Am. J. Clin. Nutr.* 42: 1099–1123.

Reilly, K. J. and Rombeau, J. L. 1993. Metabolism and potential clinical applications of short-chain fatty acids. *Clin. Nutr.* 12: 97–105.

Rising, R., Alger, S., Boyce, V., Seagle, H., Ferraro, R., Fontvieille, A. M., and Ravussin, E. 1992. Food intake measured by an automated food-selection system: Relationship to energy expenditure. *Am. J. Clin. Nutr.* 55: 343–349.

Rolls, B. J., Hetherington, M., and Burley, V. J. 1988. The specificity of satiety: The influence of foods of different macronutrient content on the development of satiety. *Physiol. Behav.* 43: 145–153.

Rolls, B. J., Kim-Harris, S., Fischman, M. W., Foltin, R. W., Moran, T. H., and Stoner, S. A. 1994. Satiety after preloads with different amounts of fat and carbohydrate: Implications for obesity. *Am. J. Clin. Nutr.* 60: 476–487.

Rolls, B. J., Pirraglia, P. A., Jones, M. B., and Peters, J. C. 1992. Effects of Olestra, a noncaloric fat substitute, on daily energy and fat intakes in lean men. *Am. J. Clin. Nutr.* 56: 84–92.

Rozin, P. 1980. Human food selection: why do we know so little and what can we do about it? *Int. J. Obes.* 4: 333–337.

Rozin, P., Fallon, A., and Mandell, R. 1984. Family resemblance in attitudes to foods. *Dev. Psychol.* 20: 309–314.

Rozin, P. and Millman, L. 1987. Family environment, not heredity, accounts for family resemblances in food preferences and attitudes: A twin study. *Appetite* 8: 125–134.

Sclafani, A. 1992. Psychobiology of fat appetite. In *Proceedings of the Conference on Promoting Dietary Changes in Communities*, M. Henderson, D. J. Bowen, and K. K. DeRoos (Ed.), pp. 82–95. University of Washington, Seattle.

Sclafani, A. and Ackeroff, K. 1993. Deprivation alters rats' flavor preferences for carbohydrates and fats. *Physiol. Behav.* 53: 1091–1099.

Schutz, Y., Flatt, J. P., and Jequier, E. 1989. Failure of dietary fat intake to promote fat oxidation: A factor favoring the development of obesity. *Am. J. Clin. Nutr.* 50: 307–314.

Shepherd, R. and Stockley, L. 1987. Nutrition knowledge, attitudes, and fat consumption. *J. Am. Diet. Assoc.* 87: 615–619.

Shide, D. J. and Blass, E. M. 1991. Opioid mediation of odor preferences induced by sugar and fat in 6-day-old rats. *Physiol. Behav.* 50: 961–966.

Smith, A., Kendrick, A., Maben, A., and Salmon, J. 1994. Effects of fat content, weight, and acceptability of the meal on postlunch changes in mood, performance, and cardiovascular function. *Physiol. Behav.* 55: 417–422.

Solheim, R. 1992. Consumer liking for sausages affected by sensory quality and information on fat content. *Appetite* 19: 285–292.

Stephen, A. M. and Wald, N. J. 1990. Trends in individual consumption of dietary fat in the United States, 1920–1984. *Am. J. Clin. Nutr.* 52: 457–469.

Sullivan, S. A. and Birch, L. L. 1994. Infant dietary experience and acceptance of solid foods. *Pediatrics* 93: 271–277.

Towler, G. and Shepherd, R. 1992. Application of Fishbein and Ajzen's expectancy-value model to understanding fat intake. *Appetite* 18: 15–27.

Triscari, J., Nelson, D., Vincent, G. P., and Li, C. H. 1989. Effect of centrally and peripherally administered β-endorphin on food intake in rats. *Int. J. Peptide Protein Res.* 34: 358–362.

Tuorila, H. and Pangborn, R. M. 1988. Prediction of reported consumption of selected fat-containing foods. *Appetite* 11: 81–95.

U.S. Department of Health and Human Services. 1988. *The Surgeon General's Report on Nutrition and Health.* U.S. Government Printing Office, Washington, DC.

Uusitupa, M., Schwab, U., Makimattila, S., Karhapaa, P., Sarkkinen, E., Maliranta, H., Agren, J., and Penttila, I. 1994. Effects of two high-fat diets with different fatty acid compositions on glucose and lipid metabolism in healthy young women. *Am. J. Clin. Nutr.* 59: 1310–1316.

Van Amelsvoort, J. M. M., Van Stratum, P., Kraal, J. H., Lussenburg, R. N., and Houtsmuller, U. M. T. 1989. Effects of varying the carbohydrate-fat ratio in a hot lunch on postprandial variables in male volunteers. *Br. J. Nutr.* 61: 267–283.

Wade, J., Milner, J., and Krondl, M. 1981. Evidence for a physiological regulation of food selection and nutrient intake in twins. *Am. J. Clin. Nutr.* 34: 143–147.

Waller, D. A., Kiser, R. S., Hardy, B. W., Fuchs, I., Feigenbaum, L. P., and Uauy, R. 1986. Eating behavior and plasma beta-endorphin in bulimia. *Am. J. Clin. Nutr.* 44: 20–23.

Warwick, Z. S., Schiffman, S. S., and Anderson, J. J. B. 1990. Relationship of dietary fat content to food preferences in young rats. *Physiol. Behav.* 48: 581–586.

Warwick, Z. S. and Weingarten, H. P. 1994. Dissociation of palatability and calorie effects on learned flavor preferences. *Physiol. Behav.* 55: 501–504.

Weidner, G., Archer, S., Healy, B., and Matarazzo, J. D. 1985. Family consumption of low-fat foods: Stated preference versus actual consumption. *J. Appl. Soc. Psychol.* 15: 773–779.

Yanovski, S. Z., Leet, M., Yanovski, J. A., Flood, M., Gold, P. W., Kissileff, H. R., and Walsh, B. T. 1992. Food selection and intake of obese women with binge-eating disorders. *Am. J. Clin. Nutr.* 56: 975–980.

Young, S. N., Pihl, R. O., and Ervin, F. R. 1988. The effect of altered tryptophan levels on mood and behavior in normal human males. *Clin. Neuropharm.* 11: 207–215.

Index